PLANS OF CARE FOR SPECIALTY PRACTICE

D1552971

Community and Home Health Nursing

IDA ANDROWICH, RN, C, PhD
Administrative Director
Nursing Education & Support Services
Associate Professor
Community & Administrative Nursing
Loyola University
Chicago, Illinois

LISA BURKHART, RN, MPH
Health Care Consultant
Evanston, Illinois

series editor
KATHY V. GETTRUST, RN, BSN
Case Manager
Midwest Medical Home Care
Milwaukee, Wisconsin

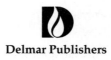

Delmar Publishers

I(T)P™ **An International Thomson Publishing Company**

Albany • Bonn • Boston • Cincinnati • Detroit • London • Madrid • Melbourne
Mexico City • New York • Pacific Grove • Paris • San Francisco • Singapore • Tokyo
Toronto • Washington

NOTICE TO THE READER

Publisher does not warrant or guarantee any of the products described herein or perform any independent analysis in connection with any of the product information contained herein. Publisher does not assume, and expressly disclaims, any obligation to obtain and include information other than that provided to it by the manufacturer.

The reader is expressly warned to consider and adopt all safety precautions that might be indicated by the activities described herein and to avoid all potential hazards. By following the instructions contained herein, the reader willingly assumes all risks in connection with such instructions.

The publisher makes no representations or warranties of any kind, including but not limited to, the warranties of fitness for particular purpose or merchantability, nor are any such representations implied with respect to the material set forth herein, and the publisher takes no responsibility with respect to such material. The publisher shall not be liable for any special, consequential or exemplary damages resulting, in whole or part, from the readers' use of, or reliance upon, this material.

Cover Illustration: Jeane Benas

Delmar Staff

Senior Acquisitions Editor: Patricia Casey
Associate Editor: Elizabeth F. Williams
Project Editor: Judith Boyd Nelson

Production Coordinator: Barbara A. Bullock
Art/Design Coordinator: Carol D. Kechane
Editorial Assistant: Tonjia Herman

COPYRIGHT © 1996 by Delmar Publishers
a division of International Thomson Publishing Inc.

The ITP logo is a trademark under license.

Printed in the United States of America

For more information, contact:

Delmar Publishers
3 Columbia Circle, Box 15015
Albany, NY 12212-5015

International Thomson Publishing Europe
Berkshire House 168-173
High Holborn
London, WC1V 7AA
England

Thomas Nelson Australia
102 Dodds Street
South Melbourne, 3205
Victoria, Australia

Nelson Canada
1120 Birchmont Road
Scarborough, Ontario
Canada, M1K 5G4

International Thomson Editores
Campos Eliseos 385, Piso 7
Col Polanco
11560 Mexico D F Mexico

International Thomson Publishing GmbH
Konigswinterer Strasse 418
53227 Bonn
Germany

International Thomson Publishing Asia
221 Henderson Road
#05-10 Henderson Building
Singapore 0315

International Thomson Publishing—Japan
Hirakawacho Kyowa Building, 3F
2-2-1 Hirakawacho
Chiyoda-ku, Tokyo 102
Japan

1 2 3 4 5 6 7 8 9 10 XXX 02 01 00 99 98 97 96

Library of Congress Cataloging-in-Publication Data

Androwich, Ida.
Community and home health nursing / Ida Androwich, Lisa Burkhart.
    p. cm. — (Plans of care for specialty practice)
Includes bibliographical references and index.
ISBN 0-8273-6227-7
1. Community health nursing. 2. Nursing care plans. I. Burkhart, Lisa II. Title. III. Series.
    [DNLM: 1. Community Health Nursing. WY 106 A576c 1996]
RT98.A54 1996
610.73'43—dc20
DNLM/DLC
for Library of Congress

95-36419
CIP

TABLE OF CONTENTS

CONTRIBUTORS

- Amy Androwich-O'Malley, BSN, RN
  Nursing Administrative Coordinator
  Childrens Memorial Medical Center
  Chicago, IL
  - Failure to Thrive
- Anne Bedlek, RN, MSN, CCRN,
  CPAN
  Nurse Clinician
  Loyola University Medical Center
  Maywood, IL
  - Congestive Heart Failure
- Lazelle Emminizer Benefield,
  PhD, RN
  Associate Professor, Harris College
  of Nursing
  Texas Christian University
  Fort Worth, TX
  - Breast Cancer/Treatment
- Marilyn E. Birchfield, RN, MA
  Assistant Professor, Niehoff School
  of Nursing
  Loyola University
  Chicago, IL
  - Ineffective Parenting
- Susan L. Breakwell, RN, MS
  Director of Home Health Services
  Columbia Home Care I—Branch 4
  Chicago, IL
  - Sensory Deficit
  - Urinary Incontinence
- Scott L. V. Chinburg, RN, MSN
  HIV/AIDS Case Manager
  Loyola University Medical Center
  Maywood, IL
  - HIV/AIDS

- Dana E. Clark, BSN, MBA
  Staff Nurse
  Loyola University Center for Home
  Care and Hospice
  Maywood, IL
  - Medication Compliance/
    Noncompliance
- Cynthia Fryhling Corbett, MN, RN
  Assistant Professor
  Pacific Lutheran University
  Tacoma, WA
  - Diabetes Mellitus
- Constance Miles Dallas, PhD, RN,
  FNP, CS
  Assistant Professor of Nursing
  Purdue University Calumet
  Hammond, ID
  - Human Sexuality
- Jennifer A. Dore, RN, MSN, CETN
  Enterostomal Clinical Nurse
  Specialist
  Rush North Shore Medical Center
  Skokie, IL
  - Ostomy Care
  - Skin Care
- Karen Egenes, RN, EdD
  Associate Professor
  Loyola University Chicago, Niehoff
  School of Nursing
  Chicago, IL
  - Altered Mental Status
  - Social Isolation
  - Substance Abuse
- Naomi E. Ervin, PhD, RN, CS
  Department of Public Health,
  Mental Health and Administrative
  Nursing
  University of Illinois at Chicago
  Chicago, IL
  - Residence Deficit

- Robin L. Evans, RN, MSN, ONC
  Clinical Research Coordinator,
  Department of Orthopaedic Surgery
  University of Pittsburgh Medical
    Center
  Pittsburgh, PA
  - Joint Replacement/Fractures

- Joan Flynn, RN, MSN
  Clinical Nurse Administrator
  Hines VA
  Hines, IL
  - Arthritis/Osteoporosis

- Dorothy Fraser, MSN, FNP
  Assistant Professor of Clinical
    Nursing
  University of Southern California
  Los Angeles, CA
  - Cardiovascular Disease
  - Hepatitis

- Elaine Small Gardner, MS, RN, CS
  Clinical Educator, VNA of Boston
  Boston, MA
  Doctoral Student, College of
    Nursing
  University of Rhode Island
  Kingston, RI
  - Caregiver Burden/Support/
    Conflict Resolution

- Barbara J. Groeschell, RN, BSN
  Staff Nurse
  Center for Children in Crisis
  Germantown, TN
  - Breastfeeding

- Diana P. Hackbarth, PhD, RN
  Professor, Community, Mental
    Health, and Administrative
    Nursing
  Loyola University
  Chicago, IL
  - Contracting

- Kevin J. Hawker, BSN, RN
  Patient Care Coordinator
  Palliative Care Center of the North
    Shore
  Evanston, IL
  - Pain

- Jackie Kareb, MS, RN
  Nurse Manager
  Loyola University, Center for
    Hospice and Home Care
  Maywood, IL
  - Infusion Therapy
  - Referral to Community Resources

- Kathleen Klauseger, MSN
  Case Manager, Cancer Services
  Loyola University Medical Center
  Maywood, IL
  - Patient and Family Rights/
    Self-Determination
  - Transplant Care

- Barbara G. Konestabo, RN, MSN
  Clinical Nurse Manager, Psychiatric
    Unit
  Lakewood Hospital
  Lakewood, OH
  - Tuberculosis

- Julie A. Loftus, RN, MSN
  Loyola Center for Home Care and
    Hospice
  Maywood, IL
  - Antepartum Home Care
  - Postpartum Home Care

- Jan McCarron, MSN, RN
  Consultant
  Home Health Care/Hospital
    Discharge Planning
  Evanston, IL
  - Peripheral Vascular Disease

- Genevieve L. Monahan, RN, MSN
  DNSc Candidate
  California State University, Long
    Beach
  Long Beach, CA
  - Pediatric Asthma

- Ruth M. Neil, PhD, RN
  Assistant Professor, School of
    Nursing
  Project Director, Denver Nursing
    Project in Human Caring
  University of Colorado
  Denver, CO
  - Death and Dying
  - Grief and Loss

- Mary Ann Noonan, RN, MSN, FNP
  Assistant Professor
  Loyola University Niehoff School of
    Nursing
  Chicago, IL
  - Cerebral Insult
- Carol J. Paulini, RN, MS
  RN Coordinator
  Evanston Hospital Corporation
  Evanston, IL
  - Adult Respiratory Diseases
- Mary Anne Revolinski, BS
  Accredited La Leche League Leader
  Milwaukee, WI
  - Breastfeeding
- Pamela K. Roark, BSN, MA, MSN
  Ambulatory Care Nurse
    Administrator
  U.S. Navy
  - Physical Activity/Exercise
  - Nutrition
  - Inadequate Personal Hygiene
  - Sleep and Rest Patterns
- Maria Elena Ruiz, RN, MSN, C-FNP
  Instructor of Clinical Nursing
  University of Southern California
  Los Angeles, CA
  - Pediatric Asthma

- Sally Schnell, RN, MSN, CNRN
  Clinical Nurse Specialist Department
    of Neurosurgery
  Loyola University Medical Center
  Maywood, IL
  - Spinal Cord Injury: Paraplegia
    and Quadriplegia
- Judith A. Scully, RNC, MSN
  Assistant Professor
  Loyola University
  Chicago, IL
  - Child Abuse/Neglect
  - Elder Abuse/Neglect
  - Parkinson's Disease
  - Violence Against Women
- Sally A. Steinhiser, RN, MSN
  Administrator, Dialysis Program
  University of Chicago Hospitals
  Chicago, IL
  - Chronic Renal Failure
- Sandra C. Swallow, BSN, MPH
  Consultant
  Select Care Services
  Wood Dale, IL
  - Environmental Infection Control

FOREWORD

This community health nursing care plan book reflects the current trend to consider community health as encompassing elements of both public health and home health. It is unique, as is community health nursing: It reflects the broad range of content that is often not included in other texts, yet is important in the care of patients in the community. Some of these topics include caregiver stress, medication noncompliance, breastfeeding, spousal abuse, contracting, environmental concerns, as well as current information on major community health problems such as human immunodeficiency virus and tuberculosis. The contributing authors are recognized for their expertise in the various content areas. This care planning book will be a useful reference for the practicing nurse in the community, including those providing home health care services.

Bianca M. Chambers, DNSc
Department Chair, Community Health Nursing, Indiana University and President, Association of Community Health Nursing Educators

PREFACE

Community health nursing as a specialty encompasses a broad and comprehensive scope of practice. Not limited to one age or population group or to one particular diagnosis, it covers all levels of prevention and care, focusing primarily on health promotion and disease prevention. It has elements of both public health and home health. It requires a blending of the skills and knowledge base of both nursing and public health science. The nurse working in the community works with individuals, families, and aggregates in settings as diverse as homes, clinics, health departments, schools, and industry. Cultural and ethnic diversity are part of the rich fabric of community care. The community health nurse must continually be sensitive to unfamiliar health beliefs and practices in order to increase the level of culturally competent care provided. Thus, where appropriate, cultural beliefs and health practices which have an impact on care delivery are addressed.

The plans of care in this book are designed to provide the experienced nurse with a reference to inform care and to assist in prioritizing activities. Since the emphasis in all community health encounters is on primary health care, patient education is an integral component of these care plans. The nurse's role in the community centers on assessment, teaching, skilled care, and appropriate referrals to other community services. Information about referrals is included in both the interventions and discharge planning sections, as referrals may be for services that will be used concurrently with nursing care, such as physical therapy and Meals on Wheels, or they may be for services that will be required by the patient after the nursing care has been terminated and thus are part of the discharge plan.

To plan, develop, implement, and evaluate the comprehensive care required in the community, patient problems are organized using the Omaha System (Martin & Sheet, 1992), a well-known community health problem taxonomy. Problems from all four of the Omaha domains are included. Primary, secondary, and tertiary prevention are included throughout. Lifestyle issues such as nutrition, exercise, substance use, sexuality, and sleep are included as separate chapters. Although both the terms *client* and *patient* are acceptable in considering community nursing care, for consistency, the term patient is used throughout this text.

SERIES INTRODUCTION

Scientific and technological developments over the past several decades have revolutionized health care and care of the sick. These rapid and extensive advancements of knowledge have occurred in all fields, necessitating an ever-increasing specialization of practice. For nurses to be effective and meet the challenge in today's specialty settings, the body of clinical knowledge and skill needs to continually expand. *Plans of Care for Specialty Practice* has been written to aid the practicing nurse in meeting this challenge. The purpose of this series is to provide comprehensive, state-of-the-art plans of care and associated resource information for patient situations most commonly seen within a specialty that will serve as a standard from which care can be individualized. These plans of care are based on the profession's scientific approach to problem solving—the nursing process. Although the books are written primarily as a guide for frontline staff nurses and clinical nurse specialists practicing in specialty settings, they have application for student nurses as well.

DOCUMENTATION OF CARE

The Joint Commission on Accreditation of Healthcare Organizations (JCAHO) assumes authority for evaluating the quality and effectiveness of the practice of nursing. In 1991, the JCAHO developed its first new nursing care standards in more than a decade. One of the changes brought about by these new standards was the elimination of the need for every patient to have a handwritten or computer-generated care plan in his or her chart detailing all or most of the care to be provided. The Joint Commission's standard that describes the documentation requirements stipulates that nursing assessments, identification of nursing diagnoses and/or patient care needs, interventions, outcomes of care, and discharge planning be permanently integrated into the clinical record. In other words, the nursing process needs to be documented. A separate care plan is no longer needed; however, planning and implementing care must continue as always, but using whatever form of documentation that has been approved by an institution. *Plans of Care for Specialty Practice* can be easily used with a wide variety of approaches to documentation of care.

ELEMENTS OF THE PLANS OF CARE

The chapter title is the presenting situation, which represents the most commonly seen conditions/disorders treated within the specialty setting. It may be a medical diagnosis (e.g., diabetes mellitus), a syndrome (e.g., acquired immunodeficiency syndrome), a surgical procedure (e.g., mastectomy), or a diagnostic/therapeutic procedure (e.g., thrombolytic therapy).

An opening paragraph provides a definition or concise overview of the presenting situation. It describes the condition and may contain pertinent physiological/psychological bases for the disorder. It is brief and not intended to replace further investigation for comprehensive understanding of the condition.

Etiologies

A listing of causative factors responsible for or contributing to the presenting situation is provided. This may include predisposing diseases, injuries or trauma, surgeries, microorganisms, genetic factors, environmental hazards, drugs, or psychosocial disorders. In presenting situations where no clear causal relationship can be established, current theories regarding the etiology may be included. For those chapters pertaining to clinical procedures, indications for the procedure are listed instead of etiologies and clinical manifestations.

Clinical Manifestations

Objective and subjective signs and symptoms that describe the particular presenting situation are included. This information is revealed as a result of a health history and physical assessment and becomes part of the data base.

Clinical/Diagnostic Findings

This component contains possible diagnostic tests and procedures which might be done to determine abnormalities associated with a particular presenting situation. The name of the diagnostic procedure and the usual abnormal findings are listed.

Nursing Diagnosis

The nursing management of the health problem commences with the planning care phase of the nursing process. This includes obtaining a comprehensive history and physical assessment and identifying the nursing diagnoses, expected outcomes, interventions, and discharge planning needs.

Diagnostic labels identified by the North American Nursing Diagnosis Association (NANDA) through the Tenth National Conference in April 1992 are being used throughout this series. (Based on NANDA 1992. *NANDA Nursing Diagnoses: Definitions and Classification 1995–1996*, Philadelphia: NANDA.) We have also identified new diagnoses not yet on the official NANDA list. We endorse NANDA's recommendation for nurses to develop new nursing diagnoses as the need arises, and we encourage nurses using this series to do the same.

"Related To" Statements

"Related to" statements suggest a link or connection to the nursing diagnosis and provide direction for identifying appropriate nursing interventions. They are termed contributing factors, causes, or etiologies. There is frequently more than one "related to" statement for a given diagnosis. For example, change in job, marital difficulties, and impending surgery may all be "related to" the nursing diagnosis of anxiety.

There is disagreement at present regarding inclusion of pathophysiological/medical diagnoses in the list of "related to" statements. A medical diagnosis often does not provide adequate direction for nursing care. For example, the nursing diagnosis of chronic pain related to rheumatoid arthritis does not readily suggest specific nursing interventions. It is more useful for the nurse to identify specific causes of the chronic pain, such as inflammation, swelling, and fatigue; these in turn suggest more specific interventions. In cases where the medical diagnosis proves the best available information, as occurs with the more medically oriented diagnoses such as "decreased cardiac output" or "impaired gas exchange," the medical terminology is included.

Defining Characteristics

Data collection is frequently the source for identifying defining characteristics, sometimes called signs and symptoms or patient behaviors. These data, both subjective and objective, are organized into meaningful patterns and used to verify the nursing diagnosis. The most commonly seen defining characteristics for a given diagnosis are included; these should not be viewed as an all-inclusive listing.

Risk Factors

Nursing diagnoses designated as high risk are supported by risk factors that direct nursing actions to reduce or prevent the problem from developing. Because these nursing diagnoses have not yet occurred, risk factors replace the listing of actual defining characteristics and "related to" statements.

Patient Outcomes

Patient outcomes are observable behaviors or data that measure changes in the condition of the patient after nursing treatment. They are objective indicators of progress toward prevention of the development of high-risk nursing diagnoses or resolution/modification of actual diagnoses. Similar to other elements of the plan of care, patient outcome statements are dynamic and must be reviewed and modified periodically as the patient progresses. Assigning realistic *target or evaluation dates* for evaluation of progress toward outcome achievement is crucial. Because so many considerations are involved in the determination of when the outcome can be achieved (e.g., varying lengths of stay, individual patient condition), these plans of care do not include evaluation dates. In each case the date needs to be individualized and assigned using the professional judgment and discretion of the nurse caring for the patient.

Nursing Interventions

Nursing interventions are the treatment options/actions the nurse employs to prevent, modify, or resolve the nursing diagnosis. They are driven by the "related to" statements and risk factors and are selected based on the outcomes to be achieved. Treatment options should be chosen only if they apply realistically to a specific patient condition. The nurse also needs to determine frequencies for each intervention based on professional judgment and individual patient need.

We have included independent, interdependent, and dependent nursing interventions as they reflect current practice. We have not made a distinction between these kinds of interventions because of institutional differences and increasing independence in nursing practice. The interventions that are interdependent or dependent will require collaboration with other professionals. The nurse will need to determine when this is necessary and take appropriate action. The interventions include assessment, therapeutic, and teaching actions.

Rationales

The rationales provide scientific explanation or theoretical bases for the interventions; interventions can then be selected more intelligently and actions can be tailored to each patient's needs.

The rationales provided may be used as a quick reference for the nurse unfamiliar with the reason for a given intervention and as a tool for patient education. These rationales may include principles, theories, and/or research findings from current literature. The rationales are intended as reference information and, as such, should not be transcribed into the permanent patient record. A rationale is not provided when the intervention is self-explanatory.

Discharge Planning/Continuity of Care

Discharge planning is the process of anticipating and planning for needs after discharge from community care. Effective discharge planning begins with the start of care and continues with ongoing assessment of the patient and family needs. Included in the discharge planning/continuity of care section are suggestions for follow-up measures, such as continuing support services; outpatient physical, occupational, speech, rehabilitation, or psychiatric therapy; spiritual counseling; social service assistance; follow-up appointments; and equipment/supplies.

References/Bibliography

A listing of references and/or bibliography appears at the conclusion of each plan of care or related group of plans. The purpose of this listing is to cite specific work used and to present background information or suggestions for further reading. Citings provided represent the most current nursing theory and/or research bases for inclusion in the plans of care.

Clinical Clips

Interspersed throughout some of the books are brief pieces of information related to the particular specialty. The intent is to blend some concept or theory tidbits with the practical nature of the books. This information not only may enrich the nurse's knowledge base but also may be used in the dissemination of patient education information.

A WORD ABOUT FAMILY

The authors and editors of this series recognize the vital role that family and/or other significant people play in the recovery of a patient. Isolation from the family unit during hospitalization may disrupt self-concept and feelings of security. Family members or persons involved in the patient's care must be included in the teaching to ensure that it is appropriate and will be followed.

ACKNOWLEDGMENTS

Any undertaking of the magnitude of this series becomes the concern of many people. I specifically thank all of the very capable nursing specialists who authored or edited the individual books. Their attention to providing state-of-the-art information in a quick, usable form will give the reader the current reference information necessary for providing excellent patient care.

Special thanks also goes to my friend Mark Gregory, for his clever coinage of the term *clinical clips*.

The editorial staff, particularly Patricia E. Casey and Elisabeth F. Williams, and the production staff at Delmar Publishers have been outstanding. Their frank criticism, comments, and encouragement have improved the quality of the series.

Finally, but most importantly, I thank my husband, John, and children, Katrina and Allison, for their sacrifices and patience during yet another publishing project.

Kathy V. Gettrust
Series Editor

*This book is dedicated to our families with appreciation for their
support, and to the many caring and competent community health
nurses with whom we have had the privilege to work.*

Environmental Conditions

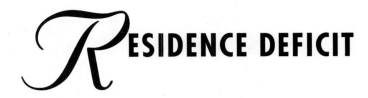

RESIDENCE DEFICIT

Naomi E. Ervin, PhD, RN, CS

A residence deficit is any situation or condition that may create an unsafe environment in the patient's home. Nurses should assess each home for deficits within the context of the patient's physical and emotional status. Since the objective of identifying residence deficits is to correct them before an adverse outcome occurs, all deficits should be noted and included in each patient's care plan.

ETIOLOGIES
- Lack of upkeep
- Poor construction
- Use of unsafe materials
- Inadequate income
- Homelessness
- Crowded living spaces
- Use of materials in unsafe manner
- High-rise apartment for elderly
- Combination of the above

CLINICAL MANIFESTATIONS
- Cluttered living space
- Inadequate/crowded living space
- Inadequate heating/cooling
- Inadequate or obstructed exits and entries
- Inadequate safety devices
- Presence of lead-based paint
- Steep stairs or unsafe stairs, decks, or railings, with children and elderly
- Structurally unsound home
- Unsafe gas/electrical appliances
- Unsafe or inadequate water supply
- Unsafe mats/throw rugs

3

- Unsafe storage of dangerous objects or substances
- Presence of rodents, insect infestation
- Presence of environmental hazards

CLINICAL/DIAGNOSTIC FINDINGS
None

▶ NURSING DIAGNOSIS: *High Risk for Impaired Home Maintenance Management*

Risk Factors
- Patient's advanced age
- Physical or psychological conditions which decrease patient's ability to maintain home
- Aging or deteriorating structures/neighborhood

Patient Outcomes
- Patient's home is free of vermin.
- Patient is protected from unsafe conditions in the home.

Nursing Interventions	Rationales
If rodents or insect infestation noted, assist patient to secure services of exterminator or to purchase and use commercially available products. Instruct patient/family in methods to keep food storage areas clean and free from vermin or chemical contamination.	Vermin contribute to unsanitary environment, contaminate food storage areas, and can spread disease.
Ensure home is secure from intruders by assessing home security devices and planning to upgrade as needed.	Securely fastened door and window locks provide enhanced safety and decrease the likelihood of unwanted home intruders.
Assess home heating/cooling/ventilation and develop correction plan with patient if deficiencies are noted.	Elderly are at high risk of hypothermia. Poor air ventilation can contribute to increased respiratory difficulties. Improperly functioning heating systems may cause carbon monoxide concentrations to rise to dangerous levels.

▶ NURSING DIAGNOSIS: *High Risk for Injury from Falls*

Risk Factors
- Loose throw rugs
- Cluttered living space
- Loose electrical cords
- Poorly lit or unsafe stairs, decks, and railings

Patient Outcomes
Patient is free from falls.

Nursing Interventions	Rationales
Assess patient's residence for risk factors that are known to frequently contribute to falls.	Falls in the home are a leading cause of injury. Elderly or unstable patients are especially at risk.
Assess patient and family's ability to correct deficits.	Assistance from other person or agency may be needed. If there are structural problems, refer to landlord or municipal department. If patient owns home, assist in identifying potential resources for securing needed assistance.
Refer patient for assistance and monitor correction of deficits.	It is important to follow up on the adequacy and completeness of referrals made for home repair and assistance.

▶ NURSING DIAGNOSIS: *High Risk for Injury from Residence Fire*

Risk Factors
- Smoking in bed
- Forgetfulness related to cooking
- Unsafe or improperly used heating equipment
- Unsafe electrical wiring
- Absence of smoke detectors
- Matches/lighters within the reach of young children

Patient Outcomes
Patient is free from injury from a fire in the home.

Nursing Interventions	Rationales
Assess residence and patient's behavior for potential fire hazards.	Fire hazards or high-risk behavior, such as smoking in bed, may not be apparent to patient.
Plan with patient to correct environment to decrease fire hazards.	Unless patient is willing to correct environmental hazards or behavior, change is unlikely.
Assess location, type, number, and maintenance of smoke detectors.	Smoke detectors must be functioning properly to prevent injury or fatality if a fire occurs.
Monitor correction of potential hazards or deficits.	Some corrections may require long-term solutions and/or may involve other agencies (e.g., city housing department).

DISCHARGE PLANNING/CONTINUITY OF CARE
Refer patient to appropriate community resources.
- Housing department of city or county
- Social service for financial need
- Health department
- Senior citizens
- Church or local service club for repairs
- Fire department for smoke detectors

OTHER PLANS OF CARE TO REFERENCE
- Environmental infection control
- Personal hygiene

BIBLIOGRAPHY
Hu, X., Wesson, D., & Kenney, B. (1993). Home injuries to children. *Canadian Journal of Public Health, 84*(93), 155–158.

Martin, K. S., & Scheet, N.J. (1992). *The Omaha system. Applications for community health nursing.* Philadelphia: Saunders.

Mayhew, M. S. (1991). Strategies for promoting safety and preventing injury. *Nursing Clinics of North America, 26*(4), 885–893.

Williams, M. N., & Nolan, M. (1993). Prevention of falls among older people at home. *British Journal of Nursing, 2*(12), 609–613.

Wortel, E., & de Geus, G. H. (1993). Prevention of home related injuries of pre-school children: Safety measures taken by mothers. *Health Education Research, 8*(2), 217–231.

$\mathcal{E}$NVIRONMENTAL INFECTION CONTROL

Sandra C. Swallow, BSN, MPH

Environmental infection control is the process of assessing the home environment, identifying situations which place the patient at increased risk for developing infections, and helping the patient develop effective strategies to minimize symptoms and prevent infections resulting from exposure to environmental irritants and toxins. The nurse's role is to observe the patient for sensitivity, assist in identifying the environmental toxic agent, provide physiological support, and assist the patient in minimizing the risk of infection from environmental contaminants. Because the practice setting is the patient's home, issues such as patient's and family's behavior, lifestyle, preferences, and privacy must be considered and respected.

─────── **Clinical Clip** ───────

Universal Precautions

Universal precautions are measures health care workers use to prevent the transmission of infections. The Occupational Safety and Health Administration's (OSHA) Bloodborne Pathogen Standard mandates universal precautions in health care, including community and home health, to prevent occupational transmission of human immunodeficiency virus (HIV) and hepatitis B virus (HBV) to health care workers by blood. All patients should be assumed potentially infectious for HBV and other blood-borne pathogens. Universal precautions apply to blood and other body fluids containing visible blood. If the potential for contact with blood or other potentially infectious material exists, universal precautions must be used consistently.

Body Fluid Chart

Use Universal Precautions	Universal Precautions Not Needed*
Semen	Feces
Vaginal secretions	Nasal secretions
Cerebrospinal fluid	Sputum
Synovial fluid	Sweat
Pleural fluid	Tears
Peritoneal fluid	Urine
Pericardial fluid	Vomitus
Amniotic fluid	

Unless visible blood is present.

Tips for Home Care Professional

Use personal protective equipment to reduce risks.

Practice safe handling of specimens.

Protect yourself when handling sharps.

Decontaminate blood spills.

Handle contaminated linen, sharps, and regulated waste properly.

Use frequent and proper handwashing technique.

Use correct bag technique.

Report exposure incidents immediately.

Use warning labels and signs.

Use gloves when drawing blood.

Consider hepatitis B vaccinations.

Educate patients and caregivers about universal precautions.

ETIOLOGIES
- Tobacco smoke
- Asbestos
- Formaldehyde
- Combustion byproducts, i.e., nitrous oxide
- Radon
- Pathogens and allergens
- Poor sanitation
- Contaminated water
- Poor ventilation
- Unvented cooking appliances
- Kerosene space heaters
- Unvented gas stoves
- Wood stoves
- Fireplaces
- Improperly installed or maintained chimneys and flues
- Motor vehicle exhaust
- Poorly maintained air conditioning systems
- Poorly maintained humidifiers, dehumidifiers
- Deteriorating/damaged insulation, fire-proofing, acoustical material
- Home remodeling projects
- Pet dander and/or urine
- Wet furnishings and carpeting
- Presence of insects
- Dry-cleaned items
- Homes with substantial amounts of new pressed-wood products
- Pesticide application
- Poor sanitation and waste disposal

CLINICAL MANIFESTATIONS
- Burning watery eyes
- Difficulty wearing contact lenses
- Headaches
- Drowsiness
- Nasal and throat irritation
- Dermatitis
- Difficulty breathing
- Chronic airway obstruction
- Laryngeal edema
- Nausea
- Weakness
- Dizziness

CLINICAL/DIAGNOSTIC FINDINGS
- Formaldehyde: The American Society of Heating, Refrigerating, and Air Conditioning sets the standard for controlling formaldehyde in indoor air outside the work place at 0.1 ppm (parts per million). Levels can be greater that 0.3 ppm in homes with substantial amounts of new pressed-wood products.

- Radon: Lower than 4 picocuries per liter. Normal levels are between 1 and 1.5 picocuries per liter of air. Four picocuries and greater per liter of air is considered a substantially elevated risk for lung cancer.
- Wood stoves: The Environmental Protection Agency (EPA) has specific emission standards for wood stoves.

▶ NURSING DIAGNOSIS: *Knowledge Deficit*

Related To change in behavior, lifestyle, or environment that affects health status, including starting to smoke, using new cosmetics or cleaning agents, moving into a new home, new household furnishings, and a new pet

Defining Characteristics
Patient is unaware of:
- adverse health affects triggered by environmental agents.
- symptoms of infection related to exposure to environmental pollutants.
- ways to modify environment to decrease adverse health effects.
- agencies and resources to help identify and resolve environmental hazards.

Patient Outcomes
Patient and family verbalizes understanding of adverse health effects triggered by environmental hazards.

Nursing Interventions	Rationales
Assess home environment for pollutants which could put the patient at risk for infections. (See etiology section.)	Pollutants in the environment have been identified as risk factors in developing infections.
Teach patient signs and symptoms of infection related to environmental hazards. (See clinical manifestations section.)	Reinforces importance of minimizing risk of infection. Helps identify environmental hazards.
Assess patient's ability to correct or modify hazard and risk. For example, smoking outside, encasing asbestos, ventilating for elevated radon level, exterminating insects/roaches, and avoiding using kerosene or wood-burning heaters.	In many cases, people cannot change their environment, but things can be done to make it safer. Family members' and landlord's support and cooperation may play an important role. For example, requesting family members smoke outside the house or having landlord exterminate roaches.

Nursing Interventions	Rationales
Teach the patient why the environmental problem is a hazard.	Teaching the patient about the environmental hazard may influence him or her to make appropriate changes.
Refer patient to agencies and resources that can assist with detecting hazards (e.g., the EPA Public Information Center or the drugstore for tests that can measure radon or lead).	Providing patient with tips and resources to answer questions may increase awareness of problems and can influence behavior and lifestyle changes. The EPA provides publications and lists of state agencies responsible for indoor air quality. A kit to test for radon can be purchased for a nominal fee. Analyzing the information collected must be done through a laboratory and requires an additional charge.

▶ NURSING DIAGNOSIS: *High Risk for Infection*

Risk Factors
- Environmental tobacco smoke
- Remodeling projects, sanding or cutting construction materials
- Wet carpeting or furnishings
- Mold/mildew
- Improperly maintained chimneys and flues
- Motor vehicle exhaust
- Pet dander or urine
- Unsafe heating appliances
- Poor air ventilation
- Poorly maintained air conditioners, humidifiers, dehumidifiers
- Cognitive deficits
- Inability to perceive environmental hazards or hazardous situations
- Improper handwashing technique

Patient Outcomes
The patient and family express a desire to modify behavior, lifestyle, or home to live in a safer environment.

Nursing Interventions	Rationales
Assess patient's residence, behavior, and lifestyle for potential infection risks.	Establishes level of need for education. Provides baseline to monitor progress.
Teach signs and symptoms of respiratory tract infections.	Being aware of outcomes may influence change. For example, tobacco smoke is linked to an increased risk of lower respiratory tract infections and chronic respiratory symptoms in children.
Instruct in ways to minimize the spread of infection to others.	Good handwashing technique controls the spread of organisms which produce disease.
Instruct in using protective barriers or safety aids when appropriate, for example, masks when house is under construction.	Protective barriers and safety aids will minimize risk of infection.

DISCHARGE PLANNING/CONTINUITY OF CARE
- Refer to smoking cessation clinics.
- Refer to state agencies to test air quality.
- Reinforce need for follow-up visits with physician if symptoms of infection occur.

BIBLIOGRAPHY
Buckler, G. F. (1994). The effects of indoor air quality on health. *Imprint, Apr/May*, 60–66.

Burge, H. A. (1989). Indoor air and infectious disease. *State of the Art Reviews: Occupational Medicine—Problems Buildings: Buildings Associated Illness and the Sick Building Syndrome 4*, 713–721.

The health consequences of involuntary smoking. A report of the Surgeon General, Department of Health and Human Services PHS publication [CDC] 87-8398. Rockville, MD: U.S. Government Printing Office, 1986

Kilburn, K. H. (1992). Asbestos and other fibers. *Public Health and Preventive Medicine*, 343–364.

Landrigan, P. J. (1992). Arsenic. *Environmental and Occupational Medicine*, 473–477.

Samet, J. M., & Spengler, J. D. (1992). A study of respiratory illnesses in infants and nitrogen dioxide exposure. *Archives of Environmental Health, 47*(1) 57–63.

Sinclair, B. J. (1994). *Alternative Health Care Resources: A Directory &*
   Guide, 126–139.

Psychosocial Conditions

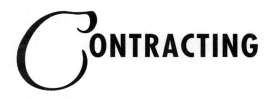

CONTRACTING

Diana P. Hackbarth, PhD, RN

Contracting with patients and families is a technique used to enhance mutual goal achievement. It can be used effectively with any nursing or medical diagnosis in almost any home care situation. Contracting requires that the home care nurse, patient, and family actively and mutually collaborate in assessing strengths and needs, in identifying mutually agreed upon goals, in specifying what each is willing and able to do, and in working actively to perform their agreed-upon activities until goals are met. The contract specifies *who* will do *what* and *when*. It is continuously evaluated and renegotiated as needs change or goals are met. (Refer to Table 3-1.)

The outcome of successful contracting is both a timely discharge from the community or home care agency and a patient and family that feel increasingly empowered, resourceful, and more able to take control of meeting their own self-care needs. Contracting is not just a method to encourage patient compliance to the therapeutic regimen. Rather, it is a way to operationalize a philosophy of collaboration between nurse, patient, and families in which each actively participates and feels a sense of achievement when mutual goals are met.

Contracting is predicated on the assumption that patients and families have the right and responsibility to participate actively in planning their own care. In community and home care, where the number of visits may be limited by the payment source or by policy, patients and families must actively participate in their self-care in a timely manner prior to discharge. The contracting process, used early on, helps delineate the nurse's role and the role of the patient and family to clearly define what is expected from each person. This notion of partnership, collaboration, mutual goal setting, and participation is congruent with the American Nurses Association (ANA) Standards of Community Health Nursing (1986) and most of the Patient Bill of Rights documents promulgated by home health care agencies.

Table 3-1 • Characteristics of a Patient Contract*

Mutual—All parties agree on goals and specific activities each will perform

Realistic—Possible, can be achieved given patient and family and resources available strengths and limitations

Measurable—How often? How much? When? Where?

Positive—Build on strengths; work *toward* goals

Time dated—When will it start? How long will it last?

Rewardable—Positive reinforcement for small steps along the way. Rewards should be individualized, low cost, culturally appropriate, and related to the target activity or behavior.

Written or Verbal—Clear, specific as to who will do what. Refer to contract and assess progress at each visit.

Evaluated—Compare criteria for success to outcomes. Modify and renegotiate as needs change or goals are met.

Based on Herje (1980).

── Clinical Clip ──

Contingency contracting is based on the work of Bandura (1977) and other social learning theorists. In its purest form, social learning theory seeks to reinforce positive behaviors through rewards and to extinguish negative or maladaptive behaviors by not rewarding them. In this model, desired behaviors are clearly specified in realistic, observable, and measurable terms. Rewards are contingent on performing the desired behaviors. Rewards can be external, such as praise or receiving a deserved object or prize, or internal, such as feelings of success or increased control over one's life.

ETIOLOGIES

- First visit or early in home care process
- Complex treatment or medication regimen involving extensive time, energy, and resources
- Treatment plan that involves difficult behavioral or lifestyle changes (e.g., diet, exercise, decreased use of alcohol, cigarettes, and drugs, change in parenting or caregiver style)
- Treatment plan that involves multiple home care providers or several agencies
- Patient newly diagnosed or patient and family unfamiliar or uncomfortable with carrying out the prescribed treatment
- Patient or family has psychosocial or environmental problems which make adherence to externally dictated treatment plans unrealistic

- Number of visits limited by third-party payors so that self-care goals need to be met quickly
- Early hospital discharge has prevented patient and family from assimilating new information related to treatment and plan of care

---
Clinical Clip

Examples of helpful contracting are:

- Changing undesirable or abusive parenting or caregiving behaviors.
- Preventing suicide among depressed persons until arrangements can be made for hospitalization.
- Helping families cope with complex drug and treatment regimens.
- Helping confused elderly patients to divide self-care tasks into manageable components.
- Teaching school-age diabetic or asthmatic children proper diet, exercise, and medication management in return for increased independence.

CLINICAL MANIFESTATIONS
- Lack of understanding or misinterpretation of the treatment plan
- Confusion, anxiety, or feelings of being overwhelmed by home care tasks
- Unwilling or unable to provide all or portions of needed care
- Disorganized, poorly maintained home environment; lack of supplies, equipment, or necessities of daily life
- Helplessness or hopelessness; inability to mobilize energy

CLINICAL/DIAGNOSTIC FINDINGS
None

▶ NURSING DIAGNOSIS: *Applies to All Nursing Diagnoses*

Defining Characteristics
See clinical manifestations section.

Patient Outcomes
Patient and family will:
- comply with care plan.
- express feelings of being empowered, resourceful, and able to take control over their self-care needs.

Nursing Interventions	Rationales
Schedule visit when primary care-giver and key family/significant others are present or available by phone.	All persons who will be involved in caregiving should participate in the contracting process so that it is truly collaborative.
Begin to develop a trusting relationship with patient and family.	Successful contracts depend on feelings of mutual trust and on sharing concerns and achievements.
Listen to patient and family. Observe, clarify, and ask for feedback and validation. Share perceptions as indicated.	Understanding the patient's caregiving situation is essential before goals can be agreed upon.
Assess patient's and family's perceptions of their needs, including what they consider priority needs. The patient's priorities may be different from the nurse's priorities or the initial treatment plan.	People are more likely to participate and feel a sense of ownership if they believe their own needs will be met.
Ask the patient and family to describe their diagnosis and treatment plan. Also elicit their feelings about the issues.	The patient and family may have varying levels of understanding related to the diagnosis and plan of care or they may have quite different feelings about similar information. It will be difficult to contract unless there is common understanding and sharing of feelings.
Assess patient's and family's perceptions of why the nurse is visiting and what they expect from home care providers and clarify patient's and family's goals.	Patients often do not know who sent the nurse, what agency employed the nurse, or why the nurse is coming to their home. Since contracting requires that each participant clearly outline what they are willing and able to do, clarifying the role of the nurse and other providers is essential. Goals often differ between patients and providers and may also differ between the patient and family members. All participants must express their goals before mutual goals can be agreed upon.

Nursing Interventions	Rationales
Explore the strengths and human, material, financial, and emotional resources the patient and family possess.	Contracts should be positive and built on existing strengths. The nurse needs to help the patient and family develop their own strengths and resources in a timely manner since home care is time limited and the family will have to be self-sufficient when visits terminate.
Assist patient and family to recognize what resources may be lacking and to identify resources in their environment which could be mobilized. Outline additional resources that could be provided by the home care agency or other community agencies.	Utilizing appropriate resources makes it easier for patients to follow the therapeutic regimen, change health-related behavior, and/or reduce the burden of care in family members.
Identify individualized motivators or rewards that could be meaningful to the patient or family and others involved in contracting.	All behavior change is difficult, especially change in lifestyle or patterns of social and emotional functioning. Contracting is based on social learning theory in which desired behaviors are rewarded and frequently reinforced.
Discuss how willing the patient and family are to share responsibility and participate in their plan of care. Encourage realistic expectations of role performance.	Contracts delineate who will do what activity. The better the match between expectations, ability, and willingness to perform activities, the more likely goals will be met and participants will feel satisfied and reinforced.
Mutually agree upon goals and specific behaviors or activities that need to be accomplished. Modify the treatment plan based on input from patient and family so that it is realistic.	Begin with concrete goals and observable behaviors that are related to known needs all can agree on.
Assist family in identifying who may be capable, affordable, and acceptable to assume responsibility for specific activities (i.e., patient, nurse,	Specific activities must be congruent with the treatment plan and possible, given the constraints of the home care agency. Patient/

Nursing Interventions	Rationales
other home care providers, family, friends, neighbors, respite care).	family caregivers' activities will depend on the treatment plan and the patient's and family members' health, level of understanding, motivation, available resources, and support systems.
Break down agreed-upon goals and tasks of patient care into smaller components and specific behaviors and activities.	Large, complex tasks often seem overwhelming. Identifying smaller, achievable activities allows for frequent positive reinforcement.
Teach the patient and family each agreed-upon activity or task so they feel safe and comfortable with the components of caregiving.	Devise achievable criteria to measure caregiving or other patient and family goals.
Specify how often, how much, where, or when tasks should be performed.	Help evaluate progress toward goal achievement.
Specify how nurse, patient, and family will feel rewarded for their efforts.	Rewards should be individualized, low cost, culturally appropriate, and related to the activity or behavior.
Specify time frame for activities included in the contract. Timing should be congruent with family lifestyle and patterns in the household. For example, caregiving could be performed before a favorite soap opera or when a neighbor is available after work to assist.	Contracts will be more likely fulfilled if they cause less disruption in daily routines.
Write or verbally agree on contracts with all participants.	Goals and directions for specific activities may be written and a copy kept by both the nurse and the patient. This contract can be referred to, modified, and rewritten as goals are achieved or needs change. Verbal contracts can be restated at each visit and renegotiated as needed.
Evaluate contract weekly or at each visit as appropriate.	Agreed-upon goals and criteria are compared for success to actual performance.

DISCHARGE PLANNING/CONTINUITY OF CARE

- Review contract and evaluate progress. Update contract as appropriate and refer to other resources if needed.
- Follow up with patient at a later date. Tickler file can be used.

SAMPLE CONTRACTS

Sample Patient Contract

Mr. R was a 69-year-old single man with peripheral vascular disease and diabetes controlled by oral medications. He lived alone in a cluttered brick bungalow in a working-class neighborhood. He was seen three times a week by a registered nurse for care of his chronic leg ulcers and received home delivered meals and homemaker services. Although he was alert and cooperative with his leg ulcer care, his lifestyle habits left much to be desired. Mr. R was overweight, had limited mobility, poor personal hygiene, ate junk food instead of his home delivered meals, and was a heavy smoker. There were many concerns about his health habits and home environment, but the immediate safety problem was the potential for injury from fire. Mr. R often sent a neighbor out to buy donuts and cigarettes and then fell asleep while smoking. His bedding, favorite armchair, and pajamas were pockmarked with cigarette burns. The nurses were very concerned about his lifestyle and some believed he should not be living alone but should be encouraged to seek institutional care instead. His primary nurse felt that contracting to change his smoking behavior was a more practical short-term goal.

The primary nurse had a trusting relationship with Mr. R and initiated the discussion of his smoking habits. Mr. R readily acknowledged that he sometimes fell asleep smoking and that this could cause a fire. He also knew that "smoking is unhealthy" but he was less informed about the specific link between poor circulation, poor wound healing, and smoking. He stated very clearly that he wanted to remain in his own home and be independent. He was initially unwilling to contract to quit smoking altogether, but he was willing to modify his smoking habits over a set period of time.

Initial Contract—First Week

- Patient agrees not to smoke in bed; will only smoke while sitting up awake in armchair or at the kitchen table for one week.
- Nurse agrees to contact the American Lung Association (ALA) to get materials on tips on quitting smoking.
- Patient and nurse agree to discuss cutting down and/or quitting smoking the following week.

In this case, the patient had several internal motivators. These were his own fear of fire and some beginning recognition that reducing smoking could speed wound healing, which was very important to him. External motivators included apprehension about possible discussion of nursing home placement if his lifestyle didn't improve and his desire to receive materials and more information on quitting smoking. He also seemed grateful for the attention and concern of the nurses and wanted to cooperate in his plan of care. His ultimate goal was healed leg ulcers, increased mobility within his home, and ability to once again participate in some outside activities. The nurse was motivated by her concerns for Mr. R's safety and her strong desire to aid patients who desired to quit smoking. She also got much support from other members of the health team who believed anybody who could help change Mr. R's lifestyle was a miracle worker!

Contract for Weeks Two and Three
- Patient agrees to reduce the amount he smokes daily from two packs to one pack by week three and write down in log book number of cigarettes he smokes each day.
- Patient agrees to only smoke while sitting up at the kitchen table which is cleared of papers and has an ashtray readily available, beginning immediately.
- Patient agrees to read, discuss, and try smoking cessation methods suggested by the ALA materials and report back each Friday visit.
- Nurse agrees to continue to support patient in quitting efforts by posting a chart of his progress.
- Nurse agrees to contact the local church to find a volunteer to help Mr. R go outside to sit in his yard within the next week.

Contract for Week Four
- Patient agrees to set quit smoking date for end of fourth week.
- Patient agrees to continue to use suggestions such as chewing gum or drinking water instead of smoking; smoking only in one place (the kitchen chair); calling one of his old poker pals who already quit smoking for emotional support, and visualizing increased blood flow and healing of his leg ulcers.
- Patient will put all smoking materials, matches, ashtrays, etc. in bag to be stored in the garage.
- Patient will put the $6.00 he used to spend daily on cigarettes in a glass jar and save up for a new television.
- Nurse will continue to encourage and support his efforts to quit smoking.
- Homemaker service will initiate a special housecleaning and "airing out" of house after the quit day.
- The church volunteer will take Mr. R out for lunch on his quit day to a smokefree restaurant.
- Mr. R's old poker pal will call everyday at 4:00 p.m. to offer support.

Contract for Weeks Five and Six
- Patient will not smoke and will continue to use techniques to aid in relieving withdrawal symptoms suggested in ALA materials.
- Nurse will monitor progress and offer support on each visit.
- Patient's physician and outpatient team will personally congratulate him on his next visit during week five. The hospital health educator will also print up a certificate to show he is a successful quitter.

- Volunteer visits and telephone calls from his old poker pal will continue for the next month.
- Nurse visits will be reduced to two times a week because leg ulcers are healing.
- Homemaker services and home delivered meals will continue.

Mr. R successfully quit smoking and his leg ulcers slowly improved. The danger of fire was diminished. His mobility increased and he was able to leave the house with assistance of the church volunteer or a neighbor. His donut consumption remained unchanged, but he did put on clean clothes for his outings. He remained in his own home and continued to live independently when home health care visits terminated.

REFERENCE

American Nurses Association, (1986). *Standards of community health nursing practice*. Washington, DC: American Nurses Association.

American Nurses Association, (1996 in press). *Standards for population-based nursing practice*. Washington, DC: American Nurses Association.

$\mathcal{P}$ATIENT AND FAMILY RIGHTS/ SELF-DETERMINATION

Kathleen Klauseger, MSN

Before the nurse begins to deliver care in the community setting, nurses and patients must set mutual goals and clarify their respective roles. They must discuss patient/caregiver rights in the health care relationship, including the right to formulate advanced directives and the right to consent to or refuse treatment.

The Patient Self-Determination Act (PSDA) is a federal legislative act. It mandates that all health care providers participating in the Medicare and Medicaid programs are responsible for informing patients of their right to formulate advance directives and their right to consent to or refuse treatment.

The PSDA is designed to encourage patients to consider treatment options and document their preferences before they are no longer capable of participating in the decision-making process. Patients are empowered through education and information to formulate advanced directives or waive their right to do so.

Advanced directives usually are written in the form of living wills and durable powers of attorney for health care. A living will is outlined in writing by a competent individual; it specifies treatment wishes. The living will becomes effective only when the individual becomes incompetent. The durable power of attorney for health care allows an individual to appoint a designated decision maker in the event of incompetence.

ETIOLOGIES
- Patient/caregiver with unrealistic goals
- Patient/caregiver unclear about their roles
- Patient mentally incompetent with no caregiver available

CLINICAL MANIFESTATIONS

- Not listening
- Not participating in care
- Anger
- Crying
- Inability to make decisions
- Depression

CLINICAL/DIAGNOSTIC FINDINGS

None

▶ NURSING DIAGNOSIS: *Knowledge Deficit*

Related To
- Right to execute advance directives
- Right to consent or refuse treatment options
- Realistic goal setting

Defining Characteristics
- Lack of knowledge regarding advanced directives and treatment options
- Unwilling or unable to set mutually agreed upon goals
- Inappropriate behavior patterns

Patient Outcomes
Patient/caregiver will be able to:
- describe advanced directives and treatment options for care.
- set goals mutually agreed upon with the nurse.

Nursing Interventions	Rationales
Discuss with patient/caregiver what advance directives are and the available treatment options related to their particular case. Encourage patients/caregiver to consider and document their treatment options before they are no longer capable of making decisions. Give written information as appropriate.	These discussions are required by law.
Discuss what the goals for care are and what is reasonable and attainable for both the patient/caregiver and the nurse. It is best to accomplish this on the admission visit.	Mutual goal setting is essential for success.

DISCHARGE PLANNING/CONTINUITY OF CARE

- Follow up with referral source if unable to mutually set goals. Care cannot be initiated until patient/caregiver is informed of their rights and agrees to goals.

Clinical Clip

Requirements of Health Care Providers

1. All adults must be furnished with written information about their rights under state law, which must include:
   - the right to accept or refuse treatment.
   - the right to execute advanced directives.
   - written policies of the facility respecting the exercise of these rights.

2. Health care providers must:
   - ensure compliance respecting advanced directives.
   - educate staff and community on issues concerning advanced directives.
   - document in the patient's medical record whether the patient has executed an advanced directive.
   - not discriminate against an individual based on whether an advanced directive has been executed.

BIBLIOGRAPHY

Davis, M. (1992). The clients right to self-determination, *Caring, 6,* 26–32.

Holly, C. (1993). Advanced directives. *Home Healthcare Nurse, 11*(5), 34–38.

Huntington, S. (1991). New provider responsibilities under the Patient Self-Determination Act. *Caring, 10*(9), 20–25.

Weber, G. (1993). Tips on implementing the Self Determination Act. *Nursing and Health Care, 14*(2), 86–91.

*R*EFERRAL TO COMMUNITY RESOURCES

Jackie Kareb, MS, RN

As case managers, home health nurses often link patients to community resources and other caregivers. Patients often need other health care providers to help them cope with receiving care at home and with health-related lifestyle changes.

Patient outcomes and eventual discharge from the home health agency depends on the ability of the patient and family to become independent in self-care and manage activities of daily living. Other professionals—including those in physical therapy, occupational therapy, social services, support groups, psychiatric counseling, spiritual counseling, and assistance with activities of daily living (ADLs)—can assure that the patient receives the optimal benefits from their care. These services may be concurrent with nursing care or continued after discharge from home care.

ETIOLOGIES

- Multiple need/providers
- New diagnosis
- Early discharge from hospital
- Complex therapeutic regimen
- Multiple caregivers

CLINICAL MANIFESTATIONS

- Unfamiliar with, uncomfortable with, or unable to carry out prescribed treatment
- Hospital readmissions or exacerbations of the same problem

CLINICAL/DIAGNOSTIC FINDINGS

None

▶ NURSING DIAGNOSIS: *Knowledge Deficit of the Referral Process*

Related To self-care skills and health maintenance

Defining Characteristics
- Early discharge prevents patient/family from assimilating new information related to diagnosis or treatment.
- Patient verbalizes need for additional services.

Patient Outcomes
- Patient and family members will be able to verbalize and demonstrate practices necessary for self-care and health maintenance.

Nursing Interventions	Rationales
Assess current level of knowledge.	Although the patient may have been taught in the past, it is important not to make assumptions about what has been learned, retained, or assimilated.
Assess willingness of patient and/or family to take responsibility for care.	Presence of an available, willing, and able caregiver is necessary for self-care.
If appropriate, assess the availability of other potential caregivers to assist.	Other family members, friends, volunteers from the local church, or paid caregivers may provide assistance when the patient or family are unable to do so.
Refer patient/family to a social worker for assistance with resources.	The home health or community care social worker can both assess patient/family coping abilities and their eligibility for resources to meet care needs.
Refer the patient to other home care team members who can assist in improving self-care capabilities.	Physical and occupational therapy can be used to upgrade functional status and endurance. A home health aide can assist the patient in becoming progressively more independent in personal care.
Provide instruction progressing from simple to complex, allowing time for return demonstration.	Use of reinforcement and return demonstration helps to improve patient/family confidence and allows the nurse to evaluate learning.

Nursing Interventions	Rationales
Begin planning for discharge from home care with the initial home visit.	Except in chronic cases, the goal of home care should be to assist the patient/family in becoming independent of the home care providers.
Periodically review with the patient his or her progress in achieving goals, updating the care plan to include progressively more patient/family involvement.	This is important in reinforcing progress and in negotiating decreasing services toward eventual discharge.

► **NURSING DIAGNOSIS:** *Impaired Communication with Community Resources*

Related To lack of knowledge, social isolation due to illness, inability to negotiate the health care delivery system

Defining Characteristics
- Hospital readmissions or exacerbations of the same problem
- Confusion regarding use of or eligibility for community assistance
- New health problem and/or change in functional status necessitating assistance

Patient Outcomes
Patient communicates with appropriate resources

Nursing Intervention	Rationales
Assess patient's current use of and experience with community resources.	This is necessary for obtaining a baseline as well as assessing if the patient has maximized use of resources.
If appropriate, initiate a care conference inviting all involved caregivers to provide input. Include the patient and family whenever appropriate.	Shared understanding and consensus regarding the plan of care is needed.
Refer the patient to the home care or community social worker for assistance with community resources.	The social worker will be able to assess eligibility and connect the patient with appropriate resources. He or she can also provide brief

Nursing Intervention	Rationales
	counseling to promote patient coping and acceptance of assistance.
Evaluate and follow up on the outcome of any referrals.	This assures patient and family follow through. It also allows the nurse to evaluate the effectiveness of the referral and patient and family satisfaction.

DISCHARGE PLANNING/CONTINUITY OF CARE

- Review current care plan and modify to ensure postdischarge needs are met.
- Coordinate care with referral to ensure ongoing participation of all appropriate providers and community resources.
- Discuss family's role in maintaining ongoing support from community resources.

BIBLIOGRAPHY

Carr, P. (1993). Discharge planning. *Home Healthcare Nurse, 11*(2), 52–53.

Helberg, J. L. (1993). Patient's status at home care discharge. *Image, 25*(2), 93–99.

Kunkler, R., & Mitchell, A. (1994). Advice over the telephone. *Nursing Times, 90*(46), 29–30.

Zalta, E. (1994). Is success spelled G-A-T-E-K-E-E-P-E-R? *Dermatology Nursing, 6*(5), 337–342.

$\mathcal{S}$OCIAL ISOLATION

Karen Egenes, RN, EdD

Social isolation occurs when an individual experiences an aloneness from an absence of anticipated relationships. The patient needs or desires contact with others but is unable to make that contact and thus experiences loneliness and unhappiness. Social isolation can develop gradually, causing a loss of all meaningful social contacts and relationships. Isolation can be self-imposed or can be due to ineffectively interacting with others. It has negative consequences when an individual feels physically or psychologically separated from others but has a desire for closer interactions. Social isolation can lead to profound feelings of depression, anger, or anxiety, which then leads to further isolation and can make others want to avoid the patient. Although not usually the primary diagnosis, the nurse in the community should be alert to manifestations of social isolation in patients when risk factors are present.

ETIOLOGIES
- Chronic illness, sensory impairment, or physical disability that results in confinement
- Depression
- Speech or hearing impediments
- Significant loss (spouse, job, etc.)
- Traumatic event (natural disaster, severe accident, etc.)
- Poor self-concept or lack of self-esteem
- Extreme poverty
- Loss of previous means of transportation
- Recent move to a different culture with unfamiliar language and customs

CLINICAL MANIFESTATIONS
Expression of feelings of being alone
- desire for increased social interaction

- feelings of loneliness
- feeling that time passes slowly

Depression
- decreased activity, physical and verbal
- difficulty making decisions
- changes in sleep patterns (constant drowsiness or insomnia)
- changes in eating patterns (overeating or anorexia)
- expression of feelings of low self-worth
- expression of feelings of helplessness or hopelessness
- mood of sadness, brooding
- drug or alcohol dependency

Anger
- blaming others for unhappiness related to social isolation
- verbally abusing or humiliating those considered responsible for the social isolation
- suicidal ideation or attempts

Anxiety
- somatic symptoms
- excessive denial to decrease anxiety and defend self against the effects of loneliness

CLINICAL/DIAGNOSTIC FINDINGS

Psychological instruments for measurement of loneliness
- the University of California at Los Angeles (UCLA) Loneliness Scale—measures the presence and degree of client loneliness
- the New York University (NYU) Loneliness Scale—measures long-term loneliness and feelings associated with the loneliness
- suicide assessment—if positive, indicates further intervention

▶ NURSING DIAGNOSIS: *High Risk for Violence—Self-Directed*

Risk Factors
- History of previous suicide attempts
- Talks about death/suicide as a solution to present problems
- Asks suspicious questions such as, "How many aspirin would it take to kill a person?"
- Seems worried and cries often
- Puts affairs in order and/or gives away prized possessions
- Has developed a realistic plan for committing suicide

Patient Outcomes
The patient will:
- refrain from impulsive acts of self-harm.

- make a verbal "no-suicide" contract.
- verbalize alternatives to suicidal behavior.
- contact a suicide intervention center or other community resource when feeling the urge to harm self.

Nursing Interventions	Rationales
Continue to assess risk for suicide (see clinical clip).	Protects the patient from harm by preventing harmful behavior.
Secure a no-suicide contract.	Demonstrates nurse's concern for the patient.
Discuss coping methods and problem-solving techniques as alternatives to suicide.	Helps the patient learn new coping methods to handle stressors.
Refer patient to crisis intervention center or other community resource.	Ensures follow-up care to provide additional support and protect patient's safety.

Clinical Clip

Eighty percent of persons attempting suicide first give behavioral or verbal clues of their intent including:
- talking about death.
- putting affairs in order, such as revising a will.
- writing a suicide note.
- saying goodby to staff members or giving away prized possessions.
- displaying sudden happiness when before they had been severely depressed.

Suicide Assessment

- Directly question the patient to clarify the meaning; "You said that death would be a welcome way to end your suffering. Are you planning to do something to hurt yourself?"
- If the patient answers "yes" to the above question, follow with another direct question: "Do you have a plan for how you will hurt yourself?"
- If the patient describes a plan, assess the lethality of the plan and the accessibility of weapons or equipment necessary to carry out the plan.
- Telephone police or family members to arrange for the patient to be escorted and admitted to a treatment facility.
- Stay with the patient until assistance arrives. A suicidal patient must never be left alone.

─────── **Clinical Clip** ───────

Suicide is the eighth leading cause of death among adults in the United States. It is the third leading cause of death among adolescents and the second leading cause of death among American college students. About 39% of all persons who commit suicide are age 65 or older. Approximately 30,000 people commit suicide each year, with an additional 250,000 suicide attempts yearly.

Suicide attempts often represent an individual's desperate attempt to communicate feelings of isolation, alienation, and worthlessness. If the individual is unable to express these feelings verbally, intense anxiety, depression, and violence directed toward the self might result. A suicide attempt might be an individual's attempt to communicate intense feelings, to resolve a painful emotional conflict, or to end a situation perceived as hopeless.

Persons most likely to commit suicide include the following:
1. White males over age 65 or between the ages of 15 and 24
2. Persons living alone, including those who are single, divorced, or widowed
3. Persons who are chronically or terminally ill
4. Persons who are psychotic or who are addicted to drugs or alcohol

▶ NURSING DIAGNOSIS: *Impaired Social Interaction*

Related To
- Absence of significant other
- Insufficient energy to initiate social interactions
- Change in role or relationship

Defining Characteristics
- Inability to establish meaningful relationships
- Marked decrease or lack of participation in social activities or relationships
- Expresses discomfort in social interactions

Patient Outcomes
Patient will:
- reestablish previous or new recreational patterns and activities.
- identify meaningful activities for times when human companionship is not available.
- establish satisfying and meaningful social relationships.

Nursing Interventions	Rationales
Provide a supportive relationship for the patient.	Increases patient self-esteem.
Encourage the patient to talk about feelings of loneliness.	Helps patient label and express feelings to define the effects of social isolation.
Involve family members and friends in escorting patients to outings and social and business activities.	A network of supportive persons increases the patient's social contacts and increases self-esteem.
Explore means of transportation available in the community.	Adequate means of transportation facilitates patient social interactions.
Identify mechanisms to provide social support and socialization, i.e., support groups and church and hobby clubs.	Increases patient opportunities for socialization.

▶ **NURSING DIAGNOSIS:** *Situational Low Self-Esteem*

Related To lack of positive feedback

Defining Characteristics
- Repeated self-deprecatory comments
- Verbalization of negative self-appraisal, i.e., perceives self as helpless or worthless
- Verbalization of inability to cope with life situations

Patient Outcomes
Patient will:
- identify positive aspects about self.
- interact socially with others.
- identify way of exerting some control over life situations.
- verbalize hope for the future.

Nursing Interventions	Rationales
Encourage patient to identify posi- tive aspects about self.	A focus on positive aspects of self decreases the likelihood of focus on negative aspects.
Assist patient to set realistic goals for self.	Enhance the likelihood of patient success.
Assist patient in planning activities in which success is likely.	Achievement/success enhance the patient's self-esteem.
Assess and activate patient's current social support network.	Reinforce satisfying, supportive relationships that build self-esteem.
Teach patient assertiveness skills.	Assertiveness helps the patient feel some control.
Praise patient for accomplishments, assertiveness, and attempts at socialization.	Recognition enhances self-esteem and encourages repeating desirable behaviors.

DISCHARGE PLANNING/CONTINUITY OF CARE
- Reinforce need for follow-up psychotherapy, as required, for treatment of depression.
- Reinforce contacting with crisis intervention center if suicidal ideation occurs/reoccurs.
- Refer patient to support groups, interest groups, and community support services. Contact social worker if necessary.
- Encourage family members and friends to maintain patient's social support network.

--- Clinical Clip ---

Support Groups

Support groups are a proven mechanism for providing social support. Self-help groups, which began with Alcoholics Anonymous in the 1930s, have demonstrated that the group process can be used effectively to change the behaviors and attitudes of group members. Support groups are usually organized around a unifying theme, such as a disabling condition or a stressful life event. Groups provide support, allow members to know they are not alone, and promote adaptive coping skills.

OTHER PLANS OF CARE TO REFERENCE

- Caregiver Burden/Support/Conflict Resolution
- Grieving and Loss
- Death and Dying

BIBLIOGRAPHY

Austin, A. (1989). Becoming immune to loneliness: Helping the elderly fill a void. *Journal of Gerontological Nursing, 15,* 25–29.

Buckwalter, K. C., & Stolley, J. (1991). Managing mentally ill elders at home. *Geriatric Nursing, 12*(3), 136–140.

Foxal, M. J., & Ekberg, J. Y. (1989). Loneliness of chronically ill adults and their spouses. *Issues in Mental Health Nursing, 10,* 44–50.

Keele-Card, G., Foxall, M. J., & Barron, C. R. (1990). Loneliness, depression, and support of patients with COPD and their spouses. *Public Health Nursing, 10*(4), 245–251.

Kinney, C. K. D., Mannetter, R., & Carpenter, M. (1985). Support groups. In G. M. Bulechek & J. C. McCloskey (Eds.), *Nursing interventions: Treatments for nursing diagnoses* (pp. 185–197). Philadelphia: W. B. Saunders.

Lehman, L., & Kelley, J. H. (1993). Nursing interventions for anxiety, depression, and suspiciousness in the home care setting. *Home Health Care Nursing, 11*(3), 35–40.

Mellick, E., Buckwalter, C., & Stolly, M. (1992). Suicide among elderly white men: Development of a profile. *Journal of Psychosocial Nursing and Mental Health Services, 30,* 30–32.

CAREGIVER BURDEN/ SUPPORT/CONFLICT RESOLUTION

Elaine Small Gardner, MS, RN, CS

Caregiving refers to the informal support provided by family members and friends for those who become dependent due to the physical and/or mental effects of chronic illness. Service providers, policymakers, and researchers have come to recognize this phenomenon as an important issue because of recent demographic, economic, and social changes (see Clinical Clip).

Many perceive caregiving as difficult, time consuming, and emotionally and physically burdensome (Given & Given, 1991). As a result, some caregivers may experience role strain, or the felt difficulty in fulfilling role obligations (Goode, 1960). The care recipient will most likely be institutionalized if role strain becomes too great.

In working with caregivers and care recipients at risk for institutionalization, nurses must utilize a broad conceptualization of health which includes such social dimensions as family functioning and resources. Additionally, the nurse's focus must include the family as well as the ill individual.

──────────────── **Clinical Clip** ────────────────

Recent Demographic, Economic, and Social Changes, Influencing Caregiving

Factors associated with the increased occurrence of caregiving:
- An increase in life expectancy and the proportion of elderly in the population
- An increase in the occurrence of chronic disease
- The Prospective Payment System (PPS) for hospital care and advancing medical technology, creating shortened hospital stays and the need for advanced care of the ill at home
- The increasing cost of institutional care for the elderly and disabled, delaying and sometimes prohibiting placement in a long-term care facility

Factors associated with burden/role strain:
- Declining birth rate, creating a reduction in the number of family members available who might provide assistance
- An increasingly mobile society whereby family members who might provide respite and support are less likely to live in the same community as the caregiver and care recipient
- A greater proportion of women, the traditional caregivers, in the labor market, decreasing their availability to provide ongoing assistance

---

ETIOLOGIES

Factors contributing to burden/role strain
- Inadequate health insurance and other financial resources to cover the cost of health care and any loss of income created by the change in roles
- Availability, continuity, and quality of services (Mui & Morrow-Howell, 1993; Small, 1987)
- Health of the care recipient and disease prognosis (Cantor, 1983)
- Onset or progression of chronic illness or disability, creating the need for assistance with activities of daily living
- Perceived health of the caregiver (Mui & Morrow-Howell, 1993)
- Reduced availability of nursing home beds, delaying admission to a nursing home and extending the period of family caregiving at home
- Role conflicts in personal, social, or occupational life (Mui & Morrow-Howell, 1993)
- Role demand overload (Mui & Morrow-Howell, 1993)
- Role incompetence
- Social isolation
- The values and motivating factors of the caregiver and care recipient, influencing the decision to keep the care recipient at home as long as possible or even past the critical point of where potential harm outweighs the potential benefit of continuing care in the home

- Type and quality of the relationship between the caregiver and care recipient
- Unmet expectations due to insufficient time, lack of resources, and/or lack of energy

CLINICAL MANIFESTATIONS

Caregiver and care recipient
- change in activity patterns
- decline in health-promoting and disease-preventing behaviors
- depression
- disease complications
- insomnia
- loss of appetite, change in eating patterns, weight change
- mood changes
- onset, exacerbation, and/or reoccurrence of disease or illness
- poor hygiene
- skin breakdown (care recipient)
- verbalizations of frustration, anxiety, guilt, inadequacy, anger (caregiver)
- withdrawal

CLINICAL/DIAGNOSTIC FINDINGS
- Blood in vomitus or stool (may indicate stress ulcer)
- High blood pressure (over 140 mm Hg systolic and 90 mm Hg diastolic)
- Increased heart rate (over 100 beats/min)
- Weight changes

▶ NURSING DIAGNOSIS: *Caregiver Role Strain*

Related To
- Complexity and quantity of caregiving activities
- Concern for finances
- Concern for the availability, continuity, and quality of services
- Concern for the health of the care recipient and disease prognosis
- Perceived health of caregiver
- Role conflicts
- Role demand overload
- Role incompetence
- Severity of the care recipient's illness
- Social isolation
- Type and quality of relationship between caregiver and care recipient
- Unmet expectations due to insufficient time, lack of resources, and/or lack of energy

Defining Characteristics
- Feelings of guilt and inadequacy in performing specific caregiving tasks
- Frustration with role and inability to meet the demands
- Lack of adequate resources to provide care
- Decline in health status
- Insomnia
- Withdrawal or depression
- Other stress-related symptoms, including constipation, diarrhea, headaches, indigestion/heartburn, and nausea/vomiting

Patient Outcomes
The caregiver and care recipient will:
- avoid and/or delay unnecessary hospitalization and institutionalization.
- communicate with the nurse and other resources regarding changes in condition and the need for assistance.
- engage in activities and strategies to promote health and prevent illness, complications, and exacerbations.
- maintain continuity in home and social life.
- maintain home care plan and treatment regimen.
- not experience preventable complications/exacerbations of the illness process.
- receive services which are coordinated, appropriate, and of high quality and provide continuity to the fullest extent possible.

The caregiver will:
- develop competencies in the caregiver role as mutually agreed upon by the caregiver and the nurse, e.g., hygiene, transferring, and wound and tube care.
- develop flexibility and decision-making skills in conducting the role on a daily basis.
- maintain own health and well-being throughout the caregiving role.
- verbalize role evolvement.
- verbalize role satisfaction.

Nursing Interventions	Rationales
Assess the severity of the care recipient's illness and disability, the home care needs, the relationship between the caregiver and care recipient, and the caregiver's ability to perform the role.	Assessment, which includes data collection and validation, is necessary when developing an appropriate and realistic plan of care.
Assess the following components of the caregiving process: 1. Instrumental (hands-on, physical assistance)	In addition to hands-on care, perceived crucial elements of the caregiving process include anticipating needs, preventing

Nursing Interventions	Rationales
2. Anticipatory (decisions based on the possible needs of the care recipient) 3. Preventive (activities to prevent deterioration) 4. Supervisory (setting up and checking on arrangements) 5. Protective (from harmful consequences and from the care recipient's self-image)	complications, supervising services, and protecting the care recipient (Bowers, 1987).
Assess the care recipient and caregiver's needs as well as their beliefs about expected outcomes. Provide necessary teaching.	Interventions for caregivers are more likely to succeed if they are tailored to the caregiver's knowledge, beliefs about expected outcomes, and ability to carry out needed care behaviors.
Determine availability and accessibility of informal and formal support systems, including family members, friends, home health aide, respite services, homemaker, Meals on Wheels, and volunteer services. Mutually develop a regular and predictable schedule for assistance. Attempt to schedule shorter periods of assistance throughout the week rather than most of the assistance in a concentrated time period.	Regular and predictable periods of assistance provide relief and respite from an experience which is otherwise intense and unending (Small, 1987).
Assess coping strategies used in this and other stressful situations. Support using those that are health promoting and effective, and encourage caregivers to discontinue harmful coping strategies.	Using coping strategies which are familiar to the caregiver and have been used effectively in the past may reduce role strain.
Discuss the caregiver's and care recipient's perceptions, goals, and priorities regarding the caregiving situation. Identify other family members or friends who might assist in decision making if it becomes necessary.	Sharing such information helps when planning care and in preventing crises.

Nursing Interventions	Rationales
Build trust and confidence in the family helping relationship by listening, discovering, and affirming strengths and by continuing to make home visits over time.	A trusting relationship must be established among the nurse, caregiver, and care recipient to maximize the effects of all other nursing interventions.
Provide the following as clinical case manager: home visits, direct care and prescribed treatments, coordinated services, assistance in mobilizing family's own network of resources, professional nursing opinion while engaging in mutual problem solving, interpretation and explanation of care plans, and support and feedback.	Case management is a valuable and versatile approach to meeting the needs of homebound elderly and others at risk of institutionalization (Steinberg and Carter, 1983). Professional assistance provided through case management reduces caregiver role demands and strain.
Role-model problem-solving and caregiving behaviors to caregiver, care recipient, and informal and formal services.	Role modeling enhances the knowledge and skills of the caregiver, which reduces role strain.
Use a medication box to reduce the likelihood of missed medications.	Medication boxes provide structure to the caregiving routine.
Encourage participation in caregiver training and support groups.	A role supplementation group focusing on communication and problem solving was found to be an effective means to understanding and gaining competence in the caregiver role (Brackley, 1992).
Monitor the caregiver and care recipient's health status, health-promoting/disease-preventing behaviors, activity level, vital signs, and medication use. Identify the health teaching and care needs of all family members.	The family should be viewed with respect and as a resource to be conserved. While the need for the home visit is based initially on the condition of an ill individual, monitoring and maintaining the other family member's health and well-being reduces caregiver role strain and enhances meeting the care recipient's needs.
Introduce changes and new services incrementally.	Introducing changes in small amounts reduces the risk of sudden role changes, role overload, and strain.

Nursing Interventions	Rationales
Maintain flexibility and responsiveness as care demands change across the care recipient's course of illness.	The illness course is characterized by periods of uncertainty, role changes, and varying care demands (Given & Given, 1991). Maintaining flexibility and responsiveness to needs helps the caregiver through periods of uncertainty and role changes, thereby reducing role strain.

DISCHARGE PLANNING/CONTINUITY OF CARE

- Determine the health status of the care recipient and caregiver, the anticipated needs after discharge, to what extent the caregiver will be able to provide the necessary care, the accessibility and availability of informal and formal support services, and the safety of the home environment (access to water, location of the bathroom, stairs).
- Clearly communicate prognosis and needs and follow up with the ill individual, caregiving family members and friends, the community health nursing agency providing follow up and case management, and other required support services. Conduct a discharge planning conference as needed and complete all required referrals in a timely manner.
- Develop a "master schedule" of who will provide assistance, at what times, and for what purposes.
- Order medications, supplies, and home care equipment. Ensure they are delivered prior to discharge.

REFERENCES/BIBLIOGRAPHY

Bowers, B. J. (1987). Intergenerational caregiving: Adult caregivers and their aging parents. *Advances in Nursing Science, 9*(2), 20–31.

Brackley, M. H. (1992). A role supplementation group pilot study: A nursing therapy for potential parental caregivers. *Clinical Nurse Specialist, 6*(1), 14–19.

Cantor, M. H. (1983). Strain among caregivers: A study of experience in the United States. *The Gerontologist, 23*(6), 597–604.

Corbin, J. M., & Strauss, A. (1992). A nursing model for chronic illness management based upon the trajectory framework. In P. Woog (Ed.), *The chronic illness trajectory framework* (pp. 9–28). New York: Springer.

Crandall, E. P. (1993). The relation of public health nursing to the public health campaign. *Public Health Nursing, 10*(3), 204–209. (Reprinted from *American Journal of Public Health,* March 1915.)

Given, B. A., & Given, C. W. (1991). Family caregiving for the elderly. In J. J. Fitzpatrick, R. L. Taunton, & A. K. Jacox (Eds.), *Annual Review of Nursing Research* (Vol. 9) (pp. 77–101). New York: Springer.

Goode, W. J. (1960). A theory of role strain. *American Sociological Review, 25*, 483–496.

Mui, A. C., & Morrow-Howell, N. (1993). Sources of emotional strain among the oldest caregivers. *Research on Aging, 15*(1), 50–69.

Pepin, J. I. (1992). Family caring and caring in nursing. *Image, 24*(2), 127–131.

Reinhard, S. C. (1994). Perspectives on the family's caregiving experience in mental illness. *Image, 26*(1), 70–74.

Sayles-Cross, S. (1993). Perceptions of familial caregivers. *Image, 25*(2), 88–92.

Small, E. (1987). The needs of nonprofessional caregivers when caring for homebound clients. Master's Thesis, Boston University School of Nursing, Boston, MA.

Steinberg, R. M., & Carter, G. W. (1983). *Case management and the elderly*. Lexington, MA: D. C. Heath and Company.

*D*EATH AND DYING

Ruth M. Neil, PhD, RN

Death and dying are described by some nurses as "the transition from life to whatever exists beyond" (Callanan & Kelley, 1992). The experience of dying and knowing one's death is imminent produces many challenging and difficult questions for the patient, family, and caregivers. The process is different for every person. Therefore, deciding on a nursing diagnosis and exact interventions has many variables, including the age of the patient, the relationships present with family and significant others, and the cause of the impending death.

Lindley-Davis (1991) reported that the experience of dying is intense and is shaped by the individual's history of illness, response to stress, the nature of the terminal illness, and the interactions with others during the dying period. The terminal phase begins when the dying individual starts to turn from the outside world and withdraws inward. This is a bodily reaction which signals that energy is being conserved.

Four types of death occur within the terminal phase:
1. Sociological death: Patient withdraws and separates from others.
2. Psychic death: The individual accepts death and regresses inward.
3. Biologic death: No consciousness.
4. Physiologic death: Vital organs no longer operate.

Variations of this death process can occur; each person is unique.

Nursing's role in health care is to "assist the individual, sick or well, in performance of those activities contributing to health or its recovery or to achieve a peaceful death." (Henderson, 1966). Supporting the patient to approach dying with a sense of dignity, understanding, and acceptance creates a more positive experience for the patient, his or her family, and support persons. The desired goal while caring for the dying patient always involves the significant other people in the patient's life.

ETIOLOGIES
- Incurable disease (e.g., cancer, overwhelming infection, immunodeficient disorders)
- Violence, trauma
- Wearing out of body systems (e.g., renal and cardiac disease)
- Genetic defects

CLINICAL MANIFESTATIONS

Physiological (preterminal, becoming more pronounced as time progresses)
- fatigue, weakness
- anorexia
- nausea/vomiting
- pain
- dyspnea

Psychological
- depression
- sense of loss or relief
- loneliness
- hopelessness
- fear
- anxiety
- grieving
- spiritual distress

CLINICAL/DIAGNOSTIC FINDINGS

Physiological (during terminal phase of dying)
- apical pulse over 100 beats/min for an adult
- respirations shallow and labored and/or periods of apnea
- secretions: increased trend in coughing, congestion, and/or adventitious lung sounds
- urinary output: decreasing in amount
- restlessness: increase in muscular activity/twitching followed by calmness
- seizures
- bowel sounds: hypoactive and/or incontinence
- blood pressure: decreasing
- body temperature: rectal temperature > 99.6
- skin temperature: cool to touch
- skin color: pale, mottled skin and lips, nails cyanotic
- edema: often present
- diaphoresis: skin often clammy, sweaty

Psychological (during terminal phase of dying)
- withdrawal: repeated periods of nonverbalization/lethargy
- mental status: blank stare, pupils fixed, responding only to deep pressure or pain
- possible loss of consciousness

─ Clinical Clip ─

Dying is a natural part of life. Working with dying patients requires that nurses examine their beliefs and feelings in order to better care for patients and to prevent feelings of frustration and failure within themselves. Callanan and Kelley (1993) suggest asking oneself questions such as the following:

- In dealing with difficult situations, how do I usually respond to stress?
- What are my strengths and weaknesses?
- Am I afraid of death? If so, do I know why?
- Have I had personal life experiences with death?
- Am I afraid of the unknown?
- What do I hope to accomplish through my involvement with the dying person?

▶ NURSING DIAGNOSIS: *Fatigue*

Related To diminished supply of nutrients to tissues

Defining Characteristics
- Verbal report of fatigue or weakness
- External discomfort or dyspnea
- Abnormal responses to activity: heart rate increased, blood pressure decreased
- Muscles of tongue and tissues of soft palate may sag back in throat, resulting in loud snoring ("death rattle")
- Sphincters may relax, resulting in incontinence during final hours of life
- Visible restlessness or struggle lasting a few seconds, followed by calmness

Patient Outcomes
- Patient and family/caregivers experience minimal discomfort, minimal anxiety, and minimal embarrassment or loss of dignity.

Nursing Interventions	Rationales
Assess patient's fatigue/weakness through general observations, conversation, and vital signs monitoring. Assist with positioning and movement to find optimum comfort	Assisting the dying person to cope with the progressive fatigue and weakness in a way that preserves dignity and minimizes anxiety improves the quality of time left

Nursing Interventions	Rationales
while preserving energy. Talk with patient and family to assure that this is a normal process. Obtain medical orders for analgesic or relaxation as needed.	for meaningful interaction with family/support persons.
Assess bowel and/or bladder incontinence. Provide appropriate schedule for using commode/bedpan/diapering or obtain an order for catheterization, depending on patient's needs.	Preserving patient's dignity is a basic goal. In addition, this intervention minimizes skin breakdown, possible infection, and an additional source of pain.

▶ **NURSING DIAGNOSIS:** *Altered Nutrition—Less Than Body Requirements*

Related To anorexia or nausea caused directly by disease process, treatment agents, environmental stimuli, and/or depression

Defining Characteristics
- Loss of appetite
- Nausea/vomiting
- Loss of weight
- Changes in elimination
- Weakness/fatigue
- Dehydration

Patient Outcomes
Patient will:
- maintain sufficient caloric intake to support activity that has meaning for the patient.
- maintain sufficient hydration to minimize discomfort from thick secretions.
- minimize discomfort and expended energy brought on by nausea and vomiting.

Nursing Interventions	Rationales
Assess food likes/dislikes with patient and offer creative options that appeal to the patient. Encourage family to prepare special homemade "favorites."	At terminal phase, food is more likely to have importance in the context of memories of when the patient felt well and enjoyed eating rather than in maintaining a healthy life.

Nursing Interventions	Rationales
Provide wide range of beverage options. Determine easiest way for patient to drink. For example, for some patients, a soft-lipped cup is easier to use than a glass and straw. As patient becomes closer to death and no longer wants to drink fluids, keep the mucous membranes of the mouth moist and the lips lubricated to increase comfort.	As with food intake, the body usually knows what it needs. Patient comfort and dignity should guide the nurse's action.

▶ NURSING DIAGNOSIS: *Reactive Depression*

Related To concerns, fears, and anxieties about impending death

Defining Characteristics
- Expressions of hopelessness, despair
- Inability to concentrate, making reading, writing, and conversation difficult
- Change (usually decrease) in physical activity, eating, sleeping, and sexual activity
- Continual questioning of self-worth (self-esteem)
- Feeling of failure (real or imagined)
- Withdrawal from others
- Threats of attempts to commit suicide
- Suspicion and sensitivity to words and actions of others related to lack of trust
- Misdirected anger (toward self)
- General irritability
- Guilt feelings
- Extreme dependency on others with related feelings of helplessness and anger

Patient Outcomes
- Patient verbalizes a sense of power and control in the situation.
- Patient and family/caregivers accept impending death with a measure of completion and comfort.

Nursing Interventions	Rationales
Encourage patient to talk and provide assurance that his or her feelings are normal.	Feelings of failure, anger toward self, guilt, and diminished self-worth are intensified when a person thinks he or she is "the only one" who has ever felt this way.
Explore with patient the meaning his or her life has had and decide on meaningful goals for the remaining time.	Being able to make decisions for oneself promotes a sense of worth and power in the situation.
If the patient is prepared, assist patient in expressing preferences for services and disposition of material resources, including messages and bequests.	For some patients, participating in this process can provide a control and a sense of accomplishment and closure.

▶ NURSING DIAGNOSIS: *Spiritual Distress*

Related To the individual trying to resolve questions about the meaning of life and death and his or her belief about "afterlife" and to resolve relationships and commitments

Defining Characteristics
- Expressed concern with meaning of life, death, and/or belief system
- Anger toward their deity
- Questioning the meaning of suffering
- Verbalizing inner conflict about beliefs
- Verbalizing concern about relationship with their deity
- Questioning meaning of own existence
- Inability to participate in usual religious practices
- Seeking spiritual assistance
- Questioning moral/ethical implications of therapeutic regimen
- Gallows humor
- Displacing anger toward religious representatives
- Nightmares/sleep disturbances
- Alterations in behavior/mood, evidenced by anger, crying, withdrawal, preoccupation, anxiety, hostility, apathy

Patient Outcomes
Patient will:
- have the opportunity to express both positive and negative feelings.

- have the opportunity to resolve conflicts.
- accept death as a transition.

Nursing Interventions	Rationales
Be willing to listen in a nonjudgmental manner.	The patient gains a sense of comfort and understanding through the process of articulating his or her fears and questions.
Share experiences from work with other dying patients and/or literature concerning "what it's like to die."	The patient feels frustrated by other people's reluctance to actually talk about what is happening. It is a relief to be able to discuss the reality that he or she is experiencing.
Offer to contact appropriate clergy, family/friends, or other spiritual counselor.	This will vary with individuals but is of great importance to both patients and families who have historically practiced a particular religion. Human beings, in general, seek to come to a sense of peace within themselves, with other people in their lives, and in their understanding of a Higher Power, God, or a Universal Meaning. The knowledge that one is dying challenges the individual to struggle with any unresolved areas in all of these realms.

DISCHARGE PLANNING/CONTINUITY OF CARE
- Notify relatives and other interested persons about cremation/burial, the memorial service/funeral, and disposition of patient's personal belongings.
- Plan with family/support persons some type of ongoing support such as a bereavement group, occasional follow-up by the nurse, or specific plans for involvement in new activities.

OTHER PLANS OF CARE TO REFERENCE
- Pain
- Grief/Loss

REFERENCES/BIBLIOGRAPHY

Callanan, M., & Kelley, P. (1993). *Final gifts. Understanding the special awareness, needs and communications of the dying.* New York: Bantam Books.

Hassler, K. (1993). Bereavement counselling. *Nursing Standard, 7*(40), 31–36.

Henderson, V. (1966). *The nature of nursing: A definition and its implications, practice, research, and education.* New York: Macmillan.

Lindley-Davis, B. (1991). Process of dying: Defining characteristics. *Cancer Nursing, 14*(6), 328–333.

Miller, R., Goldman, E., Bor, R., & Scher, I. (1992). Counselling in terminally ill patient. *British Journal of Nursing, 6*(26), 52–55.

Wyatt, P. (1992). The role of nurses in counselling the terminally ill patient. *British Journal of Nursing, 2*(14), 701–704.

Watson, J. (1985). *Nursing: The philosophy and science of caring.* Boulder, CO: Colorado Associated University Press.

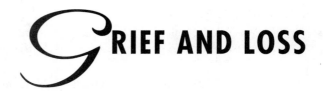

GRIEF AND LOSS

Ruth Neil, PhD, RN

Loss exists when any aspect of one's self—whether tangible, intangible, concrete, abstract, real, or imaginary—is no longer available to a person. Loss also exists when a valued object (including another person) is altered (Watson, 1985). The general categories of loss are psychological, sociocultural, and physical.

Grief and mourning are human behaviors that accompany loss. The terms *grieving, mourning, bereavement,* and *grief work* refer to the processes that follow a loss and that help the mourner give up the lost object, person, or function. The name for grieving that occurs before the loss happens is *anticipatory grieving.* "Grief work" represents a struggle to retrieve a sense of meaning that has been altered or taken away by a loss (Watson, 1985). Since grieving follows each kind of loss, the two concepts will be considered together throughout the remainder of this chapter. This process helps individuals work through their associated feeling and resolve the loss.

When caring for a patient who experienced a loss, nurses need to first recognize and identify the loss and, second, assist the patient in grieving the loss to maximize their psychological health.

ETIOLOGIES

Psychological loss
- developmental factors as one progresses through different stages of life, for example, transition from dependence to independence (childhood to adulthood), loss of independence with aging process, and role changes

Sociocultural loss
- giving up basic values or beliefs in order "to conform"
- loss of attachments
- disintegration of a predictable environment
- prospective threat to the meaning of life
- alteration of a relationship

Physical loss
- loss of external objects and possessions
- loss of usual body function, structure, or appearance [e.g., amputations, ostomy, cerebrovascular accident (CVA), burn]
- loss of a significant other person

CLINICAL MANIFESTATIONS
- Helplessness
- Loneliness
- Sadness
- Guilt
- Self-deterioration
- Anger
- Crying
- Somatic distress (especially loss of appetite, sleeplessness)
- Depression
- Withdrawal from people, events, activities
- Extreme irritability
- Restlessness
- Preoccupation with the lost object
- Inability to initiate meaningful activity
- Spiritual distress; anger or loss of faith in previously religious individual

CLINICAL/DIAGNOSTIC FINDINGS
None. Defined by subjective assessments.

▶ NURSING DIAGNOSIS: *Ineffective Individual Coping*

Related To lack of knowledge related to grieving process and care of self

Defining Characteristics
- Expressions of hopelessness, despair
- Withdrawal from others
- Misdirected anger (toward self)
- Guilt feelings
- Inability to focus on task

Patient Outcomes
Patient will:
- maintain somatic health—nutrition, sleep pattern regularity.
- verbalize increased insight into grieving process.
- resume effective behaviors for accomplishing life tasks.

Nursing Interventions	Rationales
Spend time talking with and listening to the patient or family member experiencing loss. Acknowledge the loss and emotional pain.	Loss is a highly variable personal experience, and what is loss to one person is not necessarily a loss to another. It is necessary to understand the *meaning* of the loss to the one experiencing it in order to offer constructive suggestions for getting past it.
Discuss the normal manifestations of grief—denial (shock), anger (awareness), searching (relinquishment), and reinvestment (resolution)—and encourage patient to experience these honestly.	Understanding that his or her emotions are normal helps the person needing to grieve do so with a sense of support.
Assess and provide appropriate counseling about nutrition. Obtain sedative order and/or teach relaxation techniques to encourage adequate rest.	Dealing with the psychological and emotional components of the grieving process are very stressful and proceed more smoothly if the physical body is maintained.

▶ NURSING DIAGNOSIS: *Anticipatory Grieving*

Related To an impending loss

Defining Characteristics
- Potential loss of significant object
- Verbal expression of distress at potential loss
- Anger
- Sadness, sorrow, crying
- Crying at frequent intervals, choked feeling
- Change in eating habits
- Alteration in sleep or dream patterns
- Alteration in activity level
- Altered libido
- Idealized anticipated loss
- Developmental regression
- Alterations in concentration or pursuit of tasks

Patient/Family Outcomes
Patient/family will:
- describe and discuss the process they are experiencing.

- maintain ability to experience "the present."
- communicate about the meaning of the loss/dying experience.

Nursing Interventions	Rationales
Explain the concept of anticipatory grieving in terms that the patient/family can understand.	Knowing that this is a normal process helps people understand their feelings.
Monitor the patient's and family's "progress" with the anticipatory grieving process and help them communicate about it. Attempt to prevent premature withdrawal, emotional abandonment, and disengagement from and expression of ambivalence about the loss, particularly when it involves losing a person.	Anticipatory grieving can be problematic when it involves the loss of a person. The premature withdrawal, emotional abandonment, and disengagement from and expression of the ambivalence about the loss through hostile and destructive behavior can have an emotionally distressing impact on the dying person.

DISCHARGE PLANNING/CONTINUITY OF CARE
- Refer to support groups.
- Refer to occupational/physical therapy for those experiencing changes in mobility or body function.
- Refer to outpatient counseling.
- Refer to educational programs.

OTHER PLANS OF CARE TO REFERENCE
- Death and Dying
- Social Isolation
- Nutrition
- Sleep and Rest Patterns
- Physical Activity/Exercise
- Personal Hygiene

REFERENCES/BIBLIOGRAPHY
Callanan, M., & Kelley, P. (1993). *Final gifts. Understanding the special awareness, needs and communications of the dying.* New York: Bantam Books.

Haber, J., McMahon, A. L., Price-Hoskins, P., & Sideleau, B. F. (1992). *Comprehensive psychiatric nursing* (4th ed.). St. Louis: Mosby Year-Book.

Henderson, V. (1966). *The nature of nursing: A definition and its implications, practice, research, and education.* New York: Macmillan.

Lindley-Davis, B. (1991). Process of dying: Defining characteristics. *Cancer Nursing, 14*(6), 328–333.

McIntier, T. M. (1995). Nursing the family when a child dies. *RN, 58*(2), 50–55.

Watson, J. (1985). *Nursing: The philosophy and science of caring.* Boulder, CO: Colorado Associated University Press.

*A*LTERED MENTAL STATUS

Karen Egenes, RN, EdD

Patients with altered mental states experience serious disturbances in functional ability, especially in thought, mood, and behavior. These major disturbances cause an impaired ability to test reality and lead to difficulty in relating appropriately to others. Diseases related to altered mental states include schizophrenia, Alzheimer's, brain tumors, and cerebrovascular accident (CVA). The nurse's role is to orient the patient to reality, assist the family in coping with and caring for the patient's condition, and through rehabilitation, bring the patient to the highest level of functioning possible.

During the past three decades, the care of persons with mental illness has shifted from large state institutions to community-based services. Community mental health nursing includes a commitment to consumer participation, collaboration with mental health professionals in other disciplines (medicine, social work, psychology), provision of a full range of comprehensive services, and continuity of care.

The role of the community health nurse in working with patients with altered mental states includes mental health promotion, mental illness treatment, and rehabilitation.

ETIOLOGIES
- Possible genetic influences related to schizophrenia and Alzheimer's disease
- Biochemical influences causing an overproduction of dopamine in schizophrenics. Bipolar disorder might be associated with imbalances in norepinephrine and serotonin
- Organic mental disorders caused by neurophysiological, neurochemical, or structural alterations of the brain
- Ingestion of drugs, chemicals, or metal substances
- Any physical disease causing a change in mental status (e.g., hypothyroidism, hyperthyroidism, electrolyte imbalances)

- Intrapsychic influences. Schizophrenics might be predisposed to suffer personality disintegration when exposed to high levels of stress
- Learned behavior/dysfunctional family
- Faulty family communication patterns, causing inability to maintain social relationships outside the family
- Emotional fusion of family members resulting in lack of individuality in point of view, thoughts, or feelings

CLINICAL MANIFESTATIONS

Thought disturbances
- preoccupation with personal fantasies/obsessions
- delusions: fixed, false beliefs that cannot be corrected by reasoning with the patient
- hallucinations: a false sensory perception, occurring in the absence of external stimuli (i.e., seeing "visions," hearing "voices"); also abnormalities of perception and illusions

Affect disturbances
- mood swings: rapid shifts from anger to anxiety to elation without any obvious reason for the changes/depressive disorder
- bipolar disorder
- flat affect: absence of spontaneous expression of emotion; also depression and dementia in elderly
- inappropriate affect

Social/behavioral disturbances
- low self-esteem
- lack of interpersonal skills necessary to build and maintain relationships
- impulsive, repetitive, or bizarre behavior
- wandering behavior

Deficiencies in health maintenance
- weight gain or loss secondary to overeating or anorexia
- lack of attention to personal hygiene and appearance

Deficiencies in daily living skills
- excessive dependence on others to meet basic needs
- lack of hobbies, interests or diversional activities
- difficulty with home maintenance

CLINICAL/DIAGNOSTIC FINDINGS

Rule out organic cause that can be reversed with treatment:
- computerized axial tomography (CT) scan—shows abnormalities in brain structure
- magnetic resonance imaging (MRI)
- regional cerebral blood flow (CBF)

▶ NURSING DIAGNOSIS: *Altered Thought Processes*

Related To
- Disintegration of thought processes
- High levels of anxiety from psychological or environmental stressors
- Isolation from others with concomitant lack of opportunity for reality testing

Defining Characteristics
- Inaccurate interpretation of incoming information
- Preoccupation with illogical ideas, bizarre fantasies
- Disorganized, incoherent speech patterns
- Impaired ability to engage in abstract thought, reasoning, or calculation

Patient Outcomes
Patient will:
- experience a decrease in hallucinations and delusional thought.
- differentiate between reality and fantasy.
- adhere to medication regimen.

Nursing Interventions	Rationales
Speak to patient in clear, simple terms. Avoid complex, lengthy conversations. Teach caregiver these techniques.	Decreases the possibility that patient might misinterpret the message.
Discuss patient's delusions and hallucinations only as necessary to assess patient safety.	Dwelling on thought disorders might reinforce them or increase patient anxiety.
Respond to patient's thought disorders in a calm, nonchallenging manner. Teach caregiver these techniques.	Challenging the thought disorder might encourage the patient to defend it.
Praise patient for appropriate judgment, coping, or problem solving.	Praise increases patient self-esteem and encourages the patient to continue these reality-based behaviors.
Monitor patient adherence to medication and psychotherapy regimens.	Provides continued support for necessary therapies to decrease incidence of thought disorders and lessen risk of rehospitalization.

▶ NURSING DIAGNOSIS: *Ineffective Individual Coping*

Related To
- Helplessness

- Anxiety
- Low self-esteem

Defining Characteristics
- Difficulty establishing and maintaining interpersonal relationships
- Decreased problem-solving ability
- Social withdrawal/isolation of self
- Dependence on others to meet basic needs

Patient Outcomes
Patient will:
- verbalize willingness to be involved with others.
- use coping mechanisms and problem-solving techniques appropriately in meeting own needs.
- express thoughts and needs appropriately in verbal interactions.

Nursing Interventions	Rationales
Assess patient's current level of functioning and compare it with patient's level of functioning prior to the onset of the present episode of illness.	Identifies patient's potential and aid in setting realistic, achievable goals.
Acknowledge patient's difficulty in social situations/communications.	Recognizing the patient's difficulty shows understanding and decreases patient anxiety.
Practice with patient appropriate problem-solving approaches.	Problem solving is a skill the patient might have never acquired or might have lost because of his or her illness. Practicing the skill facilitates patient learning.
Calmly and directly offer patient feedback on behaviors likely to interfere with developing interpersonal relationships (i.e., blaming, cursing, threatening).	Feedback helps the patient identify the effects of maladaptive behavior on others in the environment.
Role play a situation in which the patient must ask for assistance in meeting a need (e.g., asking directions).	Asking for help is a necessary skill in daily life. Role playing helps shape patient ability in using the skill.
Praise patient for attempts at problem-solving behavior and appropriate communications.	Encourages the patient to repeat the functional behaviors and develop ease in their use.

▶ **NURSING DIAGNOSIS:** *Self-Care Deficit—Feeding, Bathing, Dressing*

Related To
- Decreased psychomotor activity
- Low self-concept
- Knowledge deficit

Defining Characteristics
- Difficulty in preparing meal, bathing self, dressing appropriately
- Inability to take responsibility for meeting basic health needs

Patient Outcomes
Patient will:
- identify resources available for help.
- perform self-care activities of daily living (ADLs) at the highest possible level of function.

Nursing Interventions	Rationales
Assess current level of self-care ability versus self-care ability prior to current episode of illness.	Assessing patient potential helps in setting realistic, attainable goals.
Assess patient for ADL skills that are absent or in need of improvement, including hygiene, grooming, bathing, shopping, cooking, arranging transportation, and accessing help through community services.	Assessing patient deficits is necessary prior to formulating a patient teaching plan.
Refer patient to community agency that can assist patient with personal hygiene/self-care until patient is able to care for self.	Helps promote patient self-respect and self-esteem.
Practice daily living skills with patient in the home environment.	Coaching the patient in ADLs helps shape behavior and promote movement toward proficiency in skill performance.
Help the patient develop a written daily schedule of ADLs.	A written schedule provides a visual prompt and encourages adherence in the same manner as a written contract.
Praise patients for attempting to improve ADL performance.	Positive reinforcement encourages patient to continue progress in performing ADLs.

Nursing Interventions	Rationales
Instruct patient in identifying specific physical symptoms that require medical attention (e.g., a temperature over 101° F) and help patient formulate a plan for seeking medical attention.	Providing specific information alerts patient to times when health care is needed and might avert an emergency situation.

▶ NURSING DIAGNOSIS: *Diversional Activity Deficit*

Related To
- No peers or friends
- Lack of motivation
- Anxiety

Defining Characteristics
- Statements of boredom/depression from inactivity
- Physical immobility

Patient Outcomes
Patient will:
- demonstrate involvement in at least one social activity each month.
- verbalize that he or she has made one or two friends.
- participate in hobbies or other diversional activities.

Nursing Interventions	Rationales
With patient, plan a structured daily routine incorporating patient's hobbies, social activities, and recreational activities.	Decreases amount of unstructured time during the day during which patients might become preoccupied with inner fantasies.
Enlist patient and family's cooperation and input in formulating the plan for structured activities. Contract with patient and family. (See also Contracting.)	Involve patient in planning to enhance patient compliance.
Encourage patient to discuss interest areas and verbalize feelings about his or her daily experiences.	Stimulates patient motivation through the nurse's interest and encouragement.
Discourage using television as a primary source of recreation.	Prevents patient from becoming comfortable with aloneness.

Nursing Interventions	Rationales
Assist patient in listing community recreational activities available.	Involving patient in plan formulation increases patient motivation.
Discuss with patient strategies for making friends and building relationships.	Practicing social skills increases patient self-esteem and increases the likelihood the patient will use the skills in social situations.
Encourage patient involvement in community recreational activities, using nurse-initiated referrals if patient indicates interest.	Increases patient social interactions with others.
Praise patient for attempting diversional activities.	Positive reinforcement encourages patient to continue diversional activities.

▶ NURSING DIAGNOSIS: *Impaired Home Maintenance Management*

Related To
- Knowledge deficit
- Limited financial resources
- Impaired perception, individual coping skills
- Lack of support systems

Defining Characteristics
- Verbalizes or expresses difficulty in maintaining home environment
- Verbalizes or expresses difficulty caring for self or family member at home
- Unwashed clothing, cooking equipment, linen
- Accumulated dirt, food wastes, or hygienic wastes
- Offensive odors

Patient Outcomes
Patient will:
- keep home clean and free of clutter and odor.
- demonstrate the ability to perform skills necessary for home maintenance.

Nursing Interventions	Rationales
Assess current level of home maintenance versus level of home maintenance prior to current episode of illness.	Assessing patient potential is helpful in setting realistic, attainable goals for the patient.
Assess patient for home maintenance skills in need of improvement.	Identifying patient areas of deficiency is necessary in formulating a plan for patient teaching.
Determine types of assistance needed in home maintenance.	Assessing needed services helps in referring patient to appropriate community services.
Discuss with patient and family members the implications of caring for a chronically ill family member at home, including time and physical requirements and possible role conflicts. (See Caregiver Burden/Support/Conflict Resolution.)	Lack of knowledge or a sense of duty might encourage caregivers in making unrealistic time and energy commitments.
Involve patient in developing a long-term plan for optimal home maintenance.	Input from all persons affected by a long-term plan increases the likelihood the plan will be a success.

DISCHARGE PLANNING/CONTINUITY OF CARE
- Negotiate with community groups or individuals to schedule activities guarding against patient loneliness and withdrawal.
- Reinforce plans for continued outpatient treatment with a plan for obtaining immediate assistance when the patient experiences a crisis.
- Give patient written information about prescribed medication and, together, devise a plan to promote medication compliance.
- Help patient maintain social contacts in the community (interest groups, church activities, etc.) to build patient's social networking skills and enhance patient's social support.
- Refer patient to appropriate community agencies for specific needs (e.g., support groups, day treatment, respite care, crisis outreach services, nutritional programs, sheltered workshops, groups homes, home health care).

OTHER PLANS OF CARE TO REFERENCE
- Social Isolation
- Caregiver Burden/Support/Conflict Resolution
- Nutrition
- Physical Activity/Exercise

- Personal Hygiene
- Contracting
- Residence Deficit

BIBLIOGRAPHY

Baier, M. (1987). Case management with the chronically mentally ill. *Journal of Psychosocial Nursing and Mental Health Services, 25*(6), 17–21.

Brooker, C., & Butterworth, C. (1991). Working with families caring for a family member with schizophrenia: The evolving role of the community psychiatric nurse. *International Journal of Nursing Studies, 28*(2), 189–200.

Buckwalter, K. C., Abraham, I. L., & Smullen, D. E. (1993). Nursing outreach to rural elderly people who are mentally ill. *Hospital and Community Psychiatry, 44*(9), 821–823.

Buckwalter, K. C., & Stolley, J. (1991). Managing mentally ill elders at home. *Geriatric Nursing, 12*(3), 136–140.

Rawlins, R. P., & Heacock. P. E. (1993). *Clinical manual of psychiatric nursing* (2nd ed.). St. Louis: Mosby Year-Book.

Thobaben, M., & Kozlak, J. (1990). Home health care's unique role in serving the elderly mentally ill. *Home Health Care Nurse, 8*(4), 37–39.

Worley, N., & Albanese, N. (1989). Independent living skills for the chronically mentally ill. *Journal of Psychosocial Nursing and Mental Health Services, 27*(9), 18–22.

$\mathcal{H}$UMAN SEXUALITY

Constance Dallas, PhD, RN, FNP, CS

Human sexuality is defined as the way an individual expresses his or her identity through interactions with others. Both internal characteristics, such as self-esteem, self-image, and perception of health, sexual orientation, and external characteristics, such as religious values, attitudes of family and peers, cultural background, and social status, influence individual expression of sexuality. Human sexuality is expressed by a diverse range of behaviors which include individual sexual thoughts and feelings and sharing physical sexual activity with others; it is not limited to sexual activity. Instead human sexuality encompasses a full range of sexual expression including but not limited to, romantic love, lust, sensuality, flirting, and beliefs about one's attractiveness to others. Developmental stage and health are just two of the factors that influence individual expressions of sexuality.

The nurses' role in addressing sexual issues of patients is to give patients permission to discuss sexual concerns that may affect their perception of health. Nurses can convey the attitude that sexuality is an important part of holistic health care.

The nurse's comfort level with discussing sexuality will strongly influence the patient's comfort level. Learning more information about sexuality is an important start but will not automatically guarantee increased comfort. Nurses are strongly encouraged to examine their own attitudes, thoughts, values, and feelings toward different aspects of sexuality prior to initiating the topic with their patients. Talking with nurse colleagues also provides opportunities to add knowledge, share professional concerns, and alleviate personal discomfort.

ETIOLOGIES (PROBLEMS)

Physical
- recent gynecological or urological surgery
- activity intolerance, fatigue, impaired mobility
- bowel/bladder incontinence

- obesity
- pain, pain associated with sexual activity
- impaired skin integrity
- medication effects and side effects
- symptoms associated with sexually transmitted diseases
- dissatisfaction with contraception
- chronic or acute illness

Psychosocial
- anxiety, depression
- stress
- body image disturbance (e.g., ostomies, mastectomies, surgeries, recent weight gain, poor self-image, poor self-esteem)
- breastfeeding
- violence/sexual abuse
- role ambiguity, changes in role status (e.g., parenthood, loss of sexual partner)
- changes in physical characteristics associated with growth and development

CLINICAL MANIFESTATIONS
- Self/significant other reports (problems) of pain during sexual activity, sexual impotence, vaginal pain or dryness with intercourse, or diminished sexual feelings and desire
- Changes in sexual patterns
- Odor, discharge, itching from sexual organs
- Rashes, lesions on sexual organs
- Absence of morning erections
- Noncompliance with contraceptive regimen

CLINICAL/DIAGNOSTIC FINDINGS (PROBLEMS)
- Laboratory tests to diagnose sexually transmitted disease
- Venereal Disease Reseach Laboratories (VDRL), human immunodeficiency virus (HIV), hepatitis blood test positive
- Obesity

▶ NURSING DIAGNOSIS: *Knowledge Deficit*

Related To inadequate information about human sexuality

Defining Characteristics
- Expressed lack of knowledge or anxiety about reproductive process or changes in sexuality related to growth and development or physical condition.

Patient Outcomes

Patient, partner, and/or family will:

- Verbalize increased knowledge of reproductive process.
- Verbalize increased knowledge of changes associated with growth and development.
- Verbalize decreased anxiety.
- Seek treatment for symptoms of sexually transmitted diseases.
- Increase compliance with medication regimen.
- Verbalize increased self-esteem related to expression of individual sexuality.

Nursing Interventions	Rationales
Identify personal, religious, and cultural values related to expression of sexuality. Assess relevant sexual history such as recent change of partners, medication history, and methods to prevent pregnancy or sexually transmitted diseases, sexual abuse, and sexual orientation. Refer to other health providers for follow-up treatment if indicated.	Knowledge of sexual history allows nurses to provide appropriate, individualized guidance. Knowledge of deviations from the norm can promote early treatment of pathological changes such as hormonal dysfunctions or sexually transmitted diseases.
Provide anticipatory guidance to parents concerning physical changes associated with normal growth and development. Refer to other health care providers if indicated.	Knowledge of normal growth and development may decrease parental anxiety and promote communication between parent and child. Knowledge of normal changes can help identify dysfunctions such as precocious or delayed physical development.
Provide anticipatory guidance to aging patients. If appropriate, offer information about alternative methods of sexual expression less dependent on penile penetration such as cuddling and romantic gestures. Refer to health care providers if indicated.	Knowledge of physical changes associated with aging may decrease anxiety and increase self-esteem. Identifying normal developmental changes can promote treatment of pathological conditions such as atrophic vaginitis or organic causes of impotence.
Provide information to adolescents and anticipatory guidance to parents about differences in sexual orientation. Refer to other health care services as indicated.	Sexual orientation may be biologically determined and is generally established by adolescence (Masters et al, 1988). There is often less information available

Nursing Interventions	Rationales
	on and less societal support for homosexuality and bi-sexuality in comparison with heterosexuality. Providing accurate information and emotional support may decrease feelings of anxiety or guilt and may promote efforts to gain additional information and support.
Provide information about methods to prevent contraception and sexually transmitted diseases to all patients who report being sexually active; include information about types, effectiveness, and expense. Refer to other health care providers if indicated.	Appropriate use of contraceptive methods decrease the risk of sexually transmitted diseases and unplanned pregnancies. Methods that meet patient needs and are congruent with their personal, cultural, and religious values are more likely to be used on a consistent basis.

▶ NURSING DIAGNOSIS: *Sexual Dysfunction*

Related To changes in physical status, including, but not limited to, surgeries, medications, illness, fatigue, aging, paralysis/weakness

Defining Characteristics
- Reports changes in sexual desire/behavior/function associated with disease process, medication, treatments, or procedures
- Complains of odor/discharge/itching/lesions from sexual organs

Patient Outcomes
- Patient will report increased satisfaction with sexual functioning.

Nursing Interventions	Rationales
Assess information about patient's perception of what is causing the dysfunction.	Identifying patient's perception about causes will guide the nurse in providing appropriate referrals for treatment.
Provide information about variations associated with developmental changes.	Patients may lack knowledge about normal sexual functioning and hold unrealistic expectations for themselves or their partners.

Nursing Interventions	Rationales
Provide emotional support that encourages patients to verbalize their concerns. Include the patient's partner in the discussion, if possible.	A nonjudgmental atmosphere will promote verbalization and may encourage patients to seek additional treatment. Including the partner gives the message the that dysfunction is a relationship issue rather than the patient's fault.
Identify recent changes in medication and compliance with regimen. Consult with physicians if appropriate.	Some medications cause changes in sexual function. Physicians may be able to prescribe an alternative medication without similar side effects. Decreased side effects also may promote better compliance with medication regimen.
Assess signs of violence such as physical or sexual abuse. Identify professional resources and local support groups as indicated, such as the National Coalition Against Sexual Assault. (See Violence Against Women.)	Causes of sexual dysfunction may be beyond the scope of practice and expertise for most nurses. Nurses can refer the patient to other professionals and supports. Health professionals are obligated to report suspected child abuse.

▶ NURSING DIAGNOSIS: *Altered Sexuality Patterns*

Related To
- Anxiety, depression
- Body image disturbance (e.g., recent surgery, illness, weight change, ostomy, mastectomy)
- Physical or sexual abuse
- Acknowledging homosexual/bisexual orientation
- Changes in sexual activity pattern

Defining Characteristics
- Verbalizes change in perception/emotions related to sexuality
- Verbalizes dissatisfaction with present sexual pattern

Patient Outcomes
- Patient verbalizes satisfaction with sexual patterns.

Nursing Interventions	Rationales
Assess patient's perception of cause of altered sexual patterns. Assess patient's level of anxiety or depression. Refer to other health care professionals as indicated.	Knowledge of patient's perceptions guides health teaching and facilitates referral to appropriate follow-up services. Changes in sexual patterns may be a symptom of clinical depression that requires additional treatment.
Discuss weight changes with patient and provide nutrition counseling, if appropriate (See nutrition chapter.). Suggest consideration of alternative sexual positions and include patient's partner in the discussion if appropriate.	Weight control often requires prolonged behavioral changes. Including the partner can provide a source of emotional support. Including the partner also defines the issue as a relationship problem for the couple rather than the patient's fault. Morbid obesity can inhibit coitus.
Encourage patients and their sexual partner to verbalize concerns about changes in sexual patterns related to changes in physical condition associated with surgery or illness. Provide appropriate, self-care information about methods to minimize discomfort or embarrassment such as emptying ostomy bags or irrigating ostomy sites. Patients with physical deficits (paraplegia, quadriplegia) may appreciate opportunities to discuss alternative methods of achieving sexual satisfaction. Cardiac patients may consider using alternative positions to conserve energy expenditure. Refer to other health care providers such as physicians, sex therapists, and local support groups as indicated.	Mutual problem-solving may promote intimacy and communication between couples. Role modeling open discussions of sexual issues and concerns related to changed physical condition can decrease feelings of anxiety or embarrassment.
Offer pamphlets or written literature relevant to the patient's concern. Nurses should assure patients of their willingness to listen to sexual concerns.	Patients who are uncomfortable discussing sensitive topics may benefit if nurses provide printed materials. Books and pamphlets provide a less invasive method to provide information and may be a safe way to introduce sensitive topics.

DISCHARGE PLANNING/CONTINUITY OF CARE

- Provide name and number of resource person(s)/agency(ies) if patients request additional information.
- Refer to support groups if appropriate.

OTHER PLANS OF CARE TO REFERENCE

- Nutrition

REFERENCES/BIBLIOGRAPHY

Althof, S. E., & Kingsberg, S. A. (1992). Books helpful to patients with sexual and marital problems: A bibliography. *Journal of Sexual and Marital Therapy, 18*(91) 70–79.

Carotenuto, R. Bullock, J. (1980). *Physical assessment of the gerontologic client.* Philadelphia: F. A. Davis.

Coleman, E., Rosser, B. R., & Strapko, N. (1992). Sexual and intimacy dysfunction among homosexual men and women. *Psychiatric Medicine, 10*(2) 257–271.

LeMone, P. (1993). Human sexuality in adults with insulin-dependent diabetes mellitus. *Image, 25*(2) 101–105.

Litt, I. F. (1990). *Evaluation of the adolescent patient.* St. Louis: Mosby.

Masters, W., Johnson, V., & Kolodny, R. (1988). *Human sexuality* (3rd ed.). Glenview, IL: Scott, Foresman, & Co.

Remafedi, G., Farrow, J. A., & Deisher, R. W. (1991). Risk factors for attempted suicide in gay and bisexual youth. *Pediatrics, 87,* 869–875.

Stewart, F., Guest, F., Stewart, G., & Hatcher, R. (1987). Understanding your body: Every woman's guide to a lifetime of health. New York: Bantam Books.

$\mathcal{I}$NEFFECTIVE PARENTING

Marilyn E. Birchfield, RN, MA

Because of the importance of parenting in a child's growth and development, community nurses should become involved in assessing parenting capacities, both before and after the birth of a child. The foundation for parenting comes from parents' own backgrounds and experiences, their nurturing as children, and the interpersonal skills they have developed. If a parent is positive about the parenting role, assistance may be needed to gain the self-confidence required to make informed choices in the actual situation of parenting. To do this, persons must know themselves, be honest about their feelings, and start from internal awareness rather than external mechanical acts (Kitzinger, 1980). Given a "facilitating environment," that is, one that gives the parents themselves emotional support and allows them to develop confidence, most parents feel competent in their roles and are able to learn from their child. Sometimes, however, nonsupportive external conditions or inappropriate techniques of child care lead to actual or potential stress and risk to the child.

ETIOLOGIES
- Maternal problems at birth: cesarean section, complicated labor/delivery, disease/illness, etc.
- Infant problems at birth: premature, congenital anomaly, multiple births, special treatment needs [e.g., hyperbilirubinemia, diagnosed genetic condition such as phenylketonuria (PKU) or hypothyroidism]
- First child: change of family dynamics, new responsibilities as caregiver
- Family with many children
- Unwanted pregnancy/child
- Inadequate assistance or support
- Limited understanding of growth and development as a continuum of changing abilities and needs
- Misunderstandings related to common behaviors of childhood: stranger anxiety, masturbation, thumb sucking, temper tantrums

- Limited understanding of developmental principles: feeding, weaning, toilet training
- Lack of awareness of individual temperament/differences: responsiveness, distractibility, biorhythms
- Parents with limited mental/emotional ability
- Stressful living circumstances: single parent, nonsupportive mate, limited financial means, poor housing/neighborhood, new immigrant

CLINICAL MANIFESTATIONS

Infant/Child
- poor weight gain and hygiene/grooming
- below average in developmental norms: psychosocial development (bonding, smiling), language skills, gross motor and fine motor ability
- passive or disruptive child
- frequent accidents/illness
- unkept appearance (e.g., skin rashes, dirty hair/teeth/fingernails, tattered and stained clothing, clothing inappropriate for climate
- not smiling, no eye contact

Parent
- feels incompetent/inadequate in nurturing role
- inappropriate caretaking practices: feeding, sleep and rest, health care needs
- labels infant/child "bad," has negative image of child
- concern about "spoiling" infant/child by meeting needs
- confines infant/child physically to limited space; minimal social interactions or exploratory opportunities
- provides minimal physical contact or closeness for infant, limited interaction with infant/child (e.g., does not hold the infant close to her body, does not enjoy touching the infant, does not rock or sing to the infant)
- treats infant/child as an adult, expects infant/child to respond like an adult
- environment shows little evidence of infant/child activity: few play materials, unsafe articles within reach
- seldom gives positive reinforcement to child, seldom talks about positive aspects of child

CLINICAL/DIAGNOSTIC FINDINGS
None

▶ NURSING DIAGNOSIS: *Altered Parenting*

Related To
- Inadequate knowledge of infant/child needs, growth, or development

- Caretaker with inadequate skills
- Inadequate role models
- Lack of supportive relationships
- Stressful home situation
- Lack of resources for child care and financial needs

Defining Characteristics
Child
- failure to thrive
- chronic illness
- accident/illness prone
- behavior disorders

Parent
- lack of eye contact with infant
- unable to comfort crying infant
- find infant feeding schedule demanding
- make negative comments about infant
- do not enjoy or have fun with infant

Risk Factors
- Single parent or nonsupportive mate/relatives
- Teenager
- Limited knowledge/skills in caring for infants/children
- Poverty

Patient Outcomes
Knowledge of infant/child development is enhanced, as evidenced by:
- improved caretaking skills.
- increased interaction and increased interest/pleasure in infant/child.
- child-safe environment.

Support in parental role provided by
- greater involvement of mate/relatives.
- utilizing social support and child care resources.

Nursing Interventions	Rationales
Assess parental reaction to infant/child: The child is perceived as a separate individual, having her or his own special characteristics and needs; there is a feeling of interest/satisfaction in parenting.	Children must be understood as individuals who require an emotional bond with an adult to develop socially.
Monitor the basic caregiving skills of the parent: the ability to feed,	Performing these skills with assurance promotes feelings of

Nursing Interventions	**Rationales**
bathe, discipline, provide play opportunities.	competence in parenting and facilitates the physical, mental, and emotional growth of the child.
Role model caregiving skills: holding, bathing, and disciplining child.	Opportunities to learn caregiving skills are often limited unless there is a relative with experience in the family; the caregiver may be overwhelmed by how to handle a crying baby or feed a baby. Competence in caregiving promotes confidence in the parenting role.
Address limitations in skills that place the infant/child at risk for health problems or accidents (e.g., propping an infant's bottle, refusal to comfort a crying or upset child, storing poisons/medicines in areas accessible to a young child).	Child care is based on an understanding, intuitive and/or learned, about the developmental level of the child and the activities which promote the child's safety and well-being. Propping a bottle places the child at risk for gagging, regurgitating, and aspirating formula. Inability to meet a child's emotional needs leads to a sense of distress and distrust in the child and feelings of lacking control. An environment that is not child-proof or appropriate to the child's level of activity and curiosity can lead to falls, poisoning, suffocation, burning, etc.
Monitor understandings of growth and development and the constantly changing needs of the infant/child. Give anticipatory guidance for changes in growth and development skills.	The parents' understanding of the child affects the way they perceive and care for the child. The child whose developmental needs are met (e.g., for love, dependency, autonomy) will feel supported in growing through childhood into adolescence. A caregiver may find different stages of development particularly difficult, but recognition of the child's need to grow and develop is essential.
Discuss individual differences with the caregiver: how the child is different from other children and	All children have their own temperaments and abilities. A parent needs to recognize how the child is

Nursing Interventions	Rationales
different from expectations. Also discuss similarities.	different and similar to others and find some pleasure in seeing the child grow in his or her unique way.
Support a young caregiver/parent by focusing on dreams and plans for the future and identifying goals essential for self-growth and parental development (e.g., high school diploma, special training/ skills).	The caregiver/parent is often a young person who has a dream of becoming someone and needs the opportunity to do so. Although this reality is primarily of importance to the caregiver/parent, it also provides an important example to the young child.
Help caregivers identify concerns and conflicts about the parenting role (e.g., cultural differences, career/work, inadequate time for child and/or self).	Current and changing norms of child care may cause intergenerational tension; parents may have jobs or seek employment outside of the home but find it difficult to balance the demands placed on them. Parents must identify these concerns and conflicts so that they can deal with them.
Identify support groups helpful to the parent.	Parents who feel isolated or insecure need information about programs that provide socialization and information about parenting (e.g., Family Focus). Unfortunately, assistance for parents of children without special needs is limited. If an older child is enrolled in a nursery school or Headstart program, a social worker can be helpful.
Assess and assist with the conditions related to single parenting and poverty, including discussing available resources for food and clothing [e.g., Women, Infants, Children (WIC) for food, thrift stores, and garage sales for moderately priced clothing and toys].	Parents raising children without a mate may or may not have supportive relationships and assistance from others. In addition, poverty limits the provision of basic needs (e.g., food, housing, clothes, health care, diapers, and supplies). Although resources are available, efforts to use them often require travel, time, and patience and choices are limited.

DISCHARGE PLANNING/CONTINUITY OF CARE

- Refer to programs for single mothers, teen mothers, or parents with disabilities (hearing impaired, vision impairment, limited cognitive potential), as appropriate.
- Refer parents with emotional disturbances to social workers, nurse therapists, or counselors.
- Refer to parent groups for problems in disciplining children and in understanding growth and development and play/activities that promote growth, language, and skill development.
- Encourage improving housing or financial means by contact with career training programs.
- Refer families with young children to place eligible children in early childhood educational programs (such as Headstart) to help the child, give parents freedom, and decrease the social isolation and stress experienced by the primary caregiver.

Clinical Clip

Low-income single-mother families were studied by Hall et al. (1993) for psychosocial predictors of maternal depressive symptoms. Almost 60% of the mothers (*n*=225) had a higher number of depressive symptoms that could be related to greater everyday stressors, fewer social resources, and greater use of avoidance coping. Although there is debate in the literature about the relationship of social support to mental and physical well-being, the authors suggest greater attention should be paid by health professionals to the potential negative consequences of these factors. Assessments of social resources, chronic stressors, coping strategies, depressive symptoms, and parenting attitudes may identify areas for intervention that will enhance the well-being of low income single-mother families (Hall, 1991).

REFERENCES/BIBLIOGRAPHY

Doenges, M., Moorhouse, M. (1988). *Nursing diagnoses with interventions* (2nd ed.). Philadelphia: F. A. Davis.

Friedman, M. M. (1992). *Family nursing. Theory and practice.* Norwalk CT: Appleton & Lange.

Geissler, E. M. (1994). *Pocket guide, cultural assessment.* St. Louis: Mosby.

Hall, L. A., Gurley, D., Sachs, B., & Krysciao, R. J. (1993). Psychosocial predictors of maternal depressive symptoms, parenting attitudes, and child behavior in single-parent families. In G. Wegner & R. J. Alexander (Eds.) *Readings in family nursing.* (pp. 234–247). Philadelphia: J. B. Lippincott.

Jackson, D. B., & Saunders, R. B. (1993). *Child health nursing. A comprehensive approach to the care of children and their families.* Philadelphia: J. B. Lippincott.

Kitzingen (1980). *Women as Mothers.* New York: Vintage Books.

Ulrich, S. P., Canale, S. W., & Wendall, S. A. (1986). *Nursing care planning guides. A nursing diagnosis approach.* Philadelphia: W. B. Saunders.

CHILD ABUSE/NEGLECT

Judith A. Scully, RNC, MSN

Child abuse is defined as committing an act detrimental to a child's health and well-being, while child neglect is omitting an act that is necessary for a child's health and well-being. Child maltreatment is a significant social and health problem that includes physical, emotional, and sexual abuse. It also includes abandonment and physical, medical, and educational neglect. The presence of child abuse/neglect in a family indicates ineffective parenting. Although children of all ages are at risk for child maltreatment, children from birth to 3 years are at particular risk. Persons who abuse children are from every socioeconomic, educational, and racial/ethnic background.

ETIOLOGIES
No one theory illustrates the multifaceted etiologies of child maltreatment. Child maltreatment is thought to be activated through the complex interaction of personal, social, and environmental factors and is described by the following models:
- Social-psychological models: The effects of parent characteristics, child characteristics, and chronic stress combine, causing child abuse and/or neglect.
- Sociological models: Child abuse is caused by stress and environmental factors, including unemployment and related financial difficulties, isolation, lack of adequate support, single parenthood, legal difficulties, inadequate living conditions, increased stress, and drug and alcohol abuse.
- Social learning models: Aggression is a learned behavior (violence becomes an acceptable means to solve problems), and poor familial role models contribute to abusive behaviors (also called the intergenerational effect).
- Ecological models: Culture, family, parent, child, and stress are major components of child abuse and neglect.

CLINICAL MANIFESTATIONS

Physical abuse (not accidental physical injury)

- physical symptoms (bruises, welts, fractures, dislocations, poisonings, burns, central nervous system injuries, bites, head injuries, subdural hematomas, retinal or subarachnoid hemorrhage, internal injuries, and/or death)
- behavioral symptoms (cognitive/language/motor developmental delays, abusive behavior toward others, role reversal with parent, inappropriate reaction to injury such as failing to cry when in pain, fear of parents, glancing at parent before responding to questions, indiscriminate friendliness and displays of affection, poor or no eye contact)

Neglect

- physical neglect (failure to thrive, pica or inappropriate ingestion of nonnutrient materials such as dirt or starch, unclean or inappropriate clothing, poor hygiene, feeding disorders, malnutrition)
- medical neglect (inadequate medical care, untreated medical conditions, not returning for needed treatment regimens, frequent injuries)
- Educational neglect (truancy)

Emotional abuse/neglect

- physical symptoms (failure to thrive, enuresis)
- psychosocial symptoms (sleep disturbances, self-stimulating behaviors including biting and rocking, developmental lags, extremes of behavior including being overcompliant and aggressive, suicide attempts, withdrawal, indicators of lack of adequate supervision and exploitation)

Sexual abuse

- physical symptoms (chronic vaginal discharge, vaginal/rectal bleeding, genital rash, presence of sexually transmitted diseases, frequent bacterial/urinary infections, pregnancy in young adolescent, difficulty in sitting or walking)
- behavioral symptoms (suicide attempts, substance abuse, running away, truancy, phobias, sexual promiscuity, psychosomatic illnesses, gestures of a sexual nature, inappropriate sexual remarks that do not fit the developmental age, difficulty in peer relationships, sudden behavior changes, weight gain or loss, clinging behaviors, decline in school performance)

CLINICAL/DIAGNOSTIC FINDINGS

- X-rays fractures (old/ recent)
- Magnetic resonance imaging (MRI) scans: may indicate internal trauma with no apparent accident
- Vaginal or rectal smears/cultures that indicate sexual abuse

▶ NURSING DIAGNOSIS: *High Risk for Injury/Violence*

Risk Factors

Parental
- difficulty in controlling aggressive impulses
- low self-esteem
- family history of abuse/neglect
- isolation
- spouse unavailable or not supportive
- misuse of alcohol/drugs
- inadequate problem-solving techniques
- perceives infant/child as "different"
- account of injury does not fit symptoms
- no medical care sought for injury
- blames third party for abuse
- refers to infant/child in a negative manner
- single parenthood
- appears nervous/hard time remembering what happened
- inappropriate developmental expectations for infant/child
- inadequate knowledge of child care/physical development

Infant/child risk factors
- inconsolable, irritable, difficult to feed
- passive/lethargic
- premature or multiple births
- congenital anomalies
- physical or mental handicaps
- chronic health problems/special needs
- all ages, with greatest risk to toddler

Family characteristics
- all socioeconomic groups with low socioeconomic groups at highest risk
- large number of children
- single parent or "blended" families
- typically have fewer links to community (e.g., church, school, or social memberships)

Patient Outcomes

Parent/parents will be able to:
- describe the importance of providing a nurturing environment to optimize growth and development of infant/child.
- demonstrate nurturing behaviors toward infant/child.
- verbalize understanding of factors/stressors contributing to episodes of abuse toward infant/child.
- identify/demonstrate nonviolent methods of dealing with anger.
- utilize appropriate community resources.
- discuss feelings/problems about infant/child being abused.

- develop realistic expectations for self and infant/child.
- provide adequate medical care for infant/child.

Infant/Child will be able to:

- be free of additional injury/abuse.
- be temporarily removed from home if the family cannot provide a safe environment.

Nursing Interventions	Rationales
Identify at-risk population.	Early identification of at-risk families reduces adverse outcomes and long-term consequences of child abuse/neglect. An increased number of risk factors limits the provision of infant/child needs and increases parental stress.
Establish a therapeutic relationship with parent/caregiver using a non-threatening, nonpunitive approach.	Some parents may not wish to change abusive behaviors; however, many abusive parents often are frightened and anxious about losing custody of their children if they continue to abuse them.
Record signs and symptoms of abuse/neglect in child/family's medical records.	Precise documentation of child/infant interactions is important if Child Protection Services initiates legal action.
Report child abuse/neglect incident to Child Protection Services, followed by a written report.	Between 1964 and 1973 all states in the United States enacted child abuse/neglect reporting laws to protect children from further abuse. These reporting statutes were amended to mandate professionals who work with children to report child abuse/neglect and to protect health professionals from civil and criminal liability.
Discuss with family the rationale of the child abuse report.	By using an open, honest manner, nurses can maintain a therapeutic relationship with the parents when discussing the abusive episode and legal requirements. It is important to maintain a therapeutic relationship because abusive families often

Nursing Interventions	Rationales
	lack trust and are suspicious of health and social professionals.
Refer parent/family to community resources including Parents Anonymous, self-help groups, day care services, emergency housing, and supplemental income and homemaker services.	Abusive parents need to be connected to health care system/resources to prevent further abuse and to decrease isolation and stress. Support groups provide friendship, focus on parental factors that contribute to abusive behaviors, and provide parents with positive role models for child care. Support groups also help parents understand the intergenerational effects of child abuse. Emergency support services alleviate stress and prevent occurrence/reoccurrence of child abuse/neglect.
Assist parent/family to develop network of friends and relatives in caring for the infant/child.	The absence of social support networks is a significant factor in child abuse/neglect situations. Parents often need assistance in assessing who they can turn to when problem situations arise.
Coordinate child protective and other social services for family.	In most states, the child protective system cannot adequately care for abusive families due to poor staffing and funding. Home visits, however, are positive factors in providing needed support to abusive families.
Continue visiting family to role model nurturing parent behaviors, teach age-appropriate techniques for child discipline, and assess for further abuse.	Oftentimes parents persist in abusing their children despite treatment interventions. Because of the complexities of child abuse/neglect behaviors, long-term interventions are necessary and important in providing a safe environment for the child.
Explore alternative ways of coping with stressful conditions, including assisting parent/family in identifying areas of conflict in parenting roles.	Parents need knowledge of what provokes abusive behaviors. It can be major events, such as financial or job losses, but are often minor

Nursing Interventions	Rationales
	events, such as irritable infant/child behaviors.
Nurture mothers by providing positive reinforcement for nurturing behaviors. Also encourage mothers to spend some time away from infant/child.	Praising positive parenting increases the probability that the behavior will continue and increases the parent's self-esteem. Because of the intergenerational effects of child abuse/neglect, mothers and grandmothers also need to be nurtured.

DISCHARGE PLANNING/CONTINUITY OF CARE
- Refer child to physician for physical examination.
- Refer parents to Parents Anonymous.
- OCFS removes child from abusive home to safe environment
  - other family members.
  - foster care placement.

BIBLIOGRAPHY
Campbell J., Humphreys J. (1993). *Nursing care of survivors of family violence.* St. Louis: Mosby.

Cohn, A., & Lee, R.(1988). Child abuse & neglect. In H. M. Wallace, G. Ryan, & A. C. Oglesby (Eds.), *Maternal and child health practices.* CA: Third Party Publishing.

Helfer, R. E. & Kempe, R. S. (1987). *The battered child.* Chicago, IL: University Press.

Jackson, D. B. & Saunders R. B. (1993). *Child health nursing: A comprehensive approach to the care of children and their families.* Philadelphia: J. B. Lippincott.

McFarland, G. K. & McFarlane, E. A. (1993). *Nursing diagnosis & intervention.* St. Louis: Mosby.

Renshaw, D. C. & Thomasma, D. C. (1988). Child abuse: The role of health professionals and the state. In D. Thomasma & J. Menagle (Eds.), *Medical ethics: A guide for health professionals.* Rockville, MD: Aspen.

$\mathcal{E}$LDER ABUSE/NEGLECT

Judith A. Scully, RNC, MSN

Elder abuse is a term used to describe actions which cause physical or emotional pain/injury to an elderly person. A community health nurse's roles include preventing abuse by identifying caregiver role strain early, early detection/care of the elderly abused person, community education, and developing policy to prevent elder abuse.

ETIOLOGIES
- Intergenerational transmission of violent behavior: an outgrowth of family strife manifested in later life
- Inequitable levels of dependency: nature of the aging process that may create dependency of an older person on the caregiver
- Situational stress: problems associated with care of the elderly that create stress and promote abusive behaviors
- Interindividual dynamics: pathological characteristics of the abuser including alcohol/drug abuse and mental/physical illnesses
- Social isolation

CLINICAL MANIFESTATIONS
- Physical abuse (bruises, sprains/fractures, abrasions, welts, scars, burns)
- Neglect (ignoring elderly person, decubitus ulcers, withholding nutrition/malnourished, lack of personal care, lack of medical care, lack of supervision)
- Psychological (verbal assaults, fear-inducing language, ridiculing behaviors, interfering with decision making)
- Sexual (presence of sexually transmitted diseases, bruises, lacerations in genital area, unusual discharges)
- Material abuse (theft/misuse of elderly's money or property)
- Violation of rights (confinement against one's will, preventing free use of an elderly person's money)

CLINICAL/DIAGNOSTIC FINDINGS
- X-rays: fractures (old/recent)
- Magnetic resonance imaging/computerized tomography (MRI/CT) scans that indicate trauma
- Cultures/smears of vaginal/rectal secretions that indicate sexual abuse

▶ NURSING DIAGNOSIS: *High Risk for Violence*

Risk Factors

Abused
- activities of daily living (ADLs) dependent
- mental/physical handicaps
- disoriented
- aggressive behavior

Abuser
- social isolation
- poor or no social support network
- increased stress
- financial dependence on elderly parent
- conflicting role demands/forced to quit job to care for elderly person
- loss of social contacts
- negative image/unrealistic perceptions of elderly person
- unrealistic perceptions of elderly
- history of strained relationships between elderly person and caregiver
- feeling exhausted/depressed

Patient Outcomes
The patient will:
- be free of injury.
- be removed to a safe environment for evaluation/treatment.

The caregiver will:
- utilize appropriate resources to relieve the stress of caregiving.
- reduce/alter social isolation.

Nursing Interventions	Rationales
Assess for abuse. Identify at-risk population.	Knowledge of risk factors helps to identify at-risk families and reduces adverse outcomes of elder abuse.
Develop a trusting, supportive relationship with elderly patient/caregiver.	Elderly patients/caregivers are more likely to discuss actual/potential abuse if they perceive the nurse as

Nursing Interventions	Rationales
	an accepting and understanding individual.
Use communication techniques that will enhance opportunities for the elderly patient to discuss abusive behaviors. Statements such as "Tell me how you spend a typical day" may elicit information on periods of time when the elderly person is left alone or is isolated from other members of the family. Direct questions such as "How did you get injured? Who did this to you?" also may be appropriate in helping patient to discuss actual abusive behavior.	Elderly persons are reluctant to discuss actual abuse because of fear of reprisal, fear of loss of relationship with the caregiver, shame, embarrassment, disorientation, fear of institutionalization, belief in the privacy of family, and lack of knowledge. Direct questions may help patients to discuss actual abusive episode.
Provide opportunities for patient to discuss abuse in privacy.	Spending time alone with the elderly patient provides the opportunity to discuss abuse, to freely express his or her feelings, and to maximize patient's feelings of security. (see Social Isolation.)
Document specific symptoms and clinical observations.	Documentation is essential in identifying elder abuse. Evidence from a variety of sources over a period of time determines actual abusive behavior. Dementia in the elderly person often makes identification difficult.
Report abuse to protective services authorities.	Nurses have a professional and legal responsibility to report abusive behavior to designated protective services. Individual state laws govern mandatory/volunteer reporting of elder abuse and protect health professionals from criminal and civil liability.
Encourage elderly person to remove self from situation and move to an emergency shelter/safe home.	Separating the elderly person from the batterer provides physical and psychological safety, helping both parties to regain perspective and needed social service interventions.

Nursing Interventions	Rationales
Refer patient/caregiver to appropriate resources, including homemaker services (housecleaning, shopping, performance of personal care tasks), respite services, adult day care, financial resources, home-delivered meals, friendly visitors, skilled nursing care, financial management, and recreation programs.	Caring for an elderly person can be a frustrating, exhausting, and draining experience, often disrupting the caregiver's life. Relieving caregivers of the day-to-day responsibilities is critical in alleviating the actual/perceived strain of caregiving. Hospitals and nursing homes often offer short-term elderly care to relieve caregiver fatigue and strain. (see Caregiver Strain/Burden.)

DISCHARGE PLANNING/CONTINUITY OF CARE
- Referrals to nursing homes, and emergency shelters enable elderly abused individuals to receive appropriate services to meet their physical/social/mental health needs.
- Refer caretakers to support groups, respite services, or follow-up with medical/psychiatric care.

OTHER PLANS OF CARE TO REFERENCE
- Caregiver Burden/Support/Conflict Resolution
- Social Isolation

BIBLIOGRAPHY
Campbell, J., & Humphreys, J. (1993). *Nursing care of survivors of family violence.* St. Louis: Mosby.

Hackbarth, D., Andresen, P., & Konestabo, B. (1989). Maltreatment of the elderly in the home: A framework for prevention and intervention. *Journal of Home Health Care Practice, 2*(1), 43–56.

McFarland, G. K., & McFarlane, E. A. (1993). *Nursing diagnosis and intervention.* St. Louis: Mosby.

Straus, M., Gelles, R., & Steinmetz S. (1980). *Behind closed doors: Violence in the American family.* New York: Doubleday.

VanHasselt, V. B., Morrison, R. I., Bellack, A. S., & Hersen, M. (1989). *Handbook of family violence.* New York: Plenum.

$\mathcal{V}$IOLENCE AGAINST WOMEN

Judith A. Scully, RNC, MSN

Violence against women has become an increasing concern in the United States and includes battering, sexual assault, rape, and incest. According to the Surgeon General, violence is the number one public health risk to women and has serious public health implications because of its great prevalence, potential for homicide, effects on children, and long-term emotional and physical consequences. Community health nurses' roles include not only early identification/care of the abused women but also family involvement to intervene and prevent the intergenerational effects of violence.

Clinical Clip

Assault within families is the most underreported of crimes. It is estimated that between 10 and 50% of heterosexual couples have been physically abused in the United States and that 40–50% of battered women are victims of sexual abuse (Campbell & Humphreys, 1993). Over 30% of women will experience sexual violence in their lifetimes. Estimates vary because abuse is difficult to uncover. Frequently, battering is initiated in pregnancy (Bobak & Jensen, 1993).

ETIOLOGIES
- Societal factors (sex role stereotyping, the devaluing of women, power imbalances and cultural and societal support of aggressive behavior)
- Community factors (unemployment, poverty)
- Intrafamilial factors (violence and victimization behaviors either witnessed or experienced, rigid role assignments, strict disciplinary beliefs, role reversals)
- Perpetrator factors (jealousy, possessiveness, poor impulse control, power issues, increased stress, poor self-esteem, isolation, weak coping skills, use

of alcohol/other drugs, brain functioning/hormones which influence aggressive tendencies)
- Victim factors (learned helplessness, poor self-esteem, isolation, poverty, depression, financial/emotional dependency, pregnancy, alcoholism/drugs, separated, divorced, or cohabitating status)

CLINICAL MANIFESTATIONS
- Physical abuse (bruises, lacerations, burns, fractures)
- Emotional abuse (aggressive behavior, verbal belting, intimidation, psychological trauma)
- Sexual abuse (rape, incest, violent or aggressive sexual act performed without consent)

CLINICAL/DIAGNOSTIC FINDINGS
- X-rays: fractures (old/recent)
- Magnetic resonance imaging/computerized tomography (MRI/CT) scans that diagnose trauma
- Cultures/smears of vaginal/rectal secretions that identify sexual abuse

▶ NURSING DIAGNOSIS: *Physical Injury*

Related To actual abuse

Defining Characteristics
- Injuries to face, chest, breast, abdomen in particular
- Vague explanations of injuries
- Bilateral injuries
- Nonspecific psychosomatic complaints
- Social isolation
- Depression, anxiety, fear, difficulty concentrating
- No eye contact with nurse
- Missed or delay in keeping medical appointments
- Husband/significant other does not want to leave patient alone with nurse
- Increased anxiety in presence of spouse

Patient Outcomes
The patient will be able to:
- have physical injuries treated.
- be protected from further abuse and removed to a safe environment.
- increase knowledge of available options: battered women's shelters, community legal and financial aid resources.
- understand that pregnancy is a period of increasing battering episodes.
- be empowered to take action in an abusive situation.
- begin to develop a sense of control in the spousal relationship.
- participate in decisions for self/children.

Nursing Interventions	Rationales
Identify abused women by assessing actual abuse, observing general physical appearance, and observing psychological symptoms/behavior.	All women in the community need to be assessed for actual/potential abuse. Failure to identify abusive behavior endangers women's and children's lives. Nurses who encounter battered women need to be alert to subtle signs of battery (avoidance of discussing the spousal relationship, fearfulness) as well as the overt signs of physical abuse. Questions on violence must be part of every routine assessment.
Assess pregnant women, in particular, for actual/potential abuse.	The stress of pregnancy may strain the marital/spousal relationship by creating jealous feelings in the male, who perceives the baby as an intrusion in the couple's relationship. Theories suggest that battery is an unconscious attempt to end the pregnancy.
Provide support/active listening by assisting victim to sort out her feelings, communicating belief in women's explanation of abuse, acknowledging seriousness of abusive episode, creating privacy by meeting at other locations other than the home (restaurant, day care center), and providing nonauthoritarian atmosphere by being sensitive but direct. Communicate messages such as: You don't deserve to be beaten. There is help for women who have been abused.	Although victims of spouse abuse rarely report their abuse, often they report a desire to tell someone about the abuse. After an acute battering episode, women often are in a state of shock and denial. A caring, nonjudgmental attitude will contribute to a trusting relationship so patients can share abusive history with the nurse.
Identify and explore options with woman by referring them to battered women's shelters or crisis intervention programs, support groups, hot-lines, employment training programs, and financial and legal services. Also provide phone numbers of shelters in the community.	Often nurses are the first and only contact women have in the home/community and are in an ideal position to provide referrals to domestic violence programs, shelters, and other services. Support groups and women's shelters provide a supportive, nonjudgmental

Nursing Interventions	Rationales
Explore personal support systems (list the names of people who could be called on for help in the present situation). Also counsel women to obtain a restraining order.	atmosphere which fosters an abused woman's independence. Shelters separate the woman from the batterer and provide physical and psychological safety, helping her to regain perspective on the spousal relationship and begin to plan for the future.
Provide an exit plan for the victim; encourage the patient to plan for escape by packing a suitcase with clothes for self and children, gathering important documents (insurance, children's birth certificates, and other important documents) in a safe available hiding place, having available the phone numbers of police and battered shelters.	Abused women often are unable to remove themselves from the abusive environment immediately. Because abusive behavior may have been occurring for a long period of time, the woman may be reluctant to leave/seek help because of fear of further abuse, fear of retaliation toward children, the stigma associated with being abused, the fear of not being believed, and financial dependency. Anticipatory guidance in planning for a woman's exit will help to empower her when she is ready to leave the abusive relationship.
Document actual abuse by naming the person who injured the woman, completing a description of old and new injuries (use a body map). Provide a subjective account of the abusive episode. Utilize questions, such as, "Many families have problems with anger; is your family like that?" or "Are you with someone who is hurting you?"	Medical record documentation may be a source of evidence in courts of law when prosecution of the abuser is warranted. If actual abuse has occurred, questions related to violence in the marital/cohabitating relationship help women to recognize the seriousness of the abusive behavior.

▶ NURSING DIAGNOSIS: *Knowledge Deficit*

Related To abusive behavior, cycle of violence, available community resources

Defining Characteristics
- Inadequate knowledge regarding cycle of abuse
- Inadequate knowledge of available resources for self/family

Patient Outcomes

The patient will be able to:

- describe the cycle of abuse and will recognize the stages of abuse.
- verbalize that she is not responsible for the perpetrator's behavior.
- state the legal, and financial resources available in the community for battered women/family members.

Nursing Interventions	Rationales
Explain the cycle of violence, including the tension-building phase, the acute battering phase, and the honeymoon phase.	Violence occurs in repeated cycles: The tension-building phase is the gradual escalation of tension, including verbal abuse, hostility without violent outbursts, anger, blaming, and arguing. The acute battering phase is when the batterer has an uncontrollable discharge of tension through physical assault, use of objects/weapons, or sexual assault. The calm, honeymoon phase is when the batterer is contrite, manifests loving behavior toward the woman, and denies the violence.
Explain the prevalence of spousal abuse in the United States.	Statistics reveal a serious, growing problem of abusive behavior directed at women. Family violence occurs in all cultures and is prevalent in all socioeconomic, racial, and ethnic groups.
Identify social behaviors that may lead to abuse, including psychiatric diagnosis, isolation, lack of social support, chronic unemployment, history of runaways, and psychosomatic complaints.	Poverty, unemployment, and low socioeconomic status increase the risk for abuse and contribute to behaviors that may lead to abuse.

▶ NURSING DIAGNOSIS: *Self-Esteem Disturbance*

Related To continuing physical, sexual, or emotional abuse and/or ineffective coping (denial, embarrassment)

Defining Characteristics
- Isolation
- Lack of eye contact
- Stooped posture
- Depression
- History of abuse in family of origin
- Complaints of chronic pain

Patient Outcomes
The patient will be able to:
- identify and verbalize her personal strengths.
- perceive herself as deserving of respect and not of further abuse.
- utilize needed community resources for self/children.
- be empowered to take action in an abusive relationship.
- seek help of professionals who may provide counseling for perpetrator to eliminate battering episodes.

Nursing Interventions	Rationales
Identify personal strengths.	Women often believe the abuse is associated with their inadequacies and feel shame, guilt, or embarrassment over the abusive episodes. Identifying personal strengths increases self-esteem and helps to empower women to take future action in removing themselves from an abusive relationship.
Assist patient to express feelings about actual abusive episodes and spousal relationship.	Expressing feelings about disappointment or terminating an intimate relationship helps the woman grieve over the lost relationship and identify potential new roles.
Empower women to regain control over their own lives by referring them to support groups with other abused women and to other community resources. Avoid telling them what to do. Praise and support women's efforts in assuming responsibility and making decisions for themselves and their family. Treat them with respect and dignity.	Abusive behavior directed at women causes a sense of powerlessness. Empowering women helps them to gain control and to understand the role violence plays in their lives. Violence against females is a pervasive societal problem that causes human suffering and physical/psychological trauma.

Nursing Interventions	Rationales
Refer the abuser to anger management support groups.	Men often learn that venting aggression toward women is a normal and acceptable behavior. Men often were abused or witnessed abusive behavior in their families, and they need interventions to break the cycle of violence.

DISCHARGE PLANNING/CONTINUITY OF CARE
- Refer to shelters and other social services, such as legal and employment services.
- Refer to physician for complete physical.

REFERENCES/BIBLIOGRAPHY

Bobak, I. M., & Jensen, M. D. (1993). *Maternity and gynecologic care: The nurse and the family.* St. Louis: Mosby.

Campbell, J., & Humphreys, J. (1993). *Nursing care of survivors of family violence.* St. Louis: Mosby.

Cleman-Stone, S., Eigsti, D. G., & McGuire, S. L. (1991). *Comprehensive family and community health nursing.* St. Louis: Mosby.

McFarland, G. K., & McFarlane, E. A. (1993). *Nursing diagnosis and intervention: Planning for patient care.* St. Louis: Mosby.

Reiss, A. J., & Roth, J. A. (1993). *Understanding and preventing violence.* Washington, DC: National Academy Press.

Stanhope, M., & Lancaster, J. (1992). *Community health nursing: Process and practice for promoting health.* St. Louis: Mosby.

VanHasselt, V. B., Morrison, R. L., Bellack, A. S., & Hersen, M. (1988). *Handbook of family violence.* New York: Plenum.

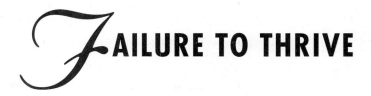

FAILURE TO THRIVE

Amy Androwich-O'Malley, BSN, RN

Failure to thrive is a syndrome in which an infant or toddler falls below the third percentile for weight and height on a standard growth chart or falls behind in growth without a known organic cause. Delays can be noted in motor, social development, and growth. Severe failure to thrive in early months may lead to permanent neurological damage or mental retardation because of protein deficits and interference with brain metabolism. The nurse's role is to teach effective parenting skills regarding nutrition and growth and development and to provide emotional support. For additional information related to normal growth and development, see the Pediatric Ambulatory Care Plan book.

ETIOLOGIES
- Lack of food
- Lack of parental knowledge about proper diet and feeding techniques
- Emotional deprivation

CLINICAL MANIFESTATIONS
- Poor muscle tone
- Lethargic appearance
- Tolerance with physical examination
- Diminished crying
- Weight loss or lack of weight gain
- Delayed developmental milestones
- Reluctant to reach for toys or initiate human contact
- Stares hungrily as if starved for human contact

CLINICAL/DIAGNOSTIC FINDINGS
None. No known organic cause.

▶ NURSING DIAGNOSIS: *Altered Growth and Development*

Related To lack of proper diet and caring environment

Defining Characteristics
- Does not meet normal developmental milestones (refer to table 16-1)
- Physical growth retarded: weight, length and head circumference not within normal limits

Patient Outcomes
- Infant/toddler will demonstrate improved personal/social, language, cognition, and motor skill behaviors appropriate to age group (see table 16-1)

Nursing Interventions	Rationales
Assess infant's/toddler's level of development by utilizing specific assessment tools (i.e., Denver Developmental Screening Tool).	Assessment tools aid in determining delays in motor, social, or growth and development.
Assess weight, length and head circumference and plot growth on chart for children under 2 years. Compare serial measurements, expecting 25 cm growth in first year of life. Birth weight usually doubles by 6 months, triples by 12 months. Head circumference increases about 12 cm in the first year.	Identifies delays in growth.
Teach parents age-related developmental tasks (see table 16-1).	Parents understanding and learning age-related developmental tasks will promote child's well-being and safety.
Teach parents to provide opportunities for an ill child to meet age-related developmental tasks. For infants (birth to 1 year), provide increased stimulation using a variety of colored toys in the crib (mobile, musical toys), provide oral experience if infant desires it (thumb or pacifier), and allow hands and feet to remain free for greater movement.	Demonstrating and explaining developmental tasks to parents will increase the probability that the child will meet those tasks.

Nursing Interventions	Rationales
Refer to an appropriate agency for a structured, ongoing stimulation program when necessary.	Provides increased structure and stimulation for child and parent.
Refer to community programs as needed based on contributing factors, such as poverty, lack of parental education, or lack of parental ability to care for child [Women, Infant, Children (WIC), social services, or counseling].	Concrete support services and assistance can help parents decrease barriers preventing child's proper diet (lack of formula or food).
Provide name of parental support group and parental education classes if needed.	Participation in a support group will allow parents to voice concerns and frustrations within a peer group. Classes will continue to educate parents on changing diet for child and changing environmental needs as child grows.
Document observations of parental interaction, teaching interventions, and changes in infant's/toddler's growth, development, weight, and height.	Such observations help identify infant/toddler and parental progress and areas which need more focus.

▶ **NURSING DIAGNOSIS:** *Altered Nutrition—Less Than Body Requirements*

Related To lack of proper diet

Defining Characteristics
- Retarded physical growth
- Evidence of malnutrition or poor nutritional status, for example, listlessness or low energy, poor skin turgor dullness of hair
- Anorexia

Patient Outcomes
- Infant/toddler will demonstrate consistent weight gain.

Nursing Interventions	Rationales
Assess factors which may contribute to nutritional deficit. In particular, assess home feeding routine, including type of formula, amount taken per feeding per day, and age when solid foods are scheduled. Also assess parent/child interactions while feeding, including positioning bottle, infant position while feeding, holding techniques/positions, verbalizing patterns, and eye contact and interactions when feeding.	Assessments identify trouble areas.
Instruct in proper infant and toddler nutrition. See table 16-2. (For breast-feeding mothers, see Breastfeeding.)	Parents may not know how much or how often to feed infant/toddler.
Instruct parents to hold infant during feedings in a relaxed environment. Avoid bottle propping.	Teaching feeding techniques will increase infant's/toddler's interest in eating, thus promoting weight gain. Bottle propping denies baby parental comfort and increases the risk of aspiration.
Instruct parents to avoid putting infant to bed with a bottle of milk or juice.	Decrease incidence of nursing bottle carries and otitis media.
Instruct parents to encourage toddler to self-feed and use a cup rather than bottle.	Promotes developmental growth.
Instruct parents to offer small frequent feedings and nutritious snacks between meals.	Increase child's tolerance for feedings. Physically, children have small stomach capacities and need small frequent feedings.
Assess infant's/toddler's food likes and dislikes. Instruct parents to provide favorite foods and fluids as appropriate. Avoid small, hard, or round foods.	Children are more apt to tolerate diets that include their favorite foods and fluids. Children can choke on small, hard foods.
Teach parents ways to make mealtime as pleasant as possible,	A pleasant environment will increase infant/toddler feedings.

Nursing Interventions	Rationales
especially to not allow mealtime to continue for extended periods of time.	Extending periods of feeding is unpleasant for child.
Ask parents to record infant/toddler meal tolerance and circumstances surrounding each meal.	Recording meal tolerance and circumstances will help pinpoint what causes problem feedings.
Ask family to obtain infant's/toddler's weight in the nude and to record results at the same time of day and using the same scale.	Demonstrates if interventions are effective.
Ask family to keep strict record of intake and output (number of wet diapers and number of stools).	Accurate intake and output will demonstrate areas of diet which are lacking and where parents may need continued education.
Monitor and document how child tolerates feedings, especially noting if child has emesis, increased stooling, refusal to eat or drink, or any other feeding difficulties as perceived by both parents and nurse.	Physical symptoms may indicate diet intolerance or introducing too many foods at one time.

▶ **NURSING DIAGNOSIS:** *High Risk for Altered Parenting*

Risk Factors
- Knowledge deficit
- Poverty
- Neglect

Defining Characteristics
- Parents exhibit low comprehension of child's emotional, developmental, and nutritional needs
- Parent/child interactions characterized by low level of parental involvement

Patient Outcomes
Parents will:
- verbalize feelings regarding child and their roles as parents.
- demonstrate a positive, effective, parent/child relationship.
- participate in child's care.

Nursing Interventions	Rationales
Closely observe parents and infant/toddler interactions and document. Pay special attention to behavioral interactions, parent and infant/toddler observations, infant's/toddler's interactions with other caretakers and nurses, and infant/toddler sleeping patterns.	Such observations help identify problem areas with parenting.
Teach play techniques appropriate for infant/toddler. See table 16-3.	Promotes infant/toddler growth and development and parental bonding.
Reinforce positive parenting techniques observed.	Promotes confidence in the parenting role.
Instruct parents to provide enough sleep/rest time. For infants, provide opportunity for 13–14 h of sleep per day and provide quiet time for morning and afternoon naps of 1–3 h. For toddlers, provide for 10–14 h of sleep per day and quiet time for an afternoon nap.	Infants/toddlers need adequate sleep and rest for proper growth and development.
Hold infant upright or place in an infant seat for infant to scan environment.	Provides infant with a stimulating environment to promote growth and development.
Instruct parents in safety techniques and devices (e.g., door locks, outlet covers, moving poisons out of reach and locking them up).	Toddlers overestimate ability to perform tasks safely. Once infants are mobile, they are curious and may poison or burn themselves or fall from heights.
Record all observations and interventions in infant's/toddler's progress notes.	Records will show progress or lack of progress based on interventions used.

DISCHARGE PLANNING/CONTINUITY OF CARE
- Ensure parents have understanding of developmental care, including age-appropriate nutritional requirement at present and future ages.
- Ensure parents have support system or refer to parental support group to decrease isolation and stress.
- Ensure parents understand when to call physician or visit emergency room if changes are noted in infant/toddler, including weight loss, persistent emesis, or diarrhea.

Table 16-1 • Physical, Cognitive, Language, Emotional, and Social Development

Age 1–3 months
- Lifts head when prone
- Eyes follow past midline
- Vocalizes (babbling)
- Smiles

Age 3–6 months
- Keeps head steady when sitting
- Reaches for objects
- Turns to follow voices
- Smiles spontaneously

Age 6–9 months
- Sits without support
- Transfers objects from hand to hand
- Imitates speech sounds
- Initially shy with strangers

Age 9–12 months
- Stands momentarily
- Uses pincher grasp
- Verbalizes mama or dada
- Mimics behavior of others

Age 1–2 years
- Feeds self
- Walks/runs
- Has vocabulary of several words
- Uses two-word phrases
- Points to body parts
- Affectionate
- Has poor self-control

Age 2–3 years
- Jumps in place
- Undresses self
- Learning bowel/bladder control
- Two- three-word sentences
- Names objects
- Sex identification
- Ritualistic

Table 16-2 • Nutritional Requirements

Infant
- Birth to 5 months: 115 kcal/kg per day
- 6–12 months: 105 kcal/kg per day
- Birth to 3 month: 2–4 oz formula every 2–4 h, gradually increasing to 5–6 oz every 4–5 h
- 4–5 months: 6–8 oz formula 4–5 times daily
- 6–12 months: 24–32 oz formula daily, gradually decreasing to 18–24 oz
- Provide iron-fortified solids after 6 months of age 1–3 times per day, depending on age.

Toddler
- 100 kcal/kg per day
- Fluid requirements are 115–135 cc/kg per day
- Provide nutrition from the following groups:
  - Milk group (including whole milk), 3–4 servings (1/2 cup each)
  - Meat group, 2 servings (1–2 oz each)
  - Fruit and vegetable group, 3–4 servings (2–3 oz each)
  - Bread and cereal group, 4 servings (2–4 servings of iron fortified cereal)
  (Whaley and Wong, 1995)

Table 16-3 • **Playing Safely**

Age 1–6 months
- Provide brightly colored objects for infant to look at
- Secure a nonbreakable mirror in infant's crib
- Provide musical toys or sing to infant
- Provide a variety of textures for infant to feel

Age 6–12 months
- Provide safe area for crawling
- Provide wagon/stroller rides if appropriate
- Infants enjoy games such as pat-a-cake and peek-a-boo
- Read simple stories/nursery rhymes
- Offer older infants push-pull toys

Age 1 year
- Offer action toys without small pieces
- Offer pull toys; large-muscle activity predominates

Age 2 years
- Prefer toys with working parts, begin to play cooperatively, interest in pretend play

For all children
- Provide toys that meet safety standards, including:
  - Unbreakable
  - No small pieces that can get lodged in throat, ear, or nose
  - No sharp corners or points
  - No parts that could pinch fingers
  - Electrical toys should be used under adult supervision

OTHER PLANS OF CARE TO REFERENCE
- Ineffective parenting
- Breastfeeding
- Child Abuse/Neglect

REFERENCES/BIBLIOGRAPHY

Dilks, S. (1991). Developmental aspects of child care. *Pediatric Clinics of North America, 38*(6). pp. 1529–1543.

Friedman, M. M. (1992). *Family nursing. Theory and practice.* Norwalk, CT: Appleton & Lange.

Greenspan, S. (1991). Clinical assessment of emotional milestones in infancy and early childhood. *Pediatric Clinics of North America, 38*(6). pp. 1371–1385.

Gulanick, M., Gradishar, D., & Pazas, M. K. (1994). *Ambulatory Pediatric Nursing.* Albany, NY: Delmar.

Smith, M. (1987). *Child and family: Concepts of nursing practice.* New York: McGraw-Hill.

Whaley, L. & Wong, D. (1995). *Nursing Care of Infants and Children* (4th ed.). St. Louis: Mosby. p. 143.

Physiological
Conditions

SENSORY DEFICIT

Susan Breakwell, RN, MS

Sensory deficits include any type of loss in vision, hearing, taste, smell, or perception. Visual deficits range from poor vision to varying degrees of blindness to loss of visual field. Hearing deficits can be minimal hearing loss or profound deafness. Taste and smell deficits are mild to severe alteration or loss in taste and/or smell. Perception deficits include diminished or absent dexterity or ability to sense pain, pressure, sensation, or temperature.

The overall nurse's role is to prevent further damage or injury, ensure a safe environment, and educate the patient to use available resources to improve sensory deficits.

ETIOLOGIES

Visual deficit
- injury/trauma
- infection
- cataracts
- retinal detachment
- corneal ulcer
- macular degeneration
- glaucoma
- diabetic retinopathy
- neurological insult resulting from diseases such as stroke and multiple sclerosis

Hearing deficit
- conductive hearing loss
- otitis media
- otosclerosis
- tympanic membrane damage or perforation
- sensorineural hearing loss
- wax buildup

Taste and smell
- injury or trauma
- agents which dry mucous membranes
- medications
- chemotherapy
- radiation therapy
- poorly balanced nutritional intake
- infection
- periodontal disease
- dentures
- tumor or mass
- tube feedings or hyperalimentation restricting oral food intake

Perception
- peripheral vascular disease
- neurological insult or trauma, including spinal cord injury
- diabetic neuropathy
- multiple sclerosis
- severe edema, including lymphedema and elephantiasis

CLINICAL MANIFESTATIONS

Visual
- blurred vision
- decreased visual field, diminished peripheral vision
- blindness
- cloudiness of lens

Hearing
- diminished ability to hear high- or low-pitched sounds
- inability to hear
- tinnitus
- deterioration of speech
- change in conversation or communication techniques (i.e., speaking more loudly, disinterest in conversation)
- change in behavior, confusion, withdrawal and isolation, depression, anger, paranoia

Taste and smell
- diminished perception of taste/odors
- alteration in taste/smell with aversion to certain foods or odors
- anorexia
- nausea
- decreased volume and increased viscosity of saliva

Perception
- pain
- paresthesias

- decreased mobility coordination, activity tolerance, or ability to perform activities of daily living (ADLs)
- decreased temperature sensitivity
- decreased ability to discern pain

CLINICAL/DIAGNOSTIC FINDINGS

Vision
- history by patient report of any visual changes or disturbances
- an inspection of the eye reveals trauma, signs of infection, cloudiness of anterior chamber or cornea, pain, or tenderness
- pupillary response to light and accommodation may be diminished or absent
- eye chart examination reveals decreased visual acuity
- assessment of the visual field indicates "blind spots"
- ophthalmoscopic examination reveals problems with retina, optic disc, macula, or retinal vessels

Hearing
- obtain history of any hearing problems from the patient
- external ear and ear canal inspected and palpated and otoscope used to inspect tympanic membrane for deformities and pain
- hearing deficits noted upon gross assessment of acuity of hearing by use of whisper, watch tick, Weber, or Rinne test; possible further evaluation of hearing loss through audiometric testing demonstrates diminished hearing acuity

Taste and smell
- dryness, lesions, periodontal disease, growths, and inflammation in mouth, oral cavity, or nose

Perception
- conditions with potential for altering perception: diabetes, cancer, human immunodeficiency virus (HIV), neurological conditions, stroke, head or spinal cord injury, surgery
- inability to perform activities of daily living involving fine and gross motor function, inability to distinguish painful stimuli, temperature, and sensation

▶ NURSING DIAGNOSIS: *Sensory/Perceptual Alteration—Vision*

Related To disease, trauma, congenital condition, or iatrogenic causes

Defining Characteristics
- Demonstrated or reported difficulty with activities such as reading or driving
- Observed or reported increased incidence of falls or accidents
- Changes in vision found during an eye examination

Patient Outcomes

Vision is maintained or enhanced, as evidenced by:

- augmenting sight with visual aids such as glasses, adequate lighting, or large-sized print.
- decreased observance or reporting of accidents related to visual problems.

Nursing Interventions	Rationales
Thoroughly assess vision for factors or diseases associated with changes in sight (e.g., diabetes, cataracts, injury, or stroke).	Visual deficits occur for a number of reasons. A thorough assessment may indicate problems or solutions related to other diseases.
Employ and teach use of equipment and techniques that enhance sight. Increase illumination to almost double the normal amount for the elderly patient. Utilize color combinations that provide adequate contrast and are most distinguishable. Use aids to vision, including glasses, contact lenses, magnifiers, and additional nonglare lighting. Special glasses or aids—such as red-tipped cane, computers, braille system, or guide dog—may be needed to correct, manage, or accommodate visual deficits.	With age, eyes need increased illumination to see objects clearly. Reds and black are generally easier to distinguish than other colors, such as greens. Enhancing sight can help to maximize the individual's sense of self-reliance and self-worth.
Teach measures to ensure safety in the individual's surroundings, including clearly marking stairs and doorways, removing loose throw rugs, and keeping things in the same place so they can be located (such as the phone). Keep clutter to a minimum. (See also Safety.)	Safety hazards should be eliminated to reduce potential for accident or injury.
Teach eye care measures individualized for the patient's needs. Include teaching importance of regular eye exams, following any prescribed medication or activity regimen, and reporting signs and symptoms for further follow-up evaluation and	Certain visual changes require immediate follow-up to minimize potential permanent damage (i.e., retinal detachment). All other health team members need to know of any eye disorders or medications to avoid potentiating

Nursing Interventions	Rationales
treatment. Notify all other health care team members of these measures.	problems related to drug interactions or contraindications.
Provide verbal cues; maximize appropriate use of touch and other senses in carrying out nursing interventions.	Other senses may be more developed.
Refer the visually impaired individual to additional resources for information or services including occupational therapy, Talking Books, the local library, and the American Foundation for the Blind.	Occupational therapy can provide specialized blind training. Enhancing the patient's efforts at communication and learning offers the opportunity for maximum independence.

▶ **NURSING DIAGNOSIS:** *Sensory/Perceptual Alteration—Hearing*

Related To disease, trauma, or congenital condition

Defining Characteristics
- Demonstrates or reports difficulty hearing
- Observes withdrawal from verbal interactions, decreased attention span, and difficulty following directions
- Changes in hearing found during hearing test
- Deterioration or lack of speech development

Patient Outcomes
Hearing is maintained or enhanced, as evidenced by:
- utilizing hearing aids, assistive listening devices, or other measures to maximize communication (lip reading, signing).
- maintaining or restoring interactive communication.

Nursing Interventions	Rationales
Thoroughly assess the level of hearing and any factors associated with changes in communication skills or hearing.	
Employ and teach measures to ensure safety in the individual's	Potential for injury is increased when a hearing deficit is present;

Nursing Interventions	Rationales
surroundings: TDD (Telecommunications device for the deaf) phone setup and a light system hooked up to the phone and door or hearing dogs.	this can be minimized by using assistive devices.
Use auxiliary techniques to enhance communication: assistive listening devices, hearing aids, appropriate use of body language, sign language, and writing.	Hard-of-hearing individuals are prone to social isolation and withdrawal. Augmenting the spoken word with other measures increases the potential for effective and meaningful communication.
Instruct in the importance of regular hearing checkups, measures to minimize exposure to potentially dangerous noise levels, and how to maximize communication through equipment and various techniques. Utilize a combination of techniques in patient teaching, including verbal and written instruction, gestures, and demonstration. Also elicit support of significant others in encouraging communication.	Hearing loss occurs with long-term exposure to certain sounds and noise levels. Something as simple as an assistive listening device may be enough to enhance the ability to hear.
Refer to additional resources such as speech therapy or organizations such as the Alexander Graham Bell Association.	Speech may be a problem in those with a hearing deficit. Speech therapy interventions may be appropriate to improve communication.

▶ **NURSING DIAGNOSIS:** *Sensory/Perceptual Alteration—Taste and Smell*

Related To disease, poor nutrition, trauma, medication/chemotherapy regimen

Defining Characteristics
- Demonstrated or reported changes in food likes or dislikes, eating habits
- Report of altered sense of taste or smell
- Weight loss, nausea, vomiting, signs/symptoms of mouth infection or periodontal disease

Patient Outcomes
Nutritional status is maintained or improved, as evidenced by:
- maintaining/gaining weight.
- report of improved tolerance of or pleasure associated with eating.

Nursing Interventions	Rationales
Assess mouth for signs and symptoms of infection or irritation, lesions, periodontal disease, poor fitting dentures, dryness. Monitor weight and other measures of nutrition status, including blood work and anthropomorphic measurements.	Thorough assessment is needed to individualize nursing care to the patient's unique needs.
Teach good routine oral hygiene measures, including brushing, mouth rinsing, flossing, and caring for dentures or other prosthesis. Refer to dentist for evaluation, if appropriate.	Poor oral hygiene can negatively affect the patient's appetite or food enjoyment.
Promote comfort by using medication, cool liquids, adequate liquid intake, hard candies, moisteners, and lubricants for lips.	Antiemetics or an analgesic mouth rinse may be beneficial in diminishing nausea or mouth pain and discomfort.
Teach measures to enhance nutritional intake, including avoiding extreme temperatures, attempting to prepare meals which appeal to the patient, and offering frequent small feedings and liquids. Encourage patient to experiment with new cooking techniques or foods, if appropriate. Allow adequate time for the meal and encourage the patient and others to eat together.	Eating a meal has a significant social and psychological component.

▶ **NURSING DIAGNOSIS:** *Sensory/Perceptual Alteration— Perception*

Related To disease, trauma

Defining Characteristics
- Report of pain or altered sensation to affected area(s)
- Abnormal findings on neurological testing for pain and pressure, such as pinprick, position sense, deep pain
- Observed changes in mobility or ADL function
- Increased incidence of injuries and accidents, such as burns and falls

Patient Outcomes

Functional ability and safety are maximized, as evidenced by:
- demonstrating independence with ADLs.
- demonstrating understanding of safety measures.
- decrease in episodes of accidents or injury related to perception deficit.

Nursing Interventions	Rationales
Assess patient's movement, sensation, temperature sensation, neurological status, and level of functioning (ADLs).	The specific problem area needs to be identified before presenting individualized interventions to the patient.
Teach safety measures that are individualized to patient's problem areas; for example, avoid temperature extremes, routinely inspect skin, wear well-fitting but not binding clothing and shoes, and exercise appropriately.	Risk of injury increases with altered perception of pressure, sensation, pain, or temperature. Teaching safety measures increases the patient's knowledge base and, therefore, decreases his or her potential for injury.
Assist with selecting assistive devices to enhance maximum level of function. Refer to physical and/or occupational therapy, as needed.	Measures to increase strength, mobility, and independence can be enhanced by appropriately using additional services.
Provide information on possible modifications to the home, including "user-friendly" door handles, ramps, uncluttered floors and pathways, and handrails on stairways. Clear paths.	Information and home modifications can increase the patient's level of independent functioning and sense of self-esteem.

DISCHARGE PLANNING/CONTINUITY OF CARE

- Refer to available resources for assistance and follow-up. Encourage or assist the patient to access those which have the potential to improve the level of independence with daily life. Resources include physical/occupational therapy, speech therapy, home health aid, homemakers, and equipment (visual aids, assistive listening devices, or hearing aids).
- Periodically reassess patient and his or her needs. The patient's needs will change over time, as do the technology and resources available.

OTHER PLANS OF CARE TO REFERENCE

- Diabetes
- Cerebral Insult
- Safety

BIBLIOGRAPHY

Brunner, L. S., Suddarth, D. S., et al. (1992). *Textbook of medical-surgical nursing.* Philadelphia, PA: J. B. Lippincott.

Gary, G. (1991). Peripheral neurologic complications and the human immunodeficiency virus: Implications for community nursing care. *Home Healthcare Nurse, 9,* 33–36.

ICMA (1994). *Membership and resource directory.* Little Rock, AR: ICMA.

Jacox, A., Carr, D. B., Payne, R., et al. (1994). *Management of cancer pain. Clinical practice guideline. no. 9.* Rockville, MD: Agency for Healthcare Policy and Research, AHCPR Publication 94-0592.

Thomason, S. S. (1990). Preventing and detecting unique complications in the spinal cord injured. *Home Healthcare Nurse, 8,* 16–21.

Wagstaff, P., & Coakley, D. (1988). *Physiotherapy and the elderly patient.* Rockville, MD: Aspen.

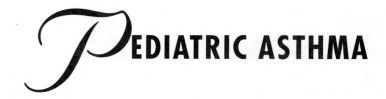

PEDIATRIC ASTHMA

Genevieve Monahan, RN, MSN, DNSc Candidate
Maria Elena Ruiz, RN, MSN, C-FNP

Pediatric asthma is a chronic lung disease causing hyperventilation when the airways of the lungs hyperrespond to stimuli and narrow and/or are obstructed due to smooth muscle spasms, mucosal tissue inflammation, and epithelial cells sloughing into the airway. Acute asthma is caused by accumulated mucus which blocks the airway and can be life threatening.

Pediatric asthma is classified into mild, moderate, and severe asthma. In mild asthma, symptoms occur less than three times per week and nocturnal symptoms occur less than three times per month. Exercise-induced asthma (EIA) is mild or absent. Normal peak expiratory function rate (PEFR) and forced expiratory volume is in one second (FEV1). There is no need for emergency care. In moderate asthma, symptoms occur more than three times per week, nocturnal symptoms occur two to three times per month, and there is mild to moderate EIA. The PEFR and/or FEV1 are 60–80% of normal. Children infrequently need emergency care. In severe asthma, symptoms occur frequently—both day and night, with marked EIA. The PEFR and/or FEV1 are less than 60% of normal. Attacks frequently require emergency care.

While there is no known cure, asthma can be controlled with appropriate treatment, education, and support. The nurse's role includes (1) monitoring asthma symptoms; (2) observing the child's response to treatment; (3) teaching the child and family about asthma symptoms, triggers, medications, and prevention techniques; and (4) supporting the child and family in their effort to effectively cope with the disease.

ETIOLOGIES
The etiology of asthma is unknown, but risk factors include:
• Lung physiology
• Family history of asthma
• Sensitivity to allergens

- Sensitivity to environmental triggers
- Low socioeconomic status

CLINICAL MANIFESTATIONS

- Cough
- Sneeze
- Itchy and/or watery eyes
- Itchy nose or throat
- Nasal congestion or stuffiness
- Chest tightness or chest pain
- Throat tightness
- Wheezing
- Shortness of breath
- Poor exercise tolerance

CLINICAL/DIAGNOSTIC FINDINGS

- History: Child has a family history of asthma or related disease, upper respiratory infections, sinusitis, rhinitis, difficulty feeding and/or elimination, history of asthma symptoms (continuous or intermittent wheezing), history of symptoms being triggered by allergens, irritants, or infections, history of treatment for asthma (e.g., emergency room, urgent care, and/or hospitalization admissions), prior intubation or life-threatening symptoms, chronic use of corticosteroids, sick days at home, symptoms interfering with play, appetite, and/or sleep, school absenteeism, poor academic achievement, and psychosocial problems.
- Physical exam: color (e.g., cyanosis or pallor), cough, abnormal respiratory sounds (e.g., prolonged expiratory wheeze, decreased air exchange), use of accessory muscles, nasal flaring, rhinitis, tonsillar hypertrophy, pulsus paradoxus, diaphoresis, anxiety, tiredness, flexural eczema, delayed growth, and development. Infants should be assessed for alertness, quality of cry (diminished with airway narrowing), and inability to feed.
- Pulmonary function studies (usually age 5 and over) indicate hyperinflation of the lungs and hypoxia (decreased PEFR and/or FEV1).
- Laboratory studies to rule out alternative diseases such as abnormal complete blood count (CBC), sputum or nasal secretion exams indicating infection, chest x-ray results indicating atelectasis, pneumomediastinum, pneumothorax, or pulmonary infiltrates.
- Abnormal pulse oximetry for infants.
- Bronchial challenge: Child's symptoms are induced after supervised exercise and/or administration of methacholine, which are reversed after using inhaled bronchodilator (e.g., albuterol).

▶ NURSING DIAGNOSIS: *Altered Health Maintenance*

Related To airway obstruction, inflammation, and hyperresponsiveness

Defining Characteristics

- Presence of asthma symptoms (see Clinical Manifestations)
- Decreased PEFR and FEV1 (or pulse oximetry in infants)

- Increased heart and respiratory rates
- Exercise intolerance

Patient Outcomes

Patient will exhibit normal pulmonary function, as evidenced by:
- absence of symptoms.
- PEFR and/or FEV1 within 70–100% of normal, or personal best, without wide fluctuations.
- respiratory rate and heart rate within normal limits.
- the ability to tolerate exercise.

Nursing Interventions	Rationales
Assess pulmonary function through spirometry or peak flow meter (infants through pulse oximetry measurement), physical appearance, lung sounds, and heart and respiratory rates. Ask child/family for presence of asthma symptoms.	Airway obstruction and inflammation may be detected hours or days before onset of symptoms using peak flow meter. Early identification of symptoms is critical to effectively manage asthma.
Monitor child's response to inhaled or oral bronchodilators (e.g., beta-2 agonists such as albuterol) and/or inhaled or oral corticosteroids, sustained-release theophylline, cromolyn sodium or other medication as needed. Monitor for adverse effects of medication (e.g., tremors and tachycardia) and theophylline level to ensure it is within therapeutic range.	Monitoring response to therapy ensures control of airway inflammation and asthma symptoms and detects adverse effects of medication.
Describe the medications' actions, possible adverse effects, and the importance of taking medications when PEFR ≤ 70% or with early symptoms. Demonstrate correct technique for using a metered dose inhaler (MDI). Explain that an MDI should not be used more than three to four times per day.	Understanding medications and equipment enhances the child/family's ability to effectively manage their care and decreases the likelihood of error in medication administration. Excessive use of MDIs increases the likelihood of adverse effects occurring.
Instruct how to use and clean spacers, nebulizers, infant masks, and other equipment used with medications.	Cleaning the equipment maintains equipment, enhances the delivery of inhaled medications, prevents infection, and decreases the secondary effects.

Nursing Interventions	Rationales
Instruct child/family in using a peak flow meter to determine green, yellow, and red zones using the child's strongest expiration on a day when they are asymptomatic to establish their "personal best." Have the child/family demonstrate how to record and interpret symptoms, medications, response to medications, and PEFR in a home diary (a.m. and p.m. for moderate and severe asthma and 3 days per week for mild asthma). Stress the importance of showing the diary to their practitioner and promptly reporting any adverse effects of medications.	Peak flow meter testing and maintaining a home diary can help children manage their asthma by detecting and treating signs of airway obstruction prior to the onset of symptoms. The home diary allows the child/family to effectively communicate with their practitioner regarding symptoms and response to treatment.
Identify signs of severe asthma symptoms (cyanosis, difficulty breathing or talking, retractions, nasal flaring, lack of response to treatment within 1 h and PEFR ≤ 50%).	Early detection and intervention is critical in managing life-threatening asthma symptoms.
Encourage children to pretreat with a bronchodilator or cromolyn sodium 5–10 min prior to exercise for EIA. Teachers, physical education teachers, and other school and/or day care personnel should be notified that the child has EIA and should be instructed in the importance of pretreating the child prior to exercise.	Pretreatment effectively prevents symptoms and allows the child to participate in all forms of exercise. School and day care personnel are an important part of the team to manage the child's asthma.

▶ **NURSING DIAGNOSIS:** *Knowledge Deficit*

Related To asthma symptoms, asthma triggers, and medication management

Defining Characteristics

Child/family
- unable to describe asthma symptoms
- unable to describe asthma triggers
- unfamiliar with environmental control measures for the home
- not pretreating with medication before exposure to unavoidable asthma triggers
- unaware of immunotherapy

Patient Outcomes

Child/family will be able to:
- describe the child's asthma symptoms.
- identify the child's major asthma triggers.
- describe ways to control or avoid exposure to asthma triggers.
- state that they understand the benefits and risks of immunotherapy.
- home will be free of environmental asthma triggers.
- child will take medication before exposure to unavoidable triggers.

Nursing Interventions	Rationales
Review common asthma symptoms with the child/family and assist them in identifying those that they experience, especially focusing on early symptoms of asthma (e.g., itchy/watery eyes, headache).	Children/families often are not aware of their early asthma symptoms, which can be used to initiate early treatment.
Assess child/family's knowledge of asthma and self-management techniques. Provide accurate information regarding diagnosis and care as needed.	Despite even lengthy contact with practitioner, child/family many have only limited understanding of asthma and asthma management.
Assess the child's sensitivity to indoor allergens (e.g., dust-mites, cockroaches, animal dander and mold) and irritants of asthma (e.g., cigarette smoke, wood smoke, household chemicals, odors, sprays, and perfumes), especially those within child's room.	Potential asthma triggers must be identified before they can be prevented.
Describe environmental control techniques as needed (e.g., encasing mattresses, washing bedding, removing bedroom carpet, keeping animals outside, changing filters, and disinfecting and fumigating the house).	Environmental control techniques may greatly reduce asthma symptoms that are sensitive to allergens.
Identify outdoor allergens (e.g., pollens, air pollution, and molds). Describe how to avoid them (e.g., playing indoors when air quality is poor) or deal with them (e.g., pretreatment).	Identifying outdoor allergens enhances the ability to avoid and/or pretreat with medication before exposure.

Nursing Interventions	Rationales
Describe other asthma triggers (e.g., strong emotions or upsets, aspirin, sulfites and preservatives, and seasonal changes).	Knowledge of other asthma triggers and prevention strategies can control symptoms.
Assess for possible referral to allergy specialist for allergy testing and/or immunotherapy for those 3 years old and over. Explain the benefits and risks associated with immunotherapy.	Immunotherapy may be recommended for those unable to control symptoms or those unwilling to take medications. Family should be informed that immunotherapy is not universally effective.
Review emergency procedures for severe shortness of breath.	It may be necessary to call 911 for severe respiratory distress.

▶ NURSING DIAGNOSIS: *Ineffective Family Coping—Compromised*

Related To impact of asthma on child/family

Defining Characteristics
- Child without a source of regular care for asthma
- Child/family unable to cope effectively with asthma symptoms, triggers, treatment, or prevention
- Child/family function adversely affected (through self-report or observation) by asthma symptoms (e.g., family activities revolve around child's symptoms)
- Child expresses low self-esteem related to asthma symptoms and loss of function
- Child not taking responsibility for asthma self-management appropriate for age/developmental level
- Expressed anxiety and sense of helplessness in child/family due to asthma symptoms

Patient Outcomes
Child/family will:
- initiate and maintain regular contact with practitioner for asthma care.
- function within normal limits despite child's asthma.
- be able to describe general aspects of asthma and self-management techniques.
- state that self-esteem has improved.
- receive additional counseling and/or support as needed.
- know and utilize relaxation and breathing techniques.

Nursing Interventions	Rationales
Assess family for need of referral to appropriate practitioner for ongoing care (specialist recommended for children whose diagnosis is not clear, who respond poorly to treatment, who experience life-threatening episodes, and/or who have severe asthma).	Family may need assistance in locating and accessing appropriate and comprehensive care.
Assess the impact of asthma on the child/family (e.g., usual activities, school attendance, academic achievement, attitudes about asthma symptoms, response of siblings/parents). Stress that usual activities can be maintained if asthma is adequately monitored and treated.	Assessing these areas helps the nurse and child/family understand how asthma is affecting their normal ability to function. The goal of preventive education and treatment is to ensure as normal a life as possible for both the child with asthma and their family.
Assess for presence of anxiety (e.g., fear of leaving child alone or with others) and available resources and social support. Determine the degree of support needed and refer to asthma education program (e.g., Asthma Care Training for Kids), support groups, or counseling as needed.	Asthma education, support groups, and counseling can support the child's/family's ability to effectively cope with asthma symptoms and self-management.
Encourage child to take as much responsibility for their asthma care as possible and to communicate with parents and other adults about their care.	Child's self-esteem and coping can improve with increasing responsibility for asthma self-management.
Provide instruction regarding breathing and relaxation exercise.	Breathing and relaxation exercises can prevent panic, maximize the effect of treatment, and enhance coping related to asthma management for child/family

DISCHARGE PLANNING/CONTINUITY OF CARE

- Monitor continuity of care with practitioner to ensure child is receiving regular evaluation and treatment.
- Refer to asthma self-management classes [e.g., Asthma Care Training (ACT) for Kids available through the Asthma and Allergy Foundation of America (AAFA)].
- Refer to asthma support groups and summer camp programs by the AAFA and the American Lung Association.
- Talk to the school nurse and/or other school or day care personnel to maintain continuity of care.
- Refer to community-based counseling services as needed.
- Refer to smoking reduction/cessation programs for smokers in contact with child.

BIBLIOGRAPHY

Asthma and Allergy Foundation of America (AAF). (1990). *Asthma Care Training (ACT) for Kids.* Washington, DC: AAF.

National Heart, Lung, and Blood Institute. (1991). Executive summary guidelines for the diagnosis and management of asthma. Washington, DC: U.S. Department of Health and Human Services, Pub. No. 91-304A.

National Asthma Education Program. (1992). Teach your patients about asthma: A clinician's guide. Washington, DC: National Heart, Lung and Blood Institute, U.S. Department of Health and Human Services, Pub. No. 92-2737.

Plout, T. F. (1988). *Children with asthma: A manual for parents.* Amherst, MA: Pedipress.

Rachelefsky, G., Fitzgerald, S., & Santamaria, B. (1993). An update on the diagnosis and management of pediatric asthma. *Nurse Practitioner, 18,* 51–62.

Tinkelman, D. G., & Naspitz, C. K. (Eds.). (1993). *Childhood asthma: Pathophysiology and treatment* (2nd ed.). New York: Marcel Dekker.

ADULT RESPIRATORY DISEASES

Carol J. Paulini, RN, MS

The common respiratory problems affecting adults include asthma, bronchitis, emphysema, and pneumonia. In asthma, the tracheobronchial tree in the lungs hyperresponds to one or more stimuli, causing bronchospasm, hypersecretion of mucus, and mucosal edema causing reversible airway obstruction and paroxysmal dyspnea.

Bronchitis is a lung disease characterized by a productive cough lasting over 3 months per year. When a person has bronchitis for two successive years, they are considered to have chronic bronchitis. With chronic bronchitis, the airway lumen narrows and secretions obstruct small bronchi with plugs of mucus causing inflammatory changes, airway edema, and fibrosis around bronchioles. Bronchitis can coexist with emphysema.

While bronchitis and asthma are airway diseases, emphysema is a disease affecting the aveoli. Emphysema is a lung condition in which irritants initiate irreversible destructive changes to the alveolar walls causing bullae formation, loss of lung elasticity, lung hyperinflation, airway collapse, and air trapping. Persons with resulting severe chronic hypoxia exhibit signs of right-sided heart failure and require increased muscle effort to exhale. Emphysema may have an asthmatic or bronchitis component.

Pneumonia, a lung infection, causes a decrease in lung volume and lung/chest compliance with a loss of functioning alveoli. Microorganisms inflame the alveoli and increase capillary permeability, causing alveoli to fill with exudate. This exudate can result in lung tissue necrosis or a lung abscess. After eradicating the infection with antimicrobial therapy, the parenchyma returns to its original condition or remains scarred.

The overall nurse's role is to identify undetected conditions, to assess diminished respiratory function that could indicate acute or exacerbation of a chronic problem, and to teach patients how to manage their disease.

ETIOLOGIES

Asthma

- Asthma is an inherited disposition to a variety of stimuli and is an allergic response to exogenous or indigenous factors.
- Asthma triggers include allergy, infections (usually of viral etiology), autonomic nervous system imbalance, and exercise and body temperature adjustment to cooling.
- Pharmacological triggers include beta-adrenergic blockade (propananol), and prostaglandin inhibitors such as acetylsalicglic acid (ASA), alcohol, and anticholinergic drugs.
- Psychological factors such as emotional upset may result in bronchospasm. Current theory does not identify this as a sole factor of asthma.

Bronchitis

- cigarette smoking
- atmospheric pollution
- lung irritants and infections

Emphysema

- exposure to lung irritants (e.g., cigarette smoke)

Pneumonia

- exposure to pathogenic organisms
- chemical irritations
- aspiration of gastric contents
- radiation therapy

CLINICAL MANIFESTATIONS

Asthma

- breathlessness
- cough
- monosyllabic speech
- use of external accessory muscles
- agitation, diaphoresis
- chest tightness
- need to stand or sit
- tachypnea, tachycardia
- wheezing
- absence of wheezes with minimal chest excursion in the presence of respiratory distress, which indicates that degree of obstruction is great enough to decrease airflow and is a medical emergency

Bronchitis

- vocal fremitus diminished or absent
- dyspnea
- increased sputum production

- cyanosis due to pulmonary vascular narrowing resulting in elevated pulmonary artery pressure
- dependent edema due to right-sided heart failure
- petechia
- stocky build
- shoulders raised
- muscles tensed from shortness of breath and increased work of breathing
- patient often described as "blue bloater" due to cyanosis from decreased oxygen

Emphysema
- dyspnea
- huffing and puffing breathing pattern
- barrel chest with muffled heart and breath sounds (results from lung hyperinflation)
- wheezing: expiratory wheezes and increased respiratory rate
- cachexia: results from appetite and weight loss
- restless sleep pattern
- decreased physical ability
- patient often described as a "pink puffer" due to rubor from hypercapnia

Pneumonia
- dyspnea
- cough (may be a productive cough with yellow/green tinged sputum)
- tachypnea
- tachycardia
- fever with or without chills
- malaise
- pleuritic chest pain
- bronchial breath sounds with expiratory rales
- increased vocal fremitus

CLINICAL/DIAGNOSTIC FINDINGS

Asthma
- complete blood count (CBC): leukocytosis with elevated eosinophils
- chest x-ray: hyperinflated lungs
- sputum culture: can indicate secondary infection
- oxygen saturation (pulse oximeter): may indicate hypoxemia

Bronchitis
- CBC: polycythemia > 50% Hct, leukocytosis
- hypokalemic: secondary to diuretic use for heart failure
- arterial Blood gases: decreased Pa oxygen, elevated Pa carbon dioxide
- chest x-ray: hyperinflation of lung, flattened diaphragm, cardiomegaly

Emphysema
- CBC: normal or secondary polycythemia, Hct > 50%
- WBC: elevated if on corticosteroids or sympathomimetic agents
- chest x-rays shows hyperinflation, superimposed secondary infection
- arterial blood gases: normal or near normal

Pneumonia
- CBC: leukocytosis
- chest x-ray: infiltrates
- sputum: purulent or blood tinged
- arterial blood gases: may be normal or indicate hypoxemia, hypocarbia

▶ NURSING DIAGNOSIS: *Ineffective Breathing Pattern*
Related To impaired gas exchange, self-care limitations (such as nutrition and activity), medication administration, and oxygen administration

Defining Characteristics
- Adventitious (abnormal or superimposed breath sounds)
- Cough
- Sputum production
- Skin coloration (pallor, cyanosis, pink tinged)
- Dyspnea
- Tachypnea, tachycardia

Patient Outcomes
Patient will exhibit:
- effective breathing patterns: respiratory rhythm control, decreased respiratory and heart rate; decreased dyspnea, decreased adventitious lung sounds (e.g., wheezes, rales).
- airway clearance by effective expectoration and appropriate sputum disposal.
- skin coloration and temperature normalization or return to baseline.
- timely, safe medication administration (inhalers, oral agents, antimicrobial agents).
- self-care ability and oxygen tolerance.
- understanding of principles of home oxygen delivery system (e.g., rationale for, safety and infection control).
- knowledge of life-style, environmental alterations necessary for optimal respiratory function.
- knowledge of respiratory triggers.

Nursing Interventions	Rationales
Teach patient how to breathe better using breathing retraining and exercises.	The focus of breathing retraining is to decrease the strenuous work of breathing, increase alveolar exchange, and provide additional space for lung expansion.
1. Deep breathing: Patient inhales slowly, pauses, and then exhales slowly. Allow patient to incrementally increase breathing retaining exercises by beginning instruction with patient at rest and then advancing to walking and other activities.	1. Deep breathing allows patient to focus and gain control of breathing patterns.
2. Pursed-lip breathing: Patient purses lips, inhales slowly through nose, and then exhales slowly. Expirations should last a minimum of twice the length of inhalation.	2. Pursed-lip breathing causes rise in intra-airway pressure and keeps airway open during exhalation, preventing air trapping.
3. Diaphragmatic breathing: Patient sits upright with head and back supported, places hand on abdomen, and inhales slowly through pursed lips. With inhalation, the patient pushes out the abdomen, pauses, and exhales slowly by gently pushing the abdomen inward and upward.	3. Patients with lung disease usually use accessory muscles (neck, shoulders, rib muscles). Using these muscles with a weakened diaphragm contributes to an increase in stress and fatigue when breathing. Diaphragmatic breathing allows the diaphragm to drop into the abdomen, providing additional space for the lungs to expand. This technique is useful for patients with severe lung hyperinflation.
4. Forced exhalations ("huffing" technique): Patient sits upright, leans slightly forward, inhales slowly with mouth and throat open, and exhales forcefully while contracting abdominal muscles. The patient relaxes and rests his or her arms and shoulders. Gradually increase ratio to 2 or 3 huffs per exhalation.	4. Huffing is used instead of coughing to manage uncontrollable coughs. It is also useful when expectorating sputum.

Nursing Interventions	Rationales
Assess heart rate and lung sounds, including rate, rhythm, and depth of respiration.	Absence of wheezes accompanied by respiratory distress may indicate airway obstruction. Heart rate and rhythm can indicate respiratory distress or a reaction to pharmacological treatments.
Assess and monitor skin color and temperature. Assess for adequate circulation and edema. Elevate extremities as appropriate. Instruct patient to use antipyretics for fever. Patients with asthma are advised not to take aspirin.	Cyanosis may indicate acute or chronic hypoxemia. In hypoxemic states, peripheral vasoconstriction occurs, shunting blood to vital organs. Fever is indicative of infection. Aspirin-induced bronchospasm occurs in 20–40% of all asthmatics. Aspirin-sensitive asthmatics may also be sensitive to non-steroidal anti-inflammatory drugs (NSAID).
Instruct patient in safe, effective administration of pulmonary drugs, including purpose and signs and symptoms of adverse reactions. Goal should be 24-h bronchodilation.	The patient may need 24-h drug coverage to maintain brochodilation. Goal of pharmacology includes relieving bronchoconstriction, promoting bronchodilation, facilitating airway patency by removing mucus, improving oxygenation by increasing alveolar ventilation, and returning normal breathing patterns.
Monitoring for therapeutic blood levels: Monitor for increased dyspnea and wheezing prior to giving maintenance doses.	This may indicate that medication dosage and frequency are ineffective and may need to be adjusted. Therapeutic theophylline range is 10–20 mg/h.
Monitor for medication noncompliance. Make sure steroids are tapered. Assure patient has adequate supply of drugs and understands schedule. Encourage patient to have Medic-Alert bracelet. Patients may require additional steroids during stressful events such as surgery and physical stress.	Sudden withdrawal from steroids may have significant adverse effects since using steroids suppresses cortical production.

Nursing Interventions

Instruct/monitor patient in safe, timely administration of metered-dose inhaler (MDI) or hand-held nebulizer (Pulmonaid). Theophylline blood levels between 30 and 50 mcg/mL are at toxic levels and is a medical emergency. Premature ventricular contractions and grand mal seizures can occur. Advise holding the next dose and contact the physician. Schedule medication administration to maximize benefits: Morning and evening treatments allow patient to clear lungs for day's activities and sleep.

Patient should demonstrate:
1. Shaking inhaler.
2. Using pursed-lip breathing.
3. Placing MDI in upright position, sealing mouth around inhaler, slowly inhaling, exhaling, and pausing. Patient then inhales slowly and depresses MDI one-third way into inhalation. Patient waits 5–10 min between puffs.
4. Preventing contamination and malfunction of equipment by cleaning mouth pieces, tubing, etc., at least every 24 h.

Placebos are available to help patient master technique.

If applicable, instruct patient in safe oxygen administration and assess for adequate tubing length to safely ambulate throughout home. Patient should assemble and test the equipment, including (1) connecting the cannula to the flowmeter, (2) securing the oxygen in the stand, (3) setting the flow to correct rate, and (4) cleaning filters, tubing, and cannula weekly. Leave the tubing to air dry. Avoid

Rationales

Chronic obstructive pulmonary disease (COPD) patients have more secretions in the morning. The goal is to promote aerosol deposition of drugs into the lungs. Minimize side effects; administer with food (crackers).

Oxygen is administered through cylinder tanks on concentrated or liquid oxygen systems. Oxygen is flammable. Equipment should be in good working order and backup systems should be available in case of equipment failure.

Nursing Interventions	Rationales
flames, smoking, electrical appliances, aerosols, and clothing that causes static electricity. Ensure that a 24-hour telephone number for the oxygen supplier is available. Assure that electrical equipment should be properly grounded and that a backup tank is usually available in the event of power failure.	

▶ **NURSING DIAGNOSIS:** *Fluid Volume Excess or Deficit*

Related To heart failure, exercise intolerance, and loss of appetite

Defining Characteristics
- Presence or absence of edema
- Diminished skin turgor
- Increased mucous viscosity
- Weight change [may be related to nutritional status or congestive heart failure (CHF)]

Patient Outcomes
Patient will:
- identify signs of fluid overload or dehydration and indicate action to resolve problem in an expedient manner (see also CHF chapter).
- describe rationale for maintaining adequate hydration.

Nursing Interventions	Rationales
Assess for and instruct patient on signs of right-sided heart failure, including increase in abdominal girth, lower extremity edema, vomiting, fullness after meals, jaundice, urine output change (decreased during the day, increased at night), and weight gain.	Progressive hypoxia results in hypoxic vasoconstriction, increased pulmonary artery pressure, and right ventricle enlargement. Backup of venous blood from the ventricle results in vascular congestion of organs (liver), dependent edema, or decreased flow to kidneys when upright or in the dependent position. Patients often require diuretics or other agents to manage heart failure.

Nursing Interventions	Rationales
Assess patient for adequate sputum production and instruct the patient in the rationale for adequate hydration. Encourage patient to drink a minimum of 2 quarts of liquid per day. Advise patient to drink a minimum of 1 glass of water with medicines.	Since individuals exhale moisture with each breath, alterations in respiratory rate, rhythm, and depth potentially can cause dehydration. Medication side effects include mouth dryness. Patients feeling ill and febrile may not drink appropriate amounts of fluid. Increased mucus viscosity from inadequate hydration makes it difficult to expectorate, causing airway obstruction.
Provide safe external humidification, by running shower, avoiding cold air, avoiding heated vaporizer, and adding a water bottle to the oxygen delivery system; the container should be emptied and changed daily with distilled water.	Warm fluid in containers is a medium for bacterial growth in heated vaporizer. Exposure to cold air may trigger asthma hyperresponse.

▶ NURSING DIAGNOSIS: *Knowledge Deficit*

Related To respiratory illness and need to control environment

Defining Characteristics
- Newly diagnosed patient
- Verbalizes questions related to disease and care
- Lives in a high-risk environment with respiratory triggers
- Medication or equipment change

Patient Outcomes
Patient will
- achieve highest capable level of functional activity.
- improve exercise tolerance and environment.
- reduce frequency and duration of hospitalization.

Nursing Interventions	Rationales
Assist patient in identifying environmental factors that contribute to respiratory disease, e.g., smoking,	Cigarette smoking and exposure to pollutants are the most frequent causes of respiratory disease.

Nursing Interventions	Rationales
dusty environments, pollution alert, or smog.	
Assist patient to develop plans to control or eliminate these factors, including attending a smoking cessation program and avoiding irritants such as insecticides, perfumes, smoke, hairsprays, deodorants, and house furnishings that collect dust, i.e., shag carpets, and open book shelves.	Smoking is the single most common risk factor in respiratory disease. Community resources in smoking cessation programs include the Lung Association and the American Cancer Society.
Assist patient in identifying signs of overexertions such as irregular breathing, fatigue, and shortness of breath.	Self-awareness of baseline abilities can allow patient to develop insight and establish goals for managing activities of daily living (ADLs).
Develop plan with patient to gradually increase activity endurance. Activities that gradually increase endurance should be coordinated with maximum oxygenation and sputum production. Upper extremity exercises can be used to increase activity.	Sputum can obstruct airways. Exercise and increased endurance can allow patient to effectively clear airways.

DISCHARGE PLANNING/CONTINUITY OF CARE

• Refer to social worker, home health aide, Meals on Wheels, pastoral care, or lung association, if needed or requested.

• Ensure that patient has access to a pharmacy and equipment supplier to refill meds or equipment (oxygen tanks).

• Ensure patient can activate emergency response system.

• Make sure patient has follow-up physician appointment.

BIBLIOGRAPHY

Clark, T. J., Godfrey, S., & Lee, T. H. (1992). *Asthma,* (3rd ed.). London: Chapman & Hall.

Critchley, D. (1993). Nurse's knowledge of nebulised therapy. *Nursing Standard, 8*(10), 37–39.

Kersten, L. D. (1989). *Comprehensive respiratory nursing, a decision making approach.* Philadelphia, PA: W. B. Saunders.

Mowad, L. & Ruhle, D. C. (1988). *Handbook of emergency nursing, the nursing process approach.* Norwalk, CT: Appleton & Lange.

Scherer, Y. K., Janelli, L. M., & Schmieder, L. (1994). The effects of pulmonary education program on quality of life in patients with chronic obstructive pulmonary disease. *Rehabilitation Nursing Research, 3*(2), 62–68.

Cardiovascular Disease

Dorothy Fraser, MSN, FNP

All patients with a history of coronary artery disease, myocardial infarction, and angina have a deficient myocardial oxygen supply caused by a decreased blood flow to the coronary arteries. Coronary artery disease is a narrowing of the coronary arteries that is sufficient to impede adequate blood supply to the myocardial muscle. Angina pectoris is pain or pressure caused by an inadequate blood supply to the myocardial muscle. A myocardial infarction occurs when reduced blood supply through one or more of the coronary arteries results in myocardial ischemia and necrosis.

Hypertension is often a coexisting or preexisting condition in patients with documented cardiovascular disease. The Joint National Committee on Detection, Evaluation, and Treatment of High Blood Pressure defines hypertension as a blood pressure greater then 140/90 mm Hg measured on three separate occasions.

Other important causes of cardiovascular disease and cardiac insufficiency are valvular disease and cardiomyopathies. In valvular disease, valve structures are damaged, causing stenosis or insufficiency. Cardiomyopathies are a group of diseases that primarily affect the myocardium and are not secondary to cardiovascular diseases, such as coronary artery disease or hypertension.

Nurses can help prevent and treat cardiovascular disease by educating patients about lifestyle changes that reduce risk factors. The nurse also can play an instrumental role in providing emotional and social support for both patients and their families.

―――――――――――――― **Clinical Clip** ――――――――――――――

Risk factors for coronary heart disease
- Hypertension
- Hyperlipidemia
- Cigarette smoking
- Diabetes mellitus
- Physical inactivity
- Stress

- Obesity
- Increasing age
- Positive family history
- Increased incidence in males
- Increased incidence in African-Americans

ETIOLOGIES

Hypertension
- primary: unknown
- secondary: renal artery stenosis, hyperaldosteronism, adrenal medulla tumors, and nephrosclerosis

Coronary artery disease/angina/myocardial infarction
- coronary atherosclerosis secondary to an abnormal deposition of lipids and fibrin in the walls of the coronary vessels
- embolus or thrombus occluding a coronary artery (partial occlusion can cause angina; complete occlusion causes myocardial infarction)

Arrhythmias
- myocardial infarction
- drug toxicity

- cardiac ischemia
- electrolyte disturbances

Cardiac insufficiency
- cardiomyopathy due to coronary artery disease or genetic factors
- valvular disease due to genetic defects, rheumatic fever, or acute or subacute bacterial endocarditis

CLINICAL MANIFESTATIONS

Hypertension
- normally asymptomatic
- headaches

Coronary artery disease
- chest pain that may radiate to jaw, teeth, arm, and neck; often described as a pressure, tightness, or feeling of a constriction
- tachycardia
- hypotension
- diaphoresis
- sense of impending doom
- nausea/vomiting

- dysrhythmias
- presence of S_3 or S_4 cardiac sounds

Dysrhythmias
- asymptomatic
- palpitations
- same as coronary artery disease, if unstable

Cardiac insufficiency
- peripheral edema [signs and symptoms of congestive heart failure (CHF)–see CHF chapter]

CLINICAL/DIAGNOSTIC FINDINGS

Hypertension
- blood pressure greater than 140 systolic or 90 diastolic

Coronary artery disease
- electrocardiogram (EKG): ST segment elevation with development of pathological Q waves is indicative of acute myocardial infarction. ST segment depression is associated with myocardial ischemia.
- elevated serum enzymes: creatine phosphokinase (CPK-MB) isoenzymes elevate within the first 4–6 h after a myocardial infarction (MI) and return to normal within 36–48 h. Lactic dehydrogenase (LDH) elevates in 24–48 h and can remain elevated for as long as 10–14 days. Aspartate amino transferase (AST) elevates within 6–12 h and returns to normal within 3–4 days.
- complete blood count (CBC): Leukocytosis occurs early in an MI and is associated with inflammatory disease of the heart.
- serum cholesterol and triglycerides: risk factor for development of coronary artery disease (CAD) and elevated levels often present in clients with history of CAD.
- chest x-ray: usually normal. Increased cardiac size seen in patients with CHF.
- coronary angiography: visualizes narrowing/occlusion of the coronary arteries. Left ventricular function measured by ejection fraction. Ejection fractions of less than 40% are associated with increased mortality.
- exercise stress testing: evaluates myocardial oxygen supply capabilities under conditions of increased need. Presence of angina and arrhythmias indicative of myocardial ischemia.
- holter monitor: ECG tracing over extended periods to evaluate for the presence of dysrhythmias during activities of daily living.

Arrhythmias
- EKG diagnoses arrhythmia

Cardiac insufficiency
- chest x-ray shows congestive heart failure.
- echocardiogram shows poor muscular movement.
- cardiac catheterization shows poor ejection fraction.

▶ NURSING DIAGNOSIS: *Decreased Cardiac Output*

Related To
- Left ventricular muscle dysfunction with decreased contractility
- Myocardial ischemia with decreased contractility
- Alterations in rate or rhythm
- Cardiac depressant effects of drugs

Defining Characteristics
- Hypotension
- Tachycardia/bradycardia
- Diaphoresis
- Apprehension, fear, sense of impending doom
- Chest pain, heaviness, or pressure that may or may not radiate
- S_3 associated with cardiac failure
- S_4 associated with decreased ventricular compliance and hypertension
- Changes in mental status
- Dysrhythmias
- Thready/weak peripheral pulses
- Complaints of increasing fatigue, weakness

Patient Outcomes
Patient will exhibit adequate cardiac output, as evidenced by:
- blood pressure within stable parameters for individual with no evidence of postural changes.
- mental status within normal parameters for patient.
- adequate urine output.
- gradually increasing activity tolerance.
- reported decreased episodes of dyspnea, chest pain, fatigue, and weakness.
- participation in activities that decrease cardiac workload.

Nursing Interventions	Rationales
Assess apical pulse for rate and rhythm.	Cardiac dysrhythmias such as premature ventricular contractions are common in individuals with CAD, hypertension (HTN), and post-surgery for CAD. Medications, such as digitalis and antihypertensives, can cause dysrhythmias.
Assess lying, sitting, and standing blood pressures.	Orthostatic blood pressure changes are associated with decreased fluid volume and decreased cardiac output. Medications used for

Nursing Interventions	Rationales
	angina—such as vasodilators and calcium channel blockers—can accentuate orthostatic changes and lead to falls.
Note presence of S_3 and S_4.	S3 is found in patients with progressive cardiac decompensation. S4 is commonly seen in clients with HTN and arteriosclerotic heart disease.
Elicit reports of chest pain, documenting location, duration, intensity, and aggravating and relieving factors.	New symptoms of chest pain or increasing incidence of complaints of chest pain can indicate worsening cardiac ischemia. Decreased symptoms may indicate less cardiac ischemia.
Auscultate breath sounds.	Congestive heart failure with development of pulmonary congestion occurs when myocardial contractility is depressed.
Evaluate response to activity by monitoring vital signs before and after activity and monitoring complaints of fatigue, weakness, and pain. Have patients describe daily activity level, noting decreased ability to perform ADLs.	Exercise increases myocardial oxygen demand. Monitoring for the presence of chest pain, increasing fatigue, and the presence of tachycardia or hypotension will provide objective data on which to base exercise program and to evaluate cardiac output.

▶ NURSING DIAGNOSIS: *Pain—Acute or Chronic*

Related To
- Myocardial ischemia
- Incisional pain postoperatively
- Altered tissue perfusion

Defining Characteristics
- Chest pain with or without radiation
- Anxiety
- Diaphoresis
- Increased or decreased blood pressure
- Restlessness

Patient Outcomes

Patient will:

- verbalize relief of pain during acute stage of anginal pain.
- verbalize decreased frequency and duration of pain.
- demonstrate use of relaxation techniques.

Nursing Intervention	Rationales
Assess and document the location, duration, quality, severity, timing, and precipitating and relieving factors associated with episodes of pain.	The characteristics, frequency, and duration of pain are important parameters used to determine the possible etiology of the pain and to determine the need for immediate referral.
Assess for restlessness, sleep deprivation, anxiety, and rapid mood changes.	Nonverbal cues can be useful indicators of the severity of the pain and the individual's specific response to pain.
Monitor vital signs.	Increased heart rate is seen with acute pain. Blood pressure often increases with acute pain. In patients with heart disease, a decrease in blood pressure may indicate decreased cardiac output secondary to diminished myocardial reserve.
Instruct patient and family on using relaxation techniques such as deep breathing, visualization, and diversional activities.	Diversional activities and relaxation techniques can promote relaxation and improve medication response by decreasing frequency and dose needed.
Instruct patient and family to maintain pain diary.	The use of a pain diary will enable the patient and family to monitor the characteristics, frequency, and duration of episodes of pain. This information will provide objective data on which to base the need for changes in medication dose and frequency as well as the need for immediate referral.
Instruct patient and family to notify health care provider immediately in each of the following cases: (1) new	Chest pain is a hallmark sign of myocardial ischemia. Changes in the characteristics of the pain

Nursing Intervention

episode of chest pain radiating to the back, jaw, or arms (call 911 for emergency services); (2) chest pain not relieved by nitroglycerine (call health care provider and 911); and (3) increasing frequency and duration of chest pain (call health care provider).

Rationales

herald a decrease in myocardial oxygen supply.

▶ NURSING DIAGNOSIS: *Activity Intolerance*

Related To
- Myocardial ischemia
- Depressant effect of cardiac medications
- Imbalance of myocardial oxygen supply and demand

Defining Characteristics
- Tachycardia/bradycardia
- Hypotension
- Chest pain associated with exercise
- Complaints of weakness, fatigue
- Dysrhythmias
- Diaphoresis

Patient Outcomes
Patient will demonstrate progressive exercise tolerance, as evidenced by stabilized vital signs and absent complaints of chest pain.

Nursing Interventions	Rationales
Monitor heart rate, blood pressure, complaints of chest pain, shortness of breath, and weakness before, during, and 10 min after exercise.	Myocardial oxygen need increases with exercise. Comparing these data before, during, and 10 min after activity can measure heart function. Stabilized vital signs, absent chest pain, and decreased fatigue indicates improving myocardial function. Unstable vital signs indicate the need to decrease activity levels and seek consultation.
Individualize patient care to allow for rest periods and activity during patient's peak energy times.	Activity at peak energy levels with periods of rest will maximize myocardial oxygen supply and energy availability.

▶ NURSING DIAGNOSIS: *Fear/Anxiety*

Related To
- Threat to physical health
- Fear of loss of role, socioeconomic status
- Threat to self-concept
- Fear of death or disability

Defining Characteristics
- Restlessness, irritability, inability to concentrate
- Palpitations
- Sleeplessness/difficulty sleeping
- Expressing anxiety, fear, feelings of helplessness
- Change in social participation and communication patterns

Patient Outcomes
Patient will:
- acknowledge fears and anxieties.
- participate in developing positive coping measures to deal with expressed fears and anxiety.
- use family and community resources available to decrease anxiety and improve communication.

Nursing Interventions	Rationales
Assess for increased heart rate, increased blood pressure, diaphoresis, irritability, and difficulty concentrating.	Fear and anxiety stimulate the sympathetic nervous system. Increased heart rate and blood pressure and increasing irritability can increase myocardial oxygen need and precipitate angina or decreased exercise tolerance.
Acknowledge patient's fears and anxieties by encouraging verbalizing in a nonthreatening environment.	The patient's expression of his or her own interpretation of the perceived threats of physical and psychological well-being is a necessary first step in assisting the patient to develop effective ways to cope with the fear and anxiety.
Evaluate patient's past coping measures and assist the patient to identify ways these coping measures can be used to deal with current concerns.	Encourage patient to use effective past coping measures to build upon personal resources already present. If current coping techniques are insufficient or unhealthy, suggest new coping methods.

Nursing Interventions	Rationales
Instruct patient and family on using relaxation techniques, such as visualization, music, massage, and meditation.	Relaxation promotes rest, increases energy, and may enhance patient's own coping measures.

▶ NURSING DIAGNOSIS: *Knowledge Deficit*

Related To
- Lack of knowledge regarding medical condition
- Lack of knowledge regarding medications
- Need for lifestyle changes
- Expressed desire to learn

Defining Characteristics
- Verbalizing misconceptions, misinformation
- Noncompliance with medical or pharmacological regimen
- Verbalizing need for lifestyle change
- Developing complications that are preventable
- Lack of information regarding new technology and its use
- Lack of familiarity with community resources

Patient Outcomes
Patient will:
- describe his or her medical condition and current medical regimen.
- describe action, reason for use, and major adverse reactions of all current medications.
- state the rationale for lifestyle changes recommended.
- state rationale and describe proper use of all new technology.
- identify community resources available.

Nursing Interventions	Rationales
Review medical condition, current medical regimen, and current medications with patient and family.	Compliance depends upon an understanding of the disease process and the recommended medical regimen. Patients and families are often not ready to incorporate this information when in an acute-care setting.

Nursing Interventions	Rationales
Describe the action, reason for use, and common adverse effects for each medication.	It is easier and more effective to monitor long-term changes in condition, recognize adverse effects of medications, and maintain compliance with the medication regimen when patients/families understand and are active participants in their care.
Review important lifestyle changes (i.e., dietary, stress reduction, exercise) that are appropriate for the individual patient.	Lifestyle changes are a cornerstone of the treatment of coronary heart disease and HTN as they can reduce risk factors that increase morbidity and mortality. These changes are the most difficult for patients and families and require ongoing evaluation and support.
Provide education information in both a verbal and written form when possible. Encourage patient and family to keep a log of questions that occur between visits.	Verbal and written instructions will enhance patient understanding and encourage active involvement. Maintaining a log will increase cooperation.

DISCHARGE PLANNING/CONTINUITY OF CARE

- Refer to the American Heart Association for educational materials regarding lifestyle changes.
- Refer to Mending Heart Clubs, the American Heart Association support group for patients recovering from heart surgery.
- Refer to a certified exercise physiologist for exercise prescription and training when medical clearance is given.
- Refer to a dietician for dietary counseling and provide information on support groups within the community to assist in weight loss and weight maintenance (i.e., Weight Watchers, Overeaters Anonymous). (See nutrition chapter.)
- Provide information on emergency procedures and when and how to contact 911. Patients living alone may contact the local emergency room to determine if life line support is provided for more rapid emergency contact.
- Instruct patient on the importance of keeping both emergency numbers and the phone number of their primary physician available. Provide emergency pad with address and phone number of closest relative.
- Provide information on cardiopulmonary resuscitation classes for family members.

BIBLIOGRAPHY

Letterer, R. et al. (1992). Learning to live with congestive heart failure. *Nursing '92*, May, 22(5). 34–41.

Merkely, K. (1991). Assessing chest pain. *RN*, June, 57(6) 58–62.

Rossi, L., & Leavy, E. (1992). Evaluating the patient with CAD. *Nursing Clinics of North America*, 27(1), 171–188.

Vickers, P. (1994). How to spot early signs of cariogenic shock. *American Journal of Nursing*, May, 94(5) 36–40.

Yacone-Morton L. A. (1991). Perfecting the art of cardiac assessment. *RN*, 54(12), 28.

$\mathcal{C}$ONGESTIVE HEART FAILURE

Anne K. Bedlek, MSN, CCRN, CPAN

Congestive heart failure (CHF) is a progressive condition of heart disease. It is commonly associated with long-term coronary artery disease and uncontrolled hypertension. CHF involves the right, left, or both sides of the heart.

With left-sided CHF, the diseased heart fails to pump blood volume from the pulmonary to the systemic circulation, causing increased pulmonary venous pressure, left atrial pressure, and left ventricular diastolic pressure. Left-sided CHF also causes decreased cardiac output from pulmonary edema and decreased O_2-CO_2 exchange.

With right-sided CHF, the diseased myocardium fails to pump blood volume to the lungs, causing an increase in lung pressure. It also impedes systemic venous return, causing fluid to accumulate in organs, resulting in liver and spleen engorgement, jugular vein distention, and lower extremity edema.

The nurses's overall role is to detect signs of impending CHF and to educate the patient and family in managing their chronic disease.

ETIOLOGIES

Left-sided CHF
- atherosclerotic heart disease
- acute myocardial infarction
- myocarditis
- fluid overload
- valvular heart disease

Right-sided CHF
- left-sided heart disease
- atherosclerotic heart disease
- acute myocardial infarction
- pulmonary valve stenosis

- mitral stenosis with pulmonary hypertension
- pulmonary emboli
- chronic obstructive pulmonary disease (COPD)
- cor pulmonale
- valvular heart disease
- atrial-septal defects

CLINICAL MANIFESTATIONS

Left-sided heart failure

- dyspnea: begins on exertion with an associated cough; progression of symptoms usually slow; may occur at rest; may include inspiratory and expiratory wheezing
- orthopnea: shortness of breath occurring when lying but that can be relieved by positioning to mid or high Fowler's position
- paroxysmal nocturnal dyspnea (PND): fluid in lungs that may awaken patient from sleep; sitting or standing may relieve symptoms but acute pulmonary edema may occur
- signs and symptoms associated with acute pulmonary edema, including cool, clammy, pale skin, anxiety, diaphoresis, gasping for breath, frothy white or pink-tinged sputum, and rales/crackles; considered a medical emergency

Right-sided heart failure

- weakness and fatigue with progressing and decreased cardiac output.
- edema: lower extremity edema, especially ankle edema. If bedridden, the fluid accumulates in the sacral, flank, and thigh areas.
- liver engorgement: liver capsular enlargement occurs due to engorgement. A right upper quadrant pain can be confused with cholecystitis.
- gastrointestinal symptoms: anorexia, bloating, and other nonspecific complaints.

CLINICAL/DIAGNOSTIC FINDINGS

- Chest x-ray reveals cardiac enlargement and interstitial density.
- Liver function tests reveal abnormal findings with hepatomegaly.
- Swan-Ganz, thallium tests, echocardiogram, and/or cardiac catherization readings detail the degree of failure.
- Pulse oximetry and arterial blood gases reveal the degree of pulmonary compromise.

▶ NURSING DIAGNOSIS: *Decreased Cardiac Output*

Related To fluid volume overload due to lack of knowledge of low-sodium diet and fluid restriction.

Defining Characteristics

- Shortness of breath
- Lower extremity edema
- Abdominal distention
- Jugular venous distention
- Fatigue
- Third heart sound
- Unilateral or bilateral rales
- Cough
- Liver enlargement

Patient Outcomes

Patient will:

- experience decreased symptoms.
- be able to verbalize an understanding of fluid and dietary restrictions.

Nursing Interventions	Rationales
Assess the patient's physical state and knowledge level. This includes assessing patient's complaints and auscultating lungs and heart for abnormal sounds. Observe for jugular venous distention, dyspnea and/or cough, fatigue, lower extremity edema, weakness, and abdominal distention. Also assess knowledge level about fluid volume overload, current condition, low-sodium diet and fluid restriction, current medications, and how to measure intake and output.	An accurate and thorough baseline assessment will identify teaching needs and other interventions.
Encourage patient's comfort and instruct in balancing rest and activities as tolerated.	Avoiding fatigue decreases the severity of symptoms.
Encourage the patient to verbalize feelings, questions, and experiences.	Often communication assists the patient in clarifying his or her reactions/feelings, encourages understanding, and promotes an atmosphere where learning can occur.
Describe those symptoms (shortness of breath, swelling, etc.) that should be reported.	Prompt attention and care allow for adjustments in therapy and can prevent or minimize harmful effects of unhealthy conditions.
Explain how to measure intake and output.	Assistance and accuracy in measurement promote wellness by decreasing the severity of the swelling and shortness of breath.

Nursing Interventions	Rationales
Instruct the patient to consume only the prescribed amounts and kinds of foods and liquids.	Indiscriminate experimentation with one's prescribed therapeutic diet may lead to an acute state of congestive heart failure.
Teach how to administer medication.	Correct medication administration increases the drug effectiveness and decreases a potential for side effects.

DISCHARGE PLANNING/CONTINUITY OF CARE

- Patient knows when to visit physician for blood draws.
- Ensure patient understands how to identify signs and symptoms of impending problems and how and when to call the physician or emergency services.
- Patient knows how to follow up with social services if financing prescriptions is a problem.

Clinical Clip

The prevalence and incidence of CHF has increased because of an increase in heart disease and an aging population. More subtle predictors are hypertension, diabetes, cigarette smoking, obesity, cardiomyopathy, familial tendencies to a low ratio of high-density lipoprotein (HDL) cholesterol, and hypercholesterolemia.

Congestive heart failure has a proven high mortality rate. In the Framingham study, within 2 years of diagnosis, 37% of men and 38% of women died from CHF. Within 6 years, 82% of men and 67% of women died from CHF.

BIBLIOGRAPHY

Funk, M. (1993). Epidemiology of heart failure. In Gould-Ahern, M. (Ed.), *Management of chronic heart failure/thoracic trauma* (Vol. 5, pp. 569–573). Philadelphia: W. B. Saunders.

$\mathcal{P}$ERIPHERAL VASCULAR DISEASE

Jan McCarron, MSN, RN

Peripheral vascular disease (PVD) refers to pathologies affecting blood vessels that supply the extremities, including arteries, veins, and lymphatics (Suddarth, 1991). These diseases are insidious at onset and are not usually diagnosed until they substantially occlude the vascular system (Herman, 1986).

The most common types of peripheral artery diseases are arterial occlusive disease and aneurysm. Arterial occlusive disease can be acute or, more commonly, chronic. In an acute attack, a thrombus or embolus suddenly blocks an artery, creating a limb-threatening emergency which needs immediate nursing and medical intervention (Blank & Irwin, 1990). In contrast, chronic arterial occlusive disease is a slowly progressive condition that gradually narrows and hardens the peripheral arteries. The second type of peripheral artery disease, aneurysm, is a localized abnormal dilation of an artery which is caused by a congenital or structural defect. The greatest percentage of aneurysms occur in the thoracic and abdominal aorta. Usually the patient reports no symptoms until the aneurysm ruptures (Bright & Georgi, 1992).

Peripheral venous disease occurs when the veins become overstretched due to increased venous pressure over time. This causes the veins to distend and prevents tight valve closure. Blood backs up and the increasing pressure makes capillary walls become more permeable, causing fluid and red blood cells to leak into the surrounding tissue, thereby causing edema (Blank & Irwin, 1990). Peripheral venous disorders also include thrombophlebitis and thrombus formation. One of the most serious is deep-vein thrombosis (DVT) because of the high risk of pulmonary embolism (Bright & Georgi, 1992).

The lymphatic system also can become obstructed. As with veins, the peripheral lymph vessels dilate from pressure, and valves become incompetent. Lymphatic obstruction causes edema and lymph node inflammation, which can reduce the node's ability to filter cellular debris and to provide protection against infection (Blank & Irwin, 1990).

In the community setting, nursing care includes monitoring the condition and helping the patient make lifestyle changes to decrease complications and exacerbations.

ETIOLOGIES

Peripheral arterial disorders

- atherosclerotic changes within arterial walls. Risk factors include genetic history, diabetes mellitus, smoking, hyperlipidemia, obesity, and hypertension.
- acute peripheral arterial occlusion caused by arterial embolism, most often originating from the heart; such an event can also be iatrogenic, resulting from poorly performed arterial blood gases or arterial line insertion (Blank & Irwin, 1990).

Peripheral vascular disorders

- thrombophlebitis: caused by venous stasis, injury to a vessel wall and/or hypercoagulability (Blank & Irwin, 1990)
- superficial thrombosis: due to carelessly inserted IV or poorly maintained IV site (Blank & Irwin, 1990)
- deep-vein thrombosis: prolonged bed rest, obesity, pregnancy, or paralyzed calf muscles after anesthesia (Blank & Irwin, 1990)
- chronic venous insufficiency: incompetent valves and linked to obesity, pregnancy, age, malignancy, and occupations that require prolonged standing (Bright & Georgi, 1992)

Peripheral lymphatic disorders (Blank & Irwin, 1990)

- swelling after mastectomy
- Hodgkin's disease
- tuberculosis
- lymphatic cancer

CLINICAL MANIFESTATIONS

Peripheral arterial disease: chronic insufficiency

- extremities are pale, especially on elevation, and turning rubor on dependency. Skin is cool to the touch, thin, shiny, and atrophic.
- toenails are thick, rigid, and slow growing.
- skin ulcers are present, especially on pressure points, including heels, toes, dorsum of the foot, or over the metatarsal heads.
- pain: intermittent claudication or rest pain, which usually occurs after lying down flat and is indicative of severe arterial occlusion.
- pulses are diminished or absent.

Peripheral arterial disease: acute occlusion

- pain: abrupt onset, severe, not relieved by rest or activity

- skin: cold (with a clear border between warm and cold zones), pallor and cyanosis when extremity is raised above level of the heart
- pulses: extremely weak or absent (Blank & Irwin, 1990)

Peripheral venous disease: chronic insufficiency
- skin: stasis dermatitis, brown-reddish pigmentation, cellulitis, varicose veins, cyanosis upon dependency
- edema: usually when dependent, reduced when extremity elevated
- pain: dull, diffused ache throughout the leg that increases with prolonged standing (Bright & Georgi, 1992)

Peripheral venous disease: thrombophlebitis
- pain and tenderness along the involved vein
- skin: redness or discoloration over the saphenous vein, local warmth and edema with induration (Kuhn & McGovern, 1992)

Peripheral venous disease: deep-vein thrombosis
- tenderness and aching pain in the calf, elevated skin temperature, swelling, and positive Homan's sign (Blank & Irwin, 1990)

Lymphatic disorders
- lymphedema not usually reduced by rest or elevation (Blank & Irwin, 1990)

CLINICAL/DIAGNOSTIC FINDINGS

Peripheral arterial disease
- Plethysmography measures blood volume changes in the legs. An abnormal tracing shows a low, round waveform with no sharp systolic peaks.
- Ankle/brachial index (ABI) [the ratio between brachial systolic blood pressure (B/P) and ankle systolic B/P] is ≥ 1.00 (ABIs decrease as the severity of the disease increases) (Kerner, 1992).
- Stress testing measures ankle pressure readings before and after a 5-min treadmill test. With arterial occlusion, ankle pressure after exercise will fall to 50 mm Hg or below.
- Angiography visually shows arterial stenosis and occlusion.

Peripheral venous disease
- Impedance plethysmography detects deep-vein thrombosis.
- Duplex scanning: Real-time imaging (ultrasound) allows scanned vessels to appear on screen as they function, while doppler capabilities measure flow and velocity within the vessel (Rudolphi, 1990).
- Venography visually shows venous stenosis and occlusion.

▶ NURSING DIAGNOSIS: *Impaired Skin Integrity*

Related To altered circulation (arterial or venous)

Defining Characteristics:
- A break in the skin of the feet or legs
- Patient reports of pain in the involved area

Patient Outcomes
Patient will experience wound healing and no new skin breakdown.

Nursing Interventions	Rationales
Assess ulcer appearance to determine wound etiology (see Table 22-1).	Interventions for arterial and venous ulcers are different.
Confer with physician as to the most appropriate wound treatment.	Prescriptions may be needed for special supplies or medications.
If possible, instruct caregiver in wound care and dressing change.	Dressing changes are daily or more frequent.
Instruct patient/family in activity permitted and special positioning of involved extremity. For arterial PVD, position leg(s) below heart level (gravity assist). For venous PVD, elevate leg(s) to increase venous return and decrease edema. Walking and range-of-motion (ROM) exercises are helpful to most patients with PVD (exercise is contraindicated in thrombophlebitis).	These activities and positions can improve circulation and promote wound healing.
Consult with/refer to physical therapy, if appropriate.	Physical therapy can teach and/or supervise a ROM program and can suggest assistive devices for correct extremity positioning, especially for bedridden and wheelchair-bound patients.
Assess patient/caregiver's educational needs regarding proper nutrition.	Establishes level of need for nutrition counseling.
Instruct high-protein, low-cholesterol diet and the role of nutrition in wound healing.	Protein provides the body with amino acids to build new tissue. Reduced levels of serum cholesterol will help prevent further plaque build-up on vessel walls.
Assess patient/caregiver knowledge regarding measures to prevent skin breakdown and infection.	Establishes level of need for patient/caregiver education.

Nursing Interventions	Rationales
Instruct patient/caregiver in measures to promote circulation. Avoid pressure on bony prominences. Use properly fitted elastic stockings (TED hose) and duration and frequency according to physician instructions. Stockings should be removed at least once a day to bathe leg and check for redness or skin breakdown. Advise patient not to cross legs and avoid the use of circular garters (compressing vessels can restrict blood flow). Take care to avoid trauma or extreme temperature changes to legs, feet, and toes. Practice good foot care (see Table 22-2). Avoid standing for long periods. Follow individualized exercise program and practice appropriate leg positioning (as specified in previous intervention).	Decreased delivery of oxygenated blood and inefficient waste product removal produce an environment conducive to skin breakdown and infection. Each of these interventions either promotes arterial flow and venous return or prevents restricted blood flow. Temperature discrimination is often diminished.
Assess patient's ability to perform activities of daily living (ADLs).	Ulcers of the lower extremities can take a long time to heal, affecting patient's ability to care for himself or herself. Establishes level of help needed from family or appropriate community resource.
Obtain a referral for a home health aide (HHA) or homemaker, if appropriate. Consider a social services referral.	A HHA or homemaker can help patient with ADLs, foot care, and exercises. A social worker may be able to help caregiver locate and use respite care.

▶ NURSING DIAGNOSIS: *Knowledge Deficit*

Related To
- New diagnosis or newly prescribed treatment
- Lack of motivation
- Cognitive deficit
- Anxiety
- Depression

Defining Characteristics
- Unable to explain or demonstrate adequate knowledge about self-care skills that are important to maintaining health and preventing exacerbation of PVD

Patient Outcome
- Patient/caregiver will verbalize/demonstrate adequate knowledge regarding diet, exercise, smoking, foot care, and identifying PVD symptoms.

Nursing Interventions	Rationales
Assess patient/caregiver knowledge about high-fat foods; consider cultural and economic influences.	Establish level of need for instruction.
Instruct patient/caregiver in low-fat diet (30% calories from fat, 10% calories from saturated fats).	Hypercholesterolemia has been identified as a major risk factor in developing arteriosclerosis obliterans.
Instruct patient/caregiver on the effects of smoking on circulation; if appropriate, attempt a mutual goal-setting plan to stop smoking.	Smoking (nicotine) has been identified as a major risk factor in PVD.
Inspect the feet and assess quality of patient's daily care routine.	Establish level of need for instruction.
Instruct patient/caregiver about good foot care as appropriate (see Table 22-2).	Peripheral arterial and venous insufficiency can cause tissue damage. Good foot care can help reduce the risk of ulcers.
Assess patient's exercise level, including kind, frequency, and duration.	Establish level of need for intervention.
If appropriate, establish an exercise plan with patient/caregiver.	Research shows that exercise promotes significant improvement in circulation in patients with PVD; 30 min of walking or stationary bike riding three times per week is optimal.
Assess patient/caregiver knowledge about symptoms of PVD and when to report them to the physician.	Reporting new symptoms quickly will hasten medical/nursing interventions, which reduces the risk of PVD exacerbation.

DISCHARGE PLANNING/CONTINUITY OF CARE

- Stress the importance of reporting new symptoms quickly to the primary health care provider. Waiting may cost a limb.
- Provide anticipatory guidance and planning by making sure patient/family knows how to contact and use community resources for personal care, meals, and shopping. Help patient identify available family and friends when more help is needed.
- Reinforce the idea that PVD is a chronic disease, and as such, lifestyle changes (diet, exercise, special foot care, smoking cessation) need to be permanent changes.
- Make sure patient/caregiver has the home health agency phone number and can call you with questions even though he or she is not receiving any more visits.
- Refer patient/caregiver to a vascular disease support group, if appropriate. These are usually sponsored by a local hospital or clinic.

Table 22-1 • Distinguishing Arterial Ulcers from Venous Stasis Ulcers

Arterial Ulcer	Venous Ulcer
1. Patient reports severe pain	1. Patient reports mild to moderate pain
2. Ulcer is deep with well-defined margins	2. Ulcer is shallow with ragged edges
3. Interior is pale and contains necrotic tissue	3. Contains granulation tissue

From Herman (1986).

Table 22-2 • Proper Foot Care

- Use lotion to prevent drying and cracking skin.
- Bathe feet daily with warm water and mild soap and pat dry (do not rub).
- Inspect skin daily for breakdown, corns, and calluses.
- Clip toenail very careful to avoid skin trauma; may need to be done by caregiver, nurse, or physician in some circumstances.
- Keep feet warm with socks; to avoid burns, do not use hot water bottles or heating pads.
- Wear shoes that are comfortable and fit well. They should not be tight, especially over bony prominences.
- Know how to care for a break in the skin and when to call the nurse or physician.
- Avoid tight or restrictive clothing, hose, socks, garters—anything that diminishes peripheral blood flow.

From Herman (1986).

PLANS OF CARE TO REFERENCE

- Social Isolation
- Pain
- Nutrition
- Physical Activity/Exercise
- Patient and Family Rights—Self-Determination
- Skin Care

REFERENCES

Blank, C., & Irwin, G. (1990). Peripheral vascular disorders: Assessment and intervention. *Nursing Clinics of North America, 25*(4), 777–793.

Bright, L., & Georgi, S. (1992). PVD: Is it arterial or venous? *American Journal of Nursing, 92*(9), 34–43.

Herman, J. (1986). Nursing assessment and nursing diagnosis in patients with peripheral vascular disease. *Nursing Clinics of North America, 21*(2), 219–231.

Kerner, M. (1992). Noninvasive testing in the evaluation of peripheral vascular disease. *Orthopaedic Nursing, 11*(2), 50–54.

Kuhn, J., & McGovern, M. (1992). Peripheral vascular assessment of the elderly client. *Journal of Gerontological Nursing, 18*(12), 35–38.

Rudolphi, D. M. (1990). Duplex scanning. *American Journal of Nursing, 90*(4), 123–124.

Suddarth, D. S. (1991). *The Lippincott manual of nursing practice* (5th ed.). Philadelphia: J. B. Lippincott.

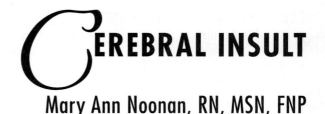

CEREBRAL INSULT

Mary Ann Noonan, RN, MSN, FNP

Cerebral insult is a complex term which involves more than a single process. It is a life-threatening situation which involves alterations in major physiological mechanisms which contribute to the brain's intricate function. Physiologically, increased intracranial pressure or cerebral edema occur as a result of direct or indirect injury to the brain's tissue. In brain edema, the brain tissue water content increases, which results in an increase in one of the three volumes of the brain [tissue, vascular, or cerebrospinal fluid (CSF)]. The Monro-Kellie hypothesis states that if one volume of the brain increases, the other volumes must decrease, or increased intracranial pressure occurs. Because the brain is confined in a nondistensible vault, the brain has limited space to expand. Therefore, cerebral swelling can cause deleterious effects.

ETIOLOGIES
- Cerebrovascular causes include either hemorrhage (intracerebral, aneurysm) or ischemia (thrombus or embolus). Cerebrovascular accident (CVA) is the third leading cause of death in the United States.
- Head injuries result from mild to extensive brain tissue damage (epidural and subdural hematoma) as a result of mechanical force causing various degrees of injuries. Head injuries account for 90% of nervous system trauma.
- Space-occupying lesions (benign or malignant intracranial tumors) within the brain result in increased intercranial pressure with symptoms dependent upon location in the brain and rate of growth.
- Infectious processes (meningitis) from viral, bacterial, or fungal organisms cause cerebral edema.
- Metabolic causes of cerebral edema are typically secondary to cardiac and renal problems.

CLINICAL MANIFESTATIONS (CHRONIC PHASE)
- Language deficits
  - aphasia
  - dysphasia (expressive, receptive, global)

- Motor deficits
  - spasticity
  - hemiplegia
  - paraplegia
  - monoplegia
  - dysphagia
  - seizures
- Sensory deficits
  - paresis
  - diminished response to sensation
  - decreased proprioception
  - decreased perception to self and others
- Bowel/bladder dysfunction
  - urinary retention/incontinence
  - fecal retention/incontinence
- Cognitive/intellectual/emotional/personality deficits
- Psychosocial deficits

CLINICAL DIAGNOSTIC FINDINGS (ACUTE PHASE)
- Blood gases: hypoxia or hypercapnia
- Skull x-ray if head injury will determine skull fracture
- Cerebral angiogram to determine cerebrovascular problem
- Computerized tomography (CT) scan, magnetic resonance imaging (MRI) definitive for tumor and/or head injury
- Lumbar puncture: bloody if bleed is subarachnoid space; intracranial pressure (ICP) elevated; protein found in CSF in tumor and infections; lumbar puncture (LP) contraindicated in some situations (e.g., some types of brain tumor, increased intracranial pressure)

▶ NURSING DIAGNOSIS: *Impaired Physical Mobility*
Related To residual physical deficits

Defining Characteristics
- Spasticity
- Paralysis
- Paresis
- Inability to move extremity
- Ataxia
- Aphasia
- Dysphasia
- Fatigue
- Inability to perform activities of daily living (ADLs)
- Change in bowel and bladder function

Patient Outcomes
Patient will:
- achieve maximum mobility and level of function as defined by limitation.
- increase ability to perform range-of-motion (ROM) and motor functions.

- participate in self-care activities (ADLs).
- identify available support systems.

Nursing Interventions	Rationales
Establish trust relationship.	Trust is basic to establish therapeutic interpersonal relationship.
Evaluate home on accessibility of stairs, entrances, doors, railings, furniture. (See Safety chapter.)	A safe and easy accessible environment promotes patient safety (preventing falls) and mobility.
Continually assess physical ability, deficits, and ADLs. Neurological assessment includes assessing (1) level of consciousness; (2) ability to move, transfer, and walk; and (3) ability to dress, feed, and toilet self.	This provides information to change the plan of care and refer for additional services, if necessary. It also provides feedback for patient and family.
Evaluate patient and caregiver in ADLs. If appropriate, teach patient and caregiver transfer techniques using good body mechanics. Move the patient from the stronger side. Make referrals as appropriate (PT, OT, home health aide). Reinforce therapy regimen.	Including additional therapies will assist patient to recover quicker.
Assess ability to swallow and speak. Refer to speech therapy as appropriate.	Speech therapy can teach muscle-strengthening exercises to assist in speech and swallowing.
If hemiplegia, approach patient on strong side. If patient has cognitive deficits, state one concept at a time. Speak slowly and clearly.	Patients with hemiplegia have limited peripheral vision on their affected side. Some patients with cerebral insults will have difficulty processing information. Speaking slowly and clearly will help them process information better.
Assess and evaluate bladder and bowel program. (See Spinal Cord Injury chapter.)	Urinary retention/incontinence and fecal constipation/incontinence frequently occur because of bladder flaccidity or hypertonicity and decreased gastrointestinal motility and lack of sphincter control.

Nursing Interventions	Rationales
Involve family in care as much as possible.	Significant other involvement is a means of support to patient, as well as permitting them to be involved in care.

▶ NURSING DIAGNOSIS: *Altered Family Processes*

Related To stroke deficits dependency and role changes within family

Defining Characteristics
- Lack of leisure and social activity
- Powerlessness
- Fear of unknown
- Role change
- Altered family relationships
- Stress
- Loss of independence
- Depression

Patient Outcomes
Patient/family will:
- communicate needs purposefully.
- express fears and concerns.
- participate in social/leisure time activities.
- identify causes of stress and ways to cope with it.
- discuss role changes within the family.

Nursing Interventions	Rationales
Facilitate and encourage patient and family to discuss frustrations, anxieties, fears, anger, and concerns.	Give patient/family permission to vent and reassure that it is normal to have those feelings. Expressing concerns promotes effective coping.
Help patient/family identify stressors by allowing them to ventilate their concerns.	Identifying problems is the best way to begin planning interventions.
Discuss concerns and help patient and family problem solve.	Problems are best solved by parties involved.
Assist patient/family in preparing for role changes within the family.	Roles are established and based on functions and activities within the family.

Nursing Interventions	Rationales
Refer patient/family to support systems (individual, family counseling, financial services, respite services).	Other professionals may help better define roles and cope with financial burdens and stressors.
Involve patient/family in deciding leisure time activities.	Increases patient and family's sense of control.

▶ NURSING DIAGNOSIS: *Knowledge Deficit*

Related To physical disability and management of care

Defining Characteristics
- Lack of knowledge and understanding of diagnosis
- Family lacks understanding of diagnosis and therapy
- Decreased memory, learning
- Decreased attention span
- Anger
- Emotional labile/flat affect
- Cries easily
- Apathy
- Frustration
- Withdrawal
- Impatience

Patient Outcomes
- Patient and family will verbalize understanding of diagnosis, therapies, and medications.
- Patient and family will problem solve and make decisions together.

Nursing Interventions	Rationales
Determine patient/family's readiness for learning by assessing their interest and motivation.	Readiness is necessary for learning to take place.
Allow sufficient time for questions.	Evaluating knowledge deficits must be determined before teaching begins.
Provide explanation to patient/family in areas of deficits (diagnosis, therapies, medications, residual deficits).	Providing information will decrease stress.

Nursing Interventions	Rationales
Teach patient/family about diagnosis (whatever the cause of the cerebral injury) and complications. Notify physician if the following occurs: (1) signs of increased intracranial pressure, including increased drowsiness/lethargy, persistent headache, or vision problems; (2) mobility and sensation decrease; (3) difficulty in eating or swallowing; (4) fever if undetermined; (5) seizures and; (6) unusual bleeding or drainage.	Identifying complications early minimizes trauma.
Teach patient/family basic health care needs, including: (1) personal hygiene and skin care (see Personal Hygiene and Skin Care chapters); (2) avoiding pressure on bony prominences to avoid skin breakdown (no more than 2 h in one position); and (3) establishing routine for toileting every 2–3 h (see Spinal Injury and Incontinence chapters).	Skin breakdown occurs with decreased mobility and irritation.
Reinforce good nutrition. Eat balanced diet high in protein and increase bulk in diet. Balance carbohydrate; decrease fat intake. Increase fluid intake.	Metabolic requirements have decreased. Bulk and fluid decrease potential for constipation, formation of renal stones, and urinary tract infections. Protein assists in tissue replacement and healing.
Allow patient/significant other to discuss sexuality issues. (See Human Sexuality chapter.)	Sexuality is often a difficult issue to discuss but is a very real problem.

DISCHARGE PLANNING/CONTINUITY OF CARE

- Ensure patient has phone number for equipment supplier and/or has supportive occupational and physical therapy supplies available.
- Refer family and patient to local support groups.
- Suggest respite services for family.
- Ensure patient and family has a plan for emergencies. Call physician if there are changes in condition or 911 for severe changes.

OTHER PLANS OF CARE TO REFERENCE
- Spinal Cord Injury
- Skin Care
- Incontinence
- Grief/Loss
- Altered Mental Status
- Caregiver Burden
- Human Sexuality
- Nutrition
- Personal Hygiene
- Safety

BIBLIOGRAPHY

Bronstein, K., Popovich, J., & Stewart-Amidei, C. (1991). *Promoting stroke recovery: A research based approach for nurses.* Chicago: Mosby.

Gulanick, M., Klopp, A., Galanes, S., Gradishar, D., & Puzas, M. (1994). *Nursing care plans: Nursing diagnoses and intervention* (3rd ed.). Chicago: Mosby.

Hickey, J. (1992). *The clinical practice of neurological and neurosurgical nursing* (3rd ed.). Philadelphia: J. B. Lippincott.

Matassarin-Jacobs, E. (1994). *Saunders review for nclex-rn* (2nd ed.). Philadelphia: W. B. Saunders.

S PINAL CORD INJURY: PARAPLEGIA AND QUADRIPLEGIA

Sally Schnell, RN, MSN, CNRN

S pinal cord injuries (SCIs) interrupt the passage of neural impulses. Complete disruption renders the patient paralyzed and without sensation below the injury. Incomplete SCI may leave the patient with some movement and/or sensation although function may not be retained. Refer to Table 24-1 for spinal cord segments and corresponding function. The role of the nurse caring for a SCI patient in the community depends on the patient's abilities and needs. A paraplegic patient may need episodic care to heal a decubitus or because of an unrelated illness such as coronary artery disease. A quadriplegic will probably need ongoing care by nurses for assessment and skilled interventions and nursing assistants for positioning, activities of daily living (ADLs), and homemaking assistance.

ETIOLOGIES
- Motor vehicle accidents
- Falls
- Diving and sporting accidents
- Violence
- Neoplasms

CLINICAL MANIFESTATIONS
- Mobility
  - loss of all or part of motor function below the level of injury
  - loss of all or part of sensory function below the level of injury
- Respiratory function
  - need for ventilatory support (C4 and above)
  - impaired cough and deep breathing, increased use of accessory muscles (T6 and above)
  - impaired cough and expiration (T12 and above)

- Bowel/bladder
  - bowel and bladder incontinence
  - bladder distention
  - frequent infections or loss of kidney function
  - need for bowel management program
- Skin breakdown/decubiti
- Disturbance in self-concept
  - changes in body image; patient may ignore personal hygiene or refuse to get dressed
  - loss of control; patient may attempt to manipulate caregivers in order to exert some control
  - fear of sexual dysfunction
  - increased reliance on others
- Social isolation
  - changes in lifestyle
  - loss of ability to work (at least temporarily)
  - depression; patient may be uncooperative with therapists and caregivers
  - potential for alcohol/substance abuse
  - difficulty with transportation and accessibility

CLINICAL/DIAGNOSTIC FINDINGS

Radiographic
- x-ray and computerized tomography (CT) for detecting bony abnormality
- magnetic resonance imaging (MRI) for detecting soft tissue abnormality

Physical exam
- absence of deep-tendon reflexes
- flaccidity or spasticity below injury

Screening for complications due to SCI
- urodynamic testing to establish baseline bladder function and to evaluate any changes in function; neurogenic bladder is usual finding
- intravenous pyelography (IVP) or renal ultrasound to evaluate for reflux of urine into kidney; normal ureter and kidney function should be found

▶ NURSING DIAGNOSIS: *Potential Complication—Autonomic Dysreflexia*

Related To bowel distention, bladder distention, urinary tract infection (UTI), decubiti, or invasive procedures below the level of the injury

Defining Characteristics

Above the lesion
- pounding headache
- flushing
- diaphoresis
- nasal congestion
- bradycardia
- vasodilation

Below the lesion
- gooseflesh
- vasoconstriction
- pale, cool skin

Patient Outcomes
- Patient will be free of or quickly relieved of autonomic dysreflexia (AD).

Nursing Interventions	Rationales
Monitor blood pressure every 5 min, if possible.	Blood pressure can elevate to dangerous levels.
Remove noxious stimuli without further irritation.	Removes cause of AD.
Place the patient in the sitting position.	Take advantage of orthostatic hypotension.
Indwelling catheters should be checked for patency and changed if necessary. If no indwelling catheter is present, the patient should be catheterized to empty the bladder. If personnel are available, monitor blood pressure during catheterization.	Relieves bladder and may remove the stimuli.
A digital exam should be done for rectal impaction. If stool is present, then anesthetic ointment should be applied to the rectum before attempting disimpaction. If personnel are available, monitor blood pressure during disimpaction.	Relieves disimpaction and removes the stimuli.
If no stimulus is identified or if condition cannot be quickly corrected, the patient may need to be transported to the emergency room for antihypertensive treatment.	Elevated blood pressure can be a life-threatening problem.
Patients should wear a bracelet identifying their potential for AD and should be taught how to direct caregivers in treatment.	Education can prevent or detect the problem early.

Clinical Clip

Autonomic Dysreflexia

Autonomic dysreflexia is a life-threatening complication of SCI, affecting patients with SCI above the T6 level. Autonomic dysreflexia is the inability of nerve impulses to descend past the level of the SCI and restore the autonomic nervous system equilibrium.

A noxious stimuli activates the sympathetic nervous system. Counterbalancing impulses from the parasympathetic system cannot descend past the cord lesion to restore the equilibrium. Blood pressure may elevate to the point of causing seizures, cerebrovascular accident (CVA), or death.

▶ **NURSING DIAGNOSIS:** *Impaired Physical Mobility*

Related To interrupted innervation

Defining Characteristics
- Lack of voluntary movement and sensation below level of injury
- Flaccidity or spasticity
- Inability to move the body below the level of injury

Patient Outcomes
The patient will exhibit the ability to compensate for altered mobility, as evidenced by:
- being able to safely transfer from bed to wheelchair to toilet (paraplegia) or to direct a caregiver in safe transfer (quadriplegia).
- utilizing wheelchair and adapted vehicle to move about.
- performing ADLs with adaptive devices and techniques (paraplegia) or directing performance of ADLs (quadriplegia).

Nursing Interventions	Rationales
Assess ability to safely perform or direct transfers using assistive devices.	Establishes safety level of present techniques.
Provide patient education if transfers are performed in an unsafe manner or positioning increases the potential for skin breakdown. Refer to physical therapy (PT) to build muscle strength and teach transfer techniques, if necessary.	Referral to PT for instruction in transfers can improve patient safety and muscle strength. Patient education regarding skin breakdown related to positioning may prevent complications related to decubiti.

Nursing Interventions	Rationales
Assess independence in using wheelchair and vehicle if applicable. If patient does not have maximum mobility, refer to PT for discussing wheelchair options and occupational therapy (OT) for driving options.	This establishes whether patient has maximum mobility. A different wheelchair and/or vehicle modification may be needed.
Assess ability to perform ADLs. Teach proper skin care and care of the urinary drainage system. Instruct caregivers that the time spent performing ADLs is an excellent opportunity to help the patient establish a preventive care routine.	This establishes amount of assistance needed so that caregivers with appropriate skills can be utilized and provides baseline for monitoring changes. Provides foundation for teaching energy and time-saving techniques. Regular skin and urinary drainage system inspection can prevent many complications.

▶ **NURSING DIAGNOSIS:** *Ineffective Airway Clearance*

Related To loss of innervation to various respiratory muscles

Defining Characteristics
• Inability to independently clear airway effectively
• Reliance on ventilatory support (C4 and above)

Patient Outcomes
Patient will have adequate respiratory function, as evidenced by:
• patient airway.
• lungs clear to auscultation.
• no signs of respiratory infection.

Nursing Interventions	Rationales
Auscultate lungs and assess respiratory patterns.	Establishes baseline for comparison. Determines need for suctioning or assisted cough and deep breathing.
Teach signs and symptoms of respiratory infection and to call health	Catching and treating respiratory infections early will quicken

Nursing Interventions	Rationales
care provider if they occur. Teach use of incentive spirometry. Perform chest PT, if ordered or necessary.	recovery. Incentive spirometry can decrease incidence of respiratory infections.
Assess for signs of respiratory infection. If necessary, suction or assist with medicated respiratory treatments or oral medications per physician order.	Determines need for further intervention. Patients may require more frequent suctioning and possibly medicated respiratory treatments to help treat infection. Aggressive pulmonary toilet may prevent the need for hospitalization.
Push fluid by mouth unless contraindicated.	Increases mucus viscosity.

▶ **NURSING DIAGNOSIS:** *Altered Bowel Elimination*

Related To decreased gastrointestinal (GI) reflexes and impaired innervation

Defining Characteristics
• Constipation
• Incontinent bowel movements

Patient Outcomes
Patient will be continent of stool, as evidenced by regular, scheduled bowel evacuation.

Nursing Interventions	Rationales
Assess patient satisfaction with current bowel function and bowel care regimen. Encourage patient to voice concerns and expectations.	Establishes baseline of bowel function. Provides teaching opportunity regarding the changes in bowel function caused by SCI. Encouraging patients to voice concerns and expectations helps them take an active part in planning a regimen.
Modify bowel care regimen as needed to fit patient and caregiver's ability and time frames. Keep regular bowel schedule. Suppository insertion and/or digital rectal stimulation	Scheduling bowel care so as not to interfere with vocational, educational, or social pursuits fosters a more independent and normal lifestyle.

Nursing Interventions	Rationales
may be performed independently by paraplegics. Quadriplegics will need assistance.	
Assess nutritional intake. Encourage drinking 3 L of fluid daily and eating a fiber-rich diet. Refer to dietician as appropriate. Discourage overeating.	Assessment provides foundation for patient education. High-fiber and high-fluid diets decrease probability of constipation. Weight gain can negatively impact functional ability.
Encourage the patient to discuss the psychosocial impact of the present bowel management and any episodes of incontinence.	Bowel incontinence, or fear thereof, is a major deterrent to an SCI patient participating in activities outside the home. The nurse recognizing this can foster open discussion and problem solving.
Encourage patient to problem solve regarding potential incontinent episodes. Suggest that patient keep a change of clothes and disposable washcloths in the vehicle.	Promotes independence and positive self-concept. Also promotes patient cooperation with bowel program and acceptance of more responsibility for bowel care.
Encourage patient and caregiver (if also the patient's sexual partner) to discuss the impact of performing bowel care on their personal relationship. Suggest having an outside caregiver perform this portion of the patient's care.	Bowel care by the partner may cause reduced feelings of intimacy and sexual desire in both the patient and partner. Patient and partner may be reluctant to discuss their feelings and will need reassurance that this is a common occurrence. Having another person perform this task may help the patient and partner to maintain their intimate relationship.

▶ NURSING DIAGNOSIS: *Altered Urinary Elimination*

Related To loss of voluntary urination and bladder reflexes

Defining Characteristics
• Urinary incontinence and/or retention
• Use of assistive devices for control of urination

Patient Outcomes
• Patient will be continent of urine.

Nursing Interventions	Rationales
Assess patient's current urinary management program.	Establishes efficacy of and satisfaction with current bladder management. Provides opportunity for teaching regarding changes in bladder function and potential complications.
Modify management program as needed and teach patient how to control incontinence. Some patients can use the crede maneuver to empty the bladder. Males with reflex emptying may use an external catheter and will need to be taught to apply it correctly to maintain skin integrity and prevent leaks. Females with reflex emptying may use intermittent or continuous catheterization, depending on dexterity, lifestyle, and frequency of voiding. Males and females with retention will require intermittent or continuous catheterization. Paraplegics and some male quadriplegics can be taught to use clean technique for intermittent catheterization. Due to truncal imbalance, it is difficult for female quadriplegics to perform self-catheterization. Women with limited use of their hands will require intermittent catheterization by a caregiver or an indwelling catheter. They should be taught to direct someone through the catheterization process.	Bladder management may need to be modified as patient lifestyle and abilities change. Controlling bladder care increases sense of self-esteem and control.
Assess fluid intake and compare it to output. Encourage patient to drink 3 L per day.	Establishes baseline. Adequate fluid intake dramatically reduces the incidence of UTI and renal calculi. Patients may be reluctant to consume the recommended 3 L per day due to increased need for catheterization or emptying of leg bag.
Assess for symptoms of UTI, including foul-smelling or cloudy urine,	Rapidly recognizing and treating infection reduce the risk of

Nursing Interventions	Rationales
large amounts of sediment in urine, and fever.	ascending infection and damaging the kidneys. Encourage patient to have urological follow-up yearly.
Assess psychosocial impact of present bladder management and any episodes of incontinence. Encourage patient to discuss concerns regarding past or potential problems. If an indwelling catheter is present, encourage the patient to decide whether to leave it in during intercourse or to remove it and reinsert it afterward.	Promotes problem solving, particularly with the sexual partner regarding the possibility of incontinence and sexual activity.

► NURSING DIAGNOSIS: *Disturbance in Self-Concept*
Related To changes in physical functioning of the body

Defining Characteristics
- Changes in self-perception
- Loss of control and increased reliance on others
- Fear of decreased sexual attractiveness and sexual dysfunction

Patient Outcomes
Patient will incorporate an adjusted self-concept into daily life, as evidenced by:
- discussing abilities and disabilities.
- setting and following through on realistic goals.
- accepting needed assistance.

Nursing Interventions	Rationales
Encourage patient to describe how he or she perceives self and the future. Refer to peer support groups and/or social worker counseling if necessary.	Provides insight into patient's perception and promotes open discussion of patient's current and future capabilities. Referrals may help promote discussion.
Assist patient in setting and following through on goals related to managing the physical aspects of SCI. Refer for vocational or	The nurse is in the unique position of knowing the patient's physical and emotional capabilities, being able to help the patient achieve the

Nursing Interventions	Rationales
educational assistance, transportation needs, and funding if necessary.	goals he or she establishes, and referring appropriately.
Assist the patient in adapting to the fact that lifestyle changes are inevitable and that some level of assistance will be needed to maintain maximum participation in life.	Most patients are young, previously healthy individuals. It is very difficult for them to have to rely on another individual for such basic functions as elimination and dressing. Accepting needed assistance while maintaining maximum independence is a sign of successful adjustment to SCI and the accompanying self-concept changes.

DISCHARGE PLANNING/CONTINUITY OF CARE
- Emphasize the need for regular health maintenance visits with a primary health care provider who is familiar with the ongoing effects of SCI.
- Periodically review patient and caregiver's physical and emotional ability to perform care.
- Refer to peer support groups, personal and family counseling, and substance abuse groups as appropriate.

Table 24-1 • Spinal Cord Segments and Corresponding Functions

C1–C3	Limited head control
C4	Diaphragmatic breathing, should shrug
C5	Shoulder abduction, partial elbow flexion
C6	Wrist extension, elbow flexion
C7	Elbow extension, finger extension
C8	Finger flexion
T1	Finger abduction and adduction
T2–T12	Deeper inhalation
T6–T12	Forceful exhalation, increased trunk stability
L1–L2	Hip flexion
L2–L3	Hip adduction
L3–L4	Knee extension
L4–L5	Ankle extension
L5	Great toe extension
S1	Plantar flexion, knee flexion
S1–S2	Toe flexion
S2–S4	Elimination

OTHER PLANS OF CARE TO REFERENCE

- Skin Care
- Grief/Loss
- Human Sexuality
- Social Isolation
- Caregiver Burden
- Substance Abuse

BIBLIOGRAPHY

Boss, B. J. (1993). The neurophysiological basis of learning: Attention and memory implications for SCI nurses. *SCI Nursing, 10*(4), 121–129.

Boss, B. J. (1994). The neurophysiological basis of learning, Part 2: Concept formation/abstraction, reasoning and executive functions: Implications for SCI nurses. *SCI Nursing, 11*(1), 3–6.

Gerhart, K. A. (1993). *Aging with spinal cord injury.* New York: Demos.

Gerhart, K. A., Bergstrom, E., Charlifue, S. W., Menter, R. R., & Whiteneck, G. G. (1993). Long-term spinal cord injury: Functional change over time. *Archives of Physical Medicine and Rehabilitation, 74*(10), 1030–1034.

Hickey, J. V. (1992). *The clinical practice of neurological and neuro-surgical nursing.* Philadelphia: Lippincott.

Miller, M. D., Steele, N. F., Nadell, J. M., Tilton, A. H., & Gates, A. J. (1993). Ventilator-assisted youth: Appraisal and nursing care. *Journal of Neuroscience Nursing, 25*(5), 287–295.

Partridge, C. (1994). Spinal cord injuries: Aspects of psychological care. *British Journal of Nursing, 3*(1), 12–14.

Tate, D. G., Maynard, F., & Forchheimer, M. (1993). Predictors of psychologic distress one year after spinal cord injury. *American Journal of Physical Medicine and Rehabilitation, 72*(5), 272–275.

White, M. J., Rintala, D. H., Hart, K. A., & Fuhrer, M. J. (1993). Sexual activities, concerns and interests of women with spinal cord injury living in the community. *American Journal of Physical Medicine and Rehabilitation, 72*(6), 372–378.

$\mathcal{P}$ARKINSON'S DISEASE

Judith A. Scully, RNC, MSN

$\mathbf{P}$arkinson's disease (PD) is a progressive disorder of the central nervous system associated with damage primarily to two areas of the brain, the substantia nigra and the striatum. The pigmented neurons in the substantia nigra degenerate and slowly decrease dopamine secretion. Deficiencies in dopamine modify both body movement and muscle tone. The onset is insidious and the progression is gradual, marked by three major sets of symptoms: tremors, rigidity, and bradycardia.

The nurse's overall role is to support individual and family coping, educate patient and family in managing the disease, monitor for complications, and make appropriate referrals.

Clinical Clip

Parkinson's disease affects between one half million to one and one half million men and women in the United States today. Although the average age of onset is 60 years of age, early onset, defined as occurring before the age of 40, is increasing and affects 5% of the PD population. Initial clinical symptoms of PD are not apparent until the deficiency is sufficiently severe (80% loss of substantia nigra pigmented cells and 80% loss of striatum dopamine content) (Paulson, 1994).

ETIOLOGIES

The causes of PD are unknown. Current theories regarding the etiologies of PD include:

- Chemical factors: Substances shown to produce PD symptoms include manganese carbon monoxide, cyanide, and carbon disulfide. Exposure to several industrial toxins including pesticides, carbon monoxide, and manganese poisoning has also been shown to produce parkinsonian symptoms.

180

- Drug-induced factors: Recently, several young people developed PD-like symptoms after using an illegal drug known as MPTP (methylphenyl tetrahydropyridine), a synthetic heroine converted to a toxin called MPP, which is taken up by brain cells in the substantia nigra where it damages the cells. Drug-induced parkinsonian syndromes also are associated with phenothiazine, serpasil, and haloperidol.
- Postencephalitic parkinsonism: PD-like symptoms were observed in many patients following the 1919–1926 worldwide epidemic of encephalitis.

CLINICAL MANIFESTATIONS
- Rigidity: stiffness and soreness; clog-wheel movements
- Tremors: trembling limbs, lips, tongue, abdomen, and/or chest, tremors increasing with stress, decreasing with purposeful movement, and absent during sleep
- Bradykinesia: slowness of bodily movements (beginning/executing movements); diminished movements such as eye blinking, "masklike" face, swinging the arms when walking, and expressive hand gesturing while talking

Other signs and symptoms
- depression
- postural deformity
- oily skin
- dysarthria with soft, low monotone voice
- constipation
- forced eyelid closure
- drooling
- difficulty with swallowing
- difficultly in voiding
- dizziness
- weight loss
- change in handwriting
- sleep disturbances
- breathing problem
- sexual problems
- masklike expressionless face
- increased perspiration
- muscle cramps
- festinating gait (shuffling, propulsive)

CLINICAL/DIAGNOSTIC FINDINGS
- Neurological examination shows signs and symptoms.
- Computerized tomography (CT) and magnetic resonance imaging (MRI) scans rule out other causes of symptoms

▶ NURSING DIAGNOSIS: *Altered Gastrointestinal Function*

Related To disease process, anti-Parkinson's medications, inadequate fluid/bulk intake, immobility

Defining Characteristics
- Accumulation of saliva
- Difficulty in swallowing
- Nausea
- Constipation/defacatory dysfunction

Patient Outcomes
Patient will:
- report decreasing episodes of drooling and nausea/vomiting.
- eat slowly without choking.
- report regular bowel patterns.
- exercise on a regular basis.

Nursing Interventions	Rationales
Assess patient's ability to swallow/chew.	The tongue often moves more slowly, causing problems swallowing. Decreased muscle function for chewing and swallowing prolongs meal time.
Review strategies to minimize aspiration: 1. Allow adequate time for eating. 2. Chew food thoroughly. 3. Cut food into small pieces. 4. Bend head forward while swallowing.	Muscle incoordination and decreased gag reflex increase the risk for aspiration.
Encourage frequent small meals.	Parkinson's disease delays stomach emptying, causing feelings of fullness and nausea/vomiting. Small meals decrease feelings of fullness/nausea.
Instruct patient to chew gum or hard candy throughout the day.	Patients with PD produce less saliva and have problems swallowing. Therefore, saliva accumulates and PD patients drool. Chewing gum or sucking on hard candy reduces saliva and encourages patients to consciously swallow. Because fluids are more difficult to swallow, they are more likely to drool out the fluid.
Assess elimination patterns.	Neuromuscular impairment slows colon motility. Between 30 and 50% of patients with PD suffer from delayed fecal movement through the colon, while 67% of patients have difficulty in evacuating fecal material.

Nursing Interventions	Rationales
Instruct patient/family to increase fiber intake (fiber-rich foods include bran, prunes) and increase fluid intake to eight (8-oz) glasses per day, discourage using laxatives, and encourage using stool softeners and regular evacuation times, eating regular meals, and maintaining a daily physical exercise program.	High-fiber diets, increased fluid intake, and stool softeners promote fecal movement through the colon, causing satisfactory bowel elimination.

▶ NURSING DIAGNOSIS: *Knowledge Deficit*

Related To
- Inadequate knowledge base regarding diagnosis, therapy, and resources
- New diagnosis for patient/family

Defining Characteristics
- Verbalization by patient/family of lack of understanding regarding diagnosis, therapy, and resources for PD

Patient Outcomes
Patient will:
- verbalize understanding of the disease process, effects, and progression.
- verbalize understanding and comply with the PD medication regimen (purpose, administration schedule, side and interaction effects of medications, and the nutritional restrictions/modifications associated with anti-Parkinson's medications).
- seek necessary support/resources.

Nursing Interventions	Rationales
Assess level of understanding of PD process and progression.	Knowledge of the disease process may help patient/family to cope with PD and understand the basis for particular medical treatments.
Monitor effects and educate patient/family on prescribed medication regimen.	The choice of medications is adapted to the individual patient. Because PD may become progressively worse and the symptoms more severe, medication dosages often need to be reevaluated.

Nursing Interventions	Rationales
	Medications may also need to be adjusted when side effects occur.
Instruct patient/family on the role of dietary restrictions for maximum effect of anti-Parkinson's drugs, particularly levodopa: (1) avoid hot spicy foods to decrease dyskinesia, (2) do not take on an empty stomach, (3) avoid high-protein meals in the morning, and (4) eat most of the protein during evening meal.	No specific diet is recommended for PD patients. Certain foods, however, may cause changes in PD symptoms or undesirable gastrointestinal (GI) effects. Protein-rich meals delay the absorption of levodopa.
Refer patient/family to local PD support group, to physical therapists for assistive devices/ equipment, and to home support services.	Parkinson's disease organizations distribute literature for patients on special needs for activities of daily living (ADLs). Support groups provide patient/family opportunities to discuss fears and concerns with others who are experiencing similar problems. As disease progresses, patient/family may require a home health aide to assist in ADLs or to relieve caregiver stress. (See also Caregiver Burden/Stress.)
Listen to patient/family's feelings regarding their concerns about PD; accept their validity.	Allowing patient/family to express their feelings of disappointment and frustration with the disease process helps to identify underlying anxieties about PD, facilitates the loss of patient's present functional abilities, and helps the patient to recognize potential new roles.

▶ NURSING DIAGNOSIS: *Injury*

Related To impaired physical mobility, tremors, weakness

Defining Characteristics
- Gait abnormalities: balancing difficulties, shuffling, slowness, limping
- Muscle rigidity
- Weakness

Patient Outcomes

Patient will:

- be free of accidental injuries.
- function as independently as possible.
- understand needed activity limitations.
- maneuver in home within physical limitations.
- employ safety measures in home to minimize injuries.
- illustrate use of adaptive devices.

Nursing Interventions	Rationales
Assess patient's physical/mental status, motor function, and level of independence in ambulation.	A thorough health history/physical assessment identifies potential and actual risk factors that cause injury. Patients with PD are more susceptible to falls and injuries due to muscle rigidity that limits mobility. Initiating movement often causes a propulsion when walking, creating further opportunities for injury.
Assess home environment for potential/actual safety hazards: (1) encourage patient/family to identify hazards and modify home, (2) remove excess furniture, (3) remove throw rugs, (4) encourage using solid shoes instead of slippers, (5) ensure adequate lighting, and (6) install safety devices (hand rails, raised toilet seat).	Ensuring a safe home environment decreases opportunities for falls/accidents. Use of adaptive devices often improves patient's mobility and independence, enhancing control over the physical environment (see Safety Hazards: Home Safety).
Encourage patient to engage in a daily exercise routine; instruct patient in active/passive range of motion (ROM); refer to physical therapist for assistance with gait training.	Regular exercise is an important part of PD treatment in helping to prevent muscle contracture/atrophy and in increasing a patient's well-being and self-esteem. Physical therapists can evaluate muscle strength and joint mobility and individualize an exercise program. If patients fall easily, exercise should be supervised.

▶ NURSING DIAGNOSIS: *Self-Care Deficit (Feeding, Bathing, Toileting, Dressing)*

Related To impaired motor ability, rigidity caused by disease process

Defining Characteristics
- Slowness and difficulty in performing ADLs
- Inability to complete ADLs

Patient Outcomes
Patient will:
- achieve the highest level of function in performing ADLs as is possible.
- modify and perform self-care tasks.
- understand the effects of the disease process on ADLs.

Nursing Interventions	Rationales
Assess patient's abilities in performing ADLs.	Rigidity, tremors, and slow movement significantly alter a patient's ability to function independently in basic needs of daily living.
Teach alternative techniques for performing tasks, including using adaptive devices to assist in ADLs.	Encouraging self-care activities and promoting functional independence foster self-reliance and decrease helplessness and isolation. Adaptive equipment will maximize patient's independence in performing ADLs (e.g., elastic thread or special buttoning devices to ease buttoning; Velcro closures in place of zippers; cups and dishes with suction cups).
Encourage caregiver to provide independence in ADLs according to patient's abilities.	Performing ADLs independently enhances self-esteem. Because PD patients' movements are slow, caregivers must provide adequate time for patients to complete self-care activities and to reduce patient's frustration (see Self-Esteem Deficit).

DISCHARGE PLANNING/CONTINUITY OF CARE
- Refer patient and family to local support groups.
- Refer to national organizations that provide information and assistance.
- Refer to Meals on Wheels, if necessary.

OTHER PLANS OF CARE TO REFERENCE
- Residence Deficit

REFERENCES/BIBLIOGRAPHY

Duvoisin, R. C. (1991). *Parkinson's disease: A guide for patient and family.* New York: Raven.

Koller, W. C. (1993). In *Epidemiology of Parkinson's disease* (pp. 1–4). The American Parkinson's Disease Association.

McFarland, G. K., McFarlane, E. A. (1993). *Nursing diagnosis and intervention: Planning for patient care.* St. Louis: Mosby.

Paulson, G. W. (1994). Management of the patient with newly-diagnosed Parkinson's disease. *Parkinson's report, 15*(4), 1–6.

Pfeiffer, R. F. (1993). *Gastrointestinal dysfunction in parkinson disease.* United Parkinson's Foundation.

Taylor, J. W., & Sallenger, S. (1980). *Neurological dysfunctions and nursing intervention.* New York: McGraw-Hill.

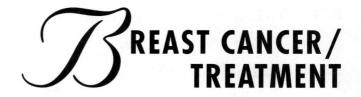

REAST CANCER/ TREATMENT

Lazelle Emminizer Benefield, PhD, RN

Breast cancer is defined as a malignant tumor within the breast. Two treatment options exist for breast cancer. The first option, breast conservation treatment, is an excision of the primary breast tumor and adjacent breast tissue. This includes lumpectomy, partial mastectomy, and segmental mastectomy. A second option is "modified radical mastectomy (or total mastectomy, axillary dissection, and preservation of the pectoralis major muscle), with or without immediate reconstruction" (Kinne, 1991). Chemotherapy, radiation treatment, and/or hormone manipulation therapy also may be included as a component of these treatment options.

Metastases may affect any body tissue. Breast cancer may spread to the axillary lymph nodes, then to the lungs, liver, bone, and/or brain. Breast self-exam, breast examination by health care providers, and mammography are valuable methods to screen for early cancer. In particular, baseline mammograms may detect cancers that are not found during palpation of breast tissue. Detecting and treating cancer early offer a better long-term prognosis.

Patients with breast cancer have varied needs that can best be met through interdisciplinary efforts of health care providers, family, and community supports. The nurse's role is to provide support to the patient and family in resuming or maintaining self-care, and the nurse facilitates the patient's sense of control over decisions regarding current and future treatment options.

Clinical Clip

Breast cancer is the most common type of cancer among American women. Thirty percent of all cancers in women are of the breast; one in nine women will develop breast cancer. There is a 93% 5-year survival rate for localized breast cancer and a 72% 5-year survival if the cancer has spread regionally (CA Facts, 1994). Men also develop breast cancer. About 300 men die of this type of cancer each year.

ETIOLOGIES
The etiology of breast cancer is unknown, but is associated with the following risk factors:

High risk
- older than 50 years of age
- North America and Northern Europe country of birth
- history of breast cancer in both a mother and a sister

Moderate risk
- high socioeconomic status
- at least 30 years old at first full-term pregnancy
- history of cancer in one breast
- history of benign proliferative lesion
- first-degree (mother or sister) relative with history of breast cancer
- mammographic parenchymal patterns (dysplastic parenchyma)
- large doses of radiation to chest

CLINICAL MANIFESTATIONS
- May see unilateral nipple discharge (clear, bloody, milky)
- Possible change in breast such as a lump, thickening, swelling, dimpling, skin irritation, and pain
- Nipple retraction

CLINICAL/DIAGNOSTIC FINDINGS
- History of risk factors
- Physical examination of breast and lymphatics that indicates a palpable lump, most often a single lump in the upper outer quadrant
- Mammography showing a mass
- Biopsy and pathology studies confirming carcinoma
- Estrogen receptor assay, chest x-rays, computerized axial tomography (CAT) scans, bone scans, liver function blood work used in staging and in follow-up posttreatment

▶ NURSING DIAGNOSIS: *Altered Health Maintenance*
Related To physical care of wound, affected arm, potential complications

Defining Characteristics
- Hospital discharge 2–5 days postsurgery
- May have incision of varying degree based on surgery performed (lumpectomy, segmented mastectomy, etc.); drain may be in place at hospital discharge, usually removed with return to physician office 2–7 days post-hospital discharge
- Limited mobility on affected side

- Potential complications: lymphedema of affected arm, motor/sensory changes on affected side, seroma/hematoma formation, necrosis of skin flap (depending on surgery performed)
- Pain at wound site

Patient Outcome

- Patient will perform physical care associated with wound/incision care and with minimizing the risk of complications.

Nursing Interventions	Rationales
Assess patient/caregiver knowledge of wound care and compliance with hospital/doctor discharge instructions.	This identifies areas for teaching.
Reinforce instructions for wound care. Discuss aseptic technique and signs and symptoms of infections. Also describe how to use emollient and when to contact the nurse.	This promotes effective healing and minimizes complications.
Assess pain; suggest comfort measures/analgesics; teach about phantom sensation in absent breast.	Patient may experience a sensation (itching, heaviness, pain, "pins and needles") in absent breast within 1 week of surgery.
Assess for potential complications. (If patient is discharged from the hospital within 2–3 days post-surgery, the next four interventions are an immediate priority and need special attention.)	This promotes healing without complications.
Assess for lymphedema, which occurs secondary to lymph node excision or radiation. Check for decrease in mobility, for sensation of heaviness, and for increased edema since hospital discharge. Measure arm 4 inches above and below elbow.	This promotes healing without complications.
Assess for motor/sensory change in affected arm/shoulder. Check range of motion (ROM) and note any numbness, tingling, or muscle weakness. Refer to physical therapy as necessary; reinforce exercises.	This promotes healing without complications.

Nursing Interventions	Rationales
Check for seroma/hematoma at surgical site. If patient had drain, check when it was removed. Assess for any amount/type of drainage from the incision. Assess for signs and symptoms of hematoma, including increased pain, edema, and discoloration. Refer the patient to the physician if the drainage is new or has increased in volume. Instruct the patient to keep her upper affected arm close to her body 1 week postsurgery.	This decreases tension on the suture line and prevents hematoma/seroma formation.
Check healing of skin flap (depending on type of surgery) by assessing skin temperature and color. Capillary refill time should be less than 3 s. Teach patient to report changes, including decreased warmth and blue, white, or red skin flap coloration. Reinforce/teach actions to promote healing: adequate nutrition, rest, activity, hygiene. Encourage no smoking.	This promotes healing without complications. Smoking increases vasoconstriction.
Assess knowledge of exercises. Request demonstration of exercises and description of the rationale for doing the exercises. Refer to Reach to Recovery at the American Cancer Society for guidelines and specific exercises. Self-referral can be done to Reach to Recovery.	Identify areas of need that improve/maintain function. Exercise prevents contractures and improves lymph/blood circulation. Patient should begin full ROM exercises when the sutures are removed. Full ROM should return within 2–3 months of surgery.
If necessary, consider incentives for following the exercise regimen, including developing a schedule with the patient for completing the exercises and documenting extension/movement improvement in a log.	This increases patient control, which increases self-esteem and maximizes the chances that patient will comply with therapy.
Teach care of affected arm if mastectomy was performed or lymph nodes were removed. Protect the arm from injury and avoid blood draws/IVs. If injured, wash the arm thoroughly with soap and water. Teach that	This helps avoid infection and potential complications.

Nursing Interventions

stiffness will decrease but armpit numbness may continue for a longer period of time if the nodes were removed.

Rationales

▶ **NURSING DIAGNOSIS:** *Knowledge Deficit*

Related To cancer diagnosis, options related to reconstruction, treatment options after surgery (radiation, chemotherapy), use of community resources

Defining Characteristics
- Verbalizes need for information
- Expresses confusion over treatments, choices
- Verbalizes misinformation
- Voices hesitancy/misconceptions about use of community resources

Patient Outcomes
The patient will:
- discuss breast cancer diagnosis, treatment, and prognosis.
- implement a plan for contacting community resources as necessary.

Nursing Interventions	Rationales
Assess patient/family knowledge of the specific cancer diagnosis, treatment expectations, and understanding of prognosis. Reinforce accuracies and clarify correct and incorrect perceptions and fears. Support realistic hope.	By learning more about the disease, treatment, and prognosis, the patient is empowered and can increase control over cancer diagnosis. This increases potential for effective coping.
Assess knowledge and use of prosthetic devices and support brassieres. Refer to local resources (American Cancer Society, specialty shops) for prosthetic fitting and Reach to Recovery for more information.	This maintains self-image and esteem. A permanent form can be fitted 4–6 weeks postsurgery.
Assess interest in and knowledge of breast reconstruction options; refer	Information will enhance understanding and control and increase

Nursing Interventions	Rationales
patient to local breast cancer center education specialist and physician for specifics.	patient's ability to make informed decisions.
Based on type and stage of tumor, assess knowledge of treatment choices postlumpectomy/mastectomy (radiation therapy, chemotherapy, hormonal therapy, autologous bone marrow transplant). Encourage patient to make informed choices.	Information will enhance understanding and control and increase patient's ability to make informed decisions.
If treatment is in progress, discuss expected side effects and reactions. Stress positive nutritional state. (See also nutrition chapter.)	Reduces potential for debilitating side effects and reactions to treatments. Adequate nutritional status will promote tissue repair.
Teach/reinforce regular follow-up examinations, including history and physical q3–4 months for first 3 years, every 6 months for years 4 and 5, and annually thereafter. Reinforce monthly breast self-examination (BSE), follow-up mammogram for affected and unaffected breast, and follow-up sonogram, if prescribed.	Increases patient control over disease and promotes early detection of recurrence. Postoperative and radiation changes to affected breast (edema, skin thickening, postoperative fluid collections) seen on mammograms are most marked in first 6 months. Then changes stabilize within 2 years. Ultrasounds differentiate between seromas and solid masses.
Supply patient/family with list of community agencies and resources listed in the Discharge Planning section. Provide written and video information. Provide age-specific materials to children.	Increasing patient's knowledge and use of resources will increase the patient's control over the disease process and coping.

▶ NURSING DIAGNOSIS: *Ineffectual Individual/Family Coping*

Related To anxiety and fear over diagnosis of cancer, grief over changed/lost body part, perceived change in individual role(s), perceived loss of control over the future

Defining Characteristics
- Feeling of "why me?" "What have I done to deserve this?"
- Crying spells

- Feeling unworthy
- Denial of loss
- Withdrawal from others
- Concern for other family members' risk for developing breast cancer
- Wanting to "maintain composure" in front of family (including children)
- Insomnia and/or constant tired feeling

Patient Outcomes
Patient will:
- maintain effective coping strategies to deal with cancer diagnosis.
- verbalize self-worth and willingness to pursue ADLs and usual roles.
- participate in social functions.

Nursing Interventions	Rationales
Assess previous coping skills and current level of coping. Facilitate venting feelings, concerns, and issues related to cancer. Acknowledge the normalcy of the grieving process (peak period of psychological distress may occur several weeks after hospitalization). Anticipate and acknowledge other stressors within the patient's life. Identify past informal and formal support systems, assist patient/family to activate or continue useful supports (see also Grief/Loss chapter).	This facilitates the grieving process.
Encourage self-care.	This reinforces/increases patient's sense of control.
Refer to Reach to Recovery, breast cancer support groups, and/or individual/family counseling as necessary.	Meeting other breast cancer survivors can inspire hope for the future.
Educate about family cancer risk. Stress monthly BSE for all females in family over 20 years of age and demonstrate BSE technique. Women over 30 should discuss having mammography screening with their physician.	There is a two to three times increased risk for developing breast cancer among patient's biological daughters/sisters.

Nursing Interventions	Rationales
Assess patient's work history and potential concerns related to returning to work; assess how much time is necessary to be away from work for treatment and rehabilitation. Assist patient to identify and contact key resource persons responsible for implementing a comprehensive work reentry program for the patient. If no program is in place, work with employer's resource person(s) to define employee's needs about reentering the work place.	Concerns for cancer survivors returning to work include facing co-workers, subordinates, and employers; feeling rejected; and fearing insurance benefit discrimination, including cancellation, increased premiums, and extended waiting prior to eligibility (Clark and Landis, 1990).

▶ NURSING DIAGNOSIS: *Altered Sexuality Patterns*

Related To change/loss in breast(s), altered self-image, self-concept disturbance, possible altered sexuality patterns associated with decreased libido secondary to hormonal therapy

Defining Characteristics
- Patient questioning and expressing uncertainty over issues related to sexuality, femininity, and self-worth
- Possible withdrawal from partner
- Verbalization of perceived loss of femininity and physical attractiveness

Patient Outcomes
Patient will:
- demonstrate beginning willingness to accept self-image and maintain relationship with partner.
- verbalize concerns and feelings about sexual identity and initiate referral to community resources as needed.

Nursing Interventions	Rationales
Assess past/current relationships with significant others. Encourage the patient and partner to discuss the meaning of the loss and surgery/diagnosis.	Promotes patient's/partner's adjustment to the effects of change/loss of breast/body image on sexuality.

Nursing Interventions	Rationales
Facilitate communication between patient/partner.	Promotes patient's/partner's adjustment to the effects of change/loss of breast/body image on sexuality.
Facilitate patient's/partner's supportive behaviors by discussing feeling with patient and encouraging both of them to look at and care for breast wound site if appropriate for this diad.	Promotes patient's/partner's adjustment to the effects of change/loss of breast/body image on sexuality.
Educate patient about sexual side effects of breast cancer treatment, potential side effects of medications (adriamycin more likely to trigger menopause than the combination cytoxin, methotrexate, 5-FU (CMF), and discuss estrogen replacement therapy if menopausal symptoms are severe. Often physicians will avoid estrogen replacement treatment because studies show that estrogen increases the risk of cancer recurrence; however, this is being rethought. Also discuss the psychological issues associated with breast cancer and treatment.	Chemotherapy may cause menopause with accompanying drop in estrogen, which may dampen sex drive and reduce the lubrication, elasticity, and size of the vagina.
Talk through and/or role play with the patient about potential social scenarios when the patient and partner/other discuss the cancer diagnosis and change/loss of the breast.	Tests out new self-image.
Promote patient's social contact with others.	Tests out new self-image.

DISCHARGE PLANNING/CONTINUITY OF CARE
- Ensure patient can perform ADLs.
- Ensure follow-up appointments for medical care have been made.
- Reinforce living with cancer versus cancer as a debilitating illness.

- Facilitate linkages between patient/family and community resources prior to discharge by having them contact the American Cancer Society programs [Breast Cancer Support Group, CanSurmount, Dialogue, H.U.G.S., I Can Cope, Look Good...Feel Better, and Reach to Recovery], National Cancer Institute, and local breast centers with support groups. Provide written and video information. Provide age-specific materials to/for children.

REFERENCES/BIBLIOGRAPHY

Cancer facts and figures. (1994). Atlanta, GA: American Cancer Society.

Clark, J. C., & Landis, L. L. (1990). *Reintegration and maintenance of employees with breast cancer in the workplace.* Atlanta: American Cancer Society. Adapted and reprinted from *American Association of Occupational Health Nurses Journal,* 1989, 37(5), 186–193.

Goodman, J. (1994). A scar I did not want to hide. How does one prepare for the loss of a breast? *Newsweek,* March 2, 1994.

Hymovich, D. (1993). Child-rearing concerns of parents with cancer. *Oncology Nursing Forum, 20*(9), 1355–1360.

Johnson, J. B., and Kelly, A. W. (1990). A multifaceted rehabilitation program for women with cancer. *Oncology Nursing Forum, 17*(5), 691–694.

Kinne, D. W. (1991). The surgical management of primary breast cancer. Atlanta: American Cancer Society. Reprinted from *Ca-A Cancer Journal for Clinicians,* 1991, *41,* 71–84.

Manson, H., Manderino, M., & Johnson, M. H. (1993). Chemotherapy: Thoughts and images of patients with cancer. *Oncology Nursing Forum, 20*(3), 527–531.

Walsh, J. (1993). Healing the hidden scars: Sex after breast cancer. *Health, July/August,* 94–97.

Winchester, D. P., & Cox, J. (1992). Standards for breast-conservation treatment. Atlanta: American Cancer Society. Reprinted from *Ca-A Journal for Clinicians,* 1992, *42,* 134–162.

$\mathscr{A}$RTHRITIS/OSTEOPOROSIS

Joan Flynn, RN, MSN

The word *arthritis* means inflammation of the joints; consequently, arthritis is known as a disease of the joints. Rheumatoid arthritis and osteoarthritis are two major types of arthritis. Osteoarthritis, the most common form of arthritis, is a degenerative joint disease which destroys the cartilage that covers the bones at the joint, resulting in bone-to-bone contact. Rheumatoid arthritis is a chronic autoimmune disease which affects the synovium, the membrane surrounding the joint. The synovium secretes more fluid, making the joint edematous.

Osteoporosis means porous bone. The term is used to describe a metabolic bone disease process in which bone resorption is more extensive than bone deposition. This causes an overall reduction in bone mass or density and leads to bones becoming brittle, making them susceptible to breaking.

ETIOLOGIES

Osteoarthritis
- joint injury
- overuse of joint
- obesity
- gene defect/heredity, genetic predisposition
- unknown (also called primary osteoarthritis)

Rheumatoid arthritis
- unknown, but thought to be an autoimmune disease
- possibly caused by an infectious agent

Osteoporosis
- low levels of estrogen
- lack of exercise, immobilization
- long-term steroid therapy
- idiopathic
- secondary to other disorders, such as hyperparathyroidism and thyrotoxicosis

CLINICAL MANIFESTATIONS

Osteoarthritis

- restricted motion in joint
- deep aching pain in movable joints during movement and at night
- joints that may become enlarged
- crepitation that may be present on movement
- changes in alignment of extremity
- bony protuberances of the interphalangeal joints of the fingers, Heverden's nodes, and Bouchards nodes
- varus or valgus deformity of knees

Rheumatoid arthritis

- morning stiffness in one or more joints
- swelling and loss of function in one or more joints
- tingling or prickling sensation in hands or feet
- tiredness, weight loss, and a feeling of ill health
- swan-neck deformities of fingers
- color changes of fingers or toes (Raynaud's phenomenon)
- low-grade fever

Osteoporosis

- stooped appearance or outward curvature of the back
- fractures without history of trauma
- loss of height
- back pain

CLINICAL/DIAGNOSTIC FINDINGS

Osteoarthritis

- abnormal findings in synovial fluid [white blood cell (WBC) count 700, neutrophils 15%]
- arthrography that shows abnormalities in the joint capsule
- computerized tomography (CT) that shows abnormalities in spinal canal, such as stenosis
- x-ray that shows obliterated joint spaces and/or calcified ligaments
- magnetic resonance imaging (MRI) that confirms x-ray and CT results

Rheumatoid arthritis

- hematocrit (Hct) 35%, hemoglobin (Hb) 12g
- red blood cell (RBC) count 3.5 million cells/mL
- WBC elevated in all differential cells
- estimated sediment rate (ESR) elevated to 15 mm/h in males, 256 mm/h in females
- positive rheumatoid factor, found in serum, in 95% of patients with rheumatoid arthritis
- serum complement decreased, particularly in exacerbation

- immunologic assays, HLA-DR4 marker present in 55–69% of persons with rheumatoid arthritis
- synovial tissue biopsy, possibly presence of calcium hydroxyapatite crystals
- abnormal findings in synovial fluid, WBC 20,000, neutrophils 70%
- x-rays that show bone erosion, bone cysts, and partial joint dislocations
- MRI that shows changes in femoral head and inflammation of carpal tunnel
- CT that shows synovial cysts

Osteoporosis
- CT that reveals bone loss
- bone loss detected on absorptiometry, a specialized x-ray technique
- x-rays that show bone loss

▶ NURSING DIAGNOSIS: *Impaired Physical Mobility*

Related To joint inflammation, deformity, and limited range of motion (ROM)

Defining Characteristics
- Limited ROM
- Difficulty performing ADLs
- Using assistive devices when ambulating

Patient Outcomes
- Maintains maximal joint mobility
- Purposeful movement within home environment

Nursing Interventions	Rationales
Assess ROM of joints, joint deformity, overall mobility, and use of assistive devices.	Establishes data base to develop plan of care and to measure outcome.
Arrange for consults with physical therapist.	Individualized programs are prescribed to strengthen the muscles and tissues supporting the joints and to maintain joint motion.
Instruct regarding correct posture and body mechanics. Focus on measures to rest and reduce stress on joints.	Prevents further joint destruction.
Instruct and encourage regarding the use of support shoes, nonrestrictive clothing, splints, braces, supports, and adaptive equipment.	Using assistive devices preserves functions over time.

▶ NURSING DIAGNOSIS: *Impaired Home Maintenance Management*

Related To pain, weakness, and limitations

Defining Characteristics
- Reports cannot prepare meals, clean, do laundry because of pain, weakness, and tiredness

Patient Outcomes
- Learns alternatives and is able to demonstrate the use of these alternatives to improve home management activities

Nursing Interventions	Rationales
Assess patient's ability to open jars, open cabinets, turn knobs on stove, vacuum, handle dishes, and perform other home management tasks.	Establishes base line data to plan care.
Arrange for occupational therapist.	Occupational therapists can provide exercises and adaptive utensils to assist with home maintenance.
Arrange for home health aid.	Lends supportive presence and gives assistance while the patient is participating in rehabilitation.
Instruct and encourage compliance with exercises and use of adaptive utensils.	Patient should understand need to comply so home maintenance will not decline further. Understanding why compliance is important increases the chance the patient will comply.
Mutually explore and identify alternate means of accomplishing ADLs and home maintenance.	Discussing options will help clarify available alternatives and plan for securing additional needed resources.

▶ NURSING DIAGNOSIS: *Pain*

Related To inflammation and deformity of joints

Defining Characteristics
- Reluctant to move
- Reports pain
- Moans and cries
- Guards affected joints

Patient Outcomes
- Patient will experience only minimum pain after treatments and medication.

Nursing Interventions	Rationales
Assess patient's experience of pain, including location, severity, duration, what offers relief, and what worsens pain.	Pain relates to inflammation, the joints involved, and the patient's pain tolerance. Accurately assessing the characteristics of pain assists all caregivers in developing a plan to alter the pain experience.
Encourage patient to express feelings about disease or pain experiences.	Uncovering feelings, especially negative ones, allows caregivers to help patients feel understood and helps patients learn to manage their negative feelings.
Assess patient's responses or reactions to medications; monitor for side effects, specifically gastrointestinal.	Medications have specific responses and side effects (frequently gastrointestinal); alternate drugs are available and may be prescribed because of an allergic reaction or severe side effect(s).
Assess effects of prescribed medications on patient's pain experiences.	Provides data regarding need to continue or change medications.
Teach patient to perform activities when pain free; instruct on use of diversionary activities such as music, art, games, and puzzles when pain is less.	Activities help patient maintain a positive outlook; diversionary activities assist in moving concentration from pain to other things, leading to longer pain-free periods.

▶ NURSING DIAGNOSIS: *High Risk for Injury*

Risk Factors
- Limited mobility
- Impaired gait or balance
- Loss of dexterity of interphalangeal joints
- Inability to safely carry out daily activities and ambulation

Patient Outcomes
- Patient's home environment will be safe.

Nursing Interventions	Rationales
Assess concerns or fears related to possible falls or fractures.	Patient feels relieved when able to share concerns.
Assess home environment (e.g., number of stairs; loose rugs; long, uncovered cords).	Identifies risk factors for injury.
Instruct patient in regard to having safe home area (e.g., use only large area rugs that will not slide or use rugs with nonskid undersurfaces, avoid waxing floors, use nonskid strip in shower or bathtub, install handrails on stairs and in bath area, provide adequate lighting).	Reduces risk of falls and injuries and gives patient some control over creating a safe environment.

▶ NURSING DIAGNOSIS: *Knowledge Deficit*

Related To disease process, potential complications, signs and symptoms to report to home health nurse or physician

Defining Characteristics
- Patient reports inaccurate or incomplete information related to disease process, potential complications, and signs and symptoms to the home health nurse or physician.

Patient Outcomes
- Patient verbalizes measures to effectively manage arthritic condition.
- Patient states the conditions, signs, and symptoms that need to be reported to the home health nurse or physician.

Nursing Interventions	Rationales
Assess current level of knowledge related to osteoarthritis, rheumatoid arthritis, or osteoporosis.	Reveals what patients do not know and identifies teaching topics.
Give written information and verbalize signs and symptoms of specific arthritic disease.	Increases level and understanding of disease.
Give written phone contacts and emergency numbers, and develop	Having a written plan for emergencies fosters feelings of control

Nursing Interventions	Rationales
plan patient can use in case of emergency.	over situations and aids patients and their family members to contact health team members.
Give instructions about their medications, including the name, administration, purpose, action, and side effects.	Patients must be made aware of all information regarding medications because they will be more likely to comply with the medication regimen when they understand the implications of not following it.

DISCHARGE PLANNING/CONTINUITY OF CARE
- Refer patient and family to social services for counseling.
- Provide information regarding community support systems (e.g., Arthritis Foundation, Meals on Wheels, community or village transportation for aged or disabled, area agencies on aging, support groups).
- Continue physical and occupational therapy, if needed.
- Follow up visits with physicians.
- Refer to outpatient pain clinic, if needed.
- Contact patient and family by phone within 3–4 weeks to inquire as to how discharge plan is being followed.

Clinical Clip

Approximately 1.5% of the people in the United States have been afflicted with rheumatoid arthritis, and it is estimated that 200,000 cases are diagnosed each year. Women are afflicted more often than men at a 3 : 1 ratio. Because of the extensive treatments, it is a very costly disease to treat.

The most common form of arthritis is osteoarthritis. Approximately 50 million Americans are affected by this disease. It is more common in men under the age of 45, but more common in women over the age of 55. This disease is thought to be almost universal in people over 75.

Osteoporosis occurs in 30% of women who are 45 years of age and in 70% of women over 45 who experience bone fractures.

BIBLIOGRAPHY
Comunale, D. L. (1992). Collaborative care planning with the arthritic client at home. *Journal of Home Health Care Practice, 4*(2), 8–15.

Loeb, S. (Ed.) (1994). *Illustrated guide to diagnostic tests*. Springhouse, PA: Springhouse Corporation.

Mourad, L. A. (1991). *Orthopedic disorders*. St. Louis: Mosby.

Sopko, J. S. (1992). Holostic mamagement of arthritic pain. *Journal of Home Health Care Practice, 4*(2), 16–22.

Wetherbee, L. L. (1994). Caring for the client with arthritis. *Home Healthcare Nurse, 12*(1), 8–13.

$\mathcal{J}$OINT REPLACEMENT/ FRACTURES

Robin L. Evans, RN, MSN, ONC

Total joint arthroplasty is the surgical procedure often performed after conservative medical or surgical measures have failed to improve a person's joint motion and/or decrease pain. Joint replacement involves resecting and replacing the articulating surfaces of all or part of a joint with a metal and/or polyethylene prosthetic component. The hip and knee are the two joints most commonly replaced due to their weight-bearing status; however, most other joints also can be replaced, including the shoulder, elbow, wrist, ankle, and interphalangeals. The goal of total joint arthroplasty is to improve the patient's quality of life by providing them with a functional, pain-free joint.

A fracture is a break or disruption in the continuity of a bone. When caring for a patient with a fracture, it is important to know the mechanism of injury and the exact location and type of the fracture (open or closed; transverse, spiral, or comminuted). This information will help determine how to manage each case.

When caring for an orthopedic patient, the nurse's roles are to prevent complications and to assist in restoring patients' independent functions.

ETIOLOGIES

Joint replacements
- destruction of the joint by degenerative joint disease or osteoarthritis, rheumatoid arthritis, avascular necrosis, traumatic arthritis, joint dysplasia/deformity, pseudoarthrosis, or congenital deformities/dislocations
- sepsis
- failure of previous internal fixation or joint arthroplasty
- joint instability/immobility

Fractures
- trauma
- pathologic fractures (related to osteoporosis or neoplastic disease)

CLINICAL MANIFESTATIONS
- Significant pain at the affected site
- Decreased range of motion
- Limp with ambulation or inability to bear weight
- Compromise in the patient's (ADLs)

CLINICAL/DIAGNOSTIC FINDINGS
- Plain film x-rays to determine the fracture site. In arthritis, the x-rays generally show joint space narrowing, bony spur production, and subchondral sclerosis. Complete joint destruction also can be visualized.
- Computed tomography to evaluate fractures in areas that are difficult to assess by plain x-rays. It also is useful when evaluating soft tissue.
- Tomography provides a three-dimensional picture of the joint and allows the physician to better ascertain the exact location of a lesion.
- Magnetic resonance imaging to determine the exact extent of joint destruction in preoperative total joint arthroplasty patients. Clinical findings include thinning of the articular cartilage, capsular edema, joint effusion, subchondral inflammation, and cyst formation.
- Radionuclide bone scanning to detect early changes in bone, to determine the distribution of osteoarthritis, and to assess for infection.

▶ NURSING DIAGNOSIS: *Impaired Physical Mobility*
Related To
- Postoperative total joint arthroplasty
- Immobilization devices; splints, casts, traction, braces, external fixators
- Activity or weight-bearing restrictions

Defining Characteristics
- Reluctance to attempt movement due to discomfort from surgery
- Limited range of motion
- Decreased muscle strength
- Medically imposed restrictions of movement

Patient Outcomes
Patient will:
- have restored or improved joint/limb function.
- be independent in self-care with use of assistive devices/ambulatory devices.
- maintain or increase mobility.
- demonstrate techniques to increase functional mobility.

Nursing Interventions	Rationales
Following total joint arthroplasty, reinforce joint positioning precautions. Patients who have had a total hip replacement should not rotate their leg internally, flex greater than 90°, or adduct (i.e., legcrossing). Encourage these patients to use pillows on chairs, an elevated toilet seat, and other assistive devices as needed to maintain these precautions. Patients who have had a total knee replacement should continue to use their immobilizers per their physicians instructions.	Joint dislocation is prevented.
If referred to physical therapy, assess patient's understanding of therapeutic programs.	The nurse, as a case manager and care coordinator, must communicate with other providers.
Encourage and assess compliance with home exercise program or outpatient physical therapy. Encourage use of continuous passive motion (CPM) machine if ordered by the physician.	Exercise increases joint mobility and muscle strength and prevents contractures and/or muscle atrophy caused by disuse.
Review/reinforce limitations/restrictions. Instruct patient to increase activity level gradually over 6–12 weeks. Restrictions will define weight-bearing status and use of assistive devices. Restrictions may also include whether the patient can drive, shower, or work. The physician will order these types of limitations and restrictions. The affected extremity will be immobile for at least 6 weeks, and the patient will have restrictions based on the body part involved. Following cast removal, the patient will still have restrictions until the extremity has regained mobility and muscle strength.	Much of this information is included in hospital discharge instructions, but it needs to be reinforced by the community health nurse.
Foster independence with ADLs using assistive devices as needed.	It is important that the patients be able to care for themselves

Nursing Interventions	Rationales
Refer to occupational therapy if necessary.	adequately, especially if no caregiver is available.
Promote ambulation with appropriate assistive devices (walker, crutches, cane). Assess that the patient is using the device properly.	Proper use avoids injury.
Teach the patient to recognize his or her own limits, and encourage energy conservation techniques. Encourage the patient to plan activities for the time of day when they have the most energy, and space activities throughout the day interspersed with rest periods.	This encourages the patient to remain active without becoming too tired. Following surgery or with casting, there is generally muscle weakness, and using assistive devices requires more energy than normal walking.

▶ NURSING DIAGNOSIS: *High Risk for Injury*

Risk Factors
- Immobility
- Open wound (all wounds can become infected)
- Presence of a total joint prosthesis
- Not using aseptic technique when changing dressings
- Status post fracture/total joint arthroplasty

Patient Outcomes
Patient is free from injury related to:
- infection.
- deep venous thrombosis.
- falls.

Nursing Interventions	Rationales
Use aseptic technique for dressing changes and staple removal (see also Skin Care chapter).	Prevents the risk of contaminating the wound site.
Assess wound and teach patient/caregiver how to assess the wound for signs and symptoms of infection (i.e., redness, swelling, heat over the area, drainage, fever, increased	Promptly recognizing infection allows for rapid treatment and may prevent further complications.

Nursing Interventions	Rationales
pain) (see also Skin Care chapter). Instruct them to notify the physician immediately if any of these signs or symptoms occur.	
Instruct the patient that, following total joint replacement, prophylactic antibiotics are frequently used for routine dental work or minor surgical procedures [e.g., gastrointestinal (GI) lab testing or genitourinary (GU) instrumentation].	Total joint replacements can become infected via hematogenous routes long after the initial operative procedure.
Maintain prescribed pharmacological protocol with aspirin or low-dose warfarin. Encourage using antiembolism stockings if ordered by the physician.	These agents are often continued after discharge for continued prophylaxis of deep-vein thrombosis. Research has shown that there are two "peaks" when deep-vein thrombosis is likely to occur. The first is approximately 5 days postoperatively, and the second is 2 weeks after surgery, when the patient has usually returned home.
Assess for and teach the patient the signs and symptoms of deep-vein thrombosis and pulmonary embolus (i.e., redness, swelling, and pain in the calf or thigh, shortness of breath, or difficulty breathing) (see also Peripheral Vascular Disease chapter).	Prompt recognition allows for rapid treatment and may prevent further complications.
Evaluate the patients home layout regarding steps, bathroom, and bedroom, and assess for conditions which may pose a risk to the patient. Stress home safety measures to the patient using the following guidelines: 1. Remove scatter rugs. 2. Encourage the use of well-fitting, supportive shoes. 3. Encourage use of stair rails. 4. Advise use of a night light on stairs and in the hall between the bedroom and bathroom.	Appropriate safety measures may prevent falls and, therefore, injuries.

Nursing Interventions	**Rationales**
5. Encourage use of assistive devices (i.e., grab bars, reachers, etc.) as needed.	
6. Arrange furniture so that pathways between rooms are clear, being particularly mindful of low-rise coffee tables, footrests, magazine racks, plants, as well as electric appliance and phone cords which may be in the pathways.	
7. Do not leave objects on the stairs and be sure that the tread is in good repair.	
8. Place nonskid strips on the floor of the bathtub or shower as well as encourage using a slip-resistant rug adjacent to the bathtub for safe entry and exit.	
9. Clean up spills on bare floors immediately.	

▶ **NURSING DIAGNOSIS:** *High Risk for Peripheral Neurovascular Dysfunction*

Risk Factors
- Compression from immobilization devices (casts, splints, traction, braces, ace bandages, dressings, and pillows)
- Immobilization
- Incorrect positioning
- Surgical intervention
- Soft tissue disruption from trauma
- Fracture fragments or displaced fracture
- Joint dislocation
- Edema

Patient Outcomes
Patient will:
- be free from neurovascular deficits or deficits will be quickly identified.
- demonstrate appropriate neurovascular status assessment skills.

Nursing Interventions	Rationales
Assess neurovascular status (pain, color, capillary refill time, temperature, presence of peripheral pulses, edema, sensation, and active and passive and motion, and compare the affected extremity to the unaffected side and to baseline).	Allows the nurse to identify any deficits.
Assess for signs and symptoms of neurovascular deficits, including increasing pain, decreased motion (muscle weakness), pain on passive stretch, paresthesias, decreased sensation, pallor, extremity cool to touch, and pulselessness. Teach patient these signs and symptoms and, if positive, instruct the patient to call the doctor immediately.	Identifying symptoms early allows for rapid intervention to preserve limb function. If neurovascular deficits exist and are ignored, paralysis or permanent injury may result.
Elevate extremity.	Prevents edema.
Assess appliances at regular intervals for proper fit, position, and function.	Appliance fit may change over time due to decreasing edema or changes in the patient's muscle mass from atrophy or strengthening.
Instruct/reinforce proper cast care, including: 1. Keep cast dry, unless permitted by physician and only if waterproof casting material was used. Cover the cast with a plastic bag closed tightly at the top during showering/bathing. Avoid rain and other sources of moisture. 2. Remember that the surface of a cast is frequently rough and may scratch other body parts and/or furniture. 3. Observe the cast for any cracks, softening, or flaking. Report these conditions to the physician. 4. Inspect the skin at the edges of the cast for redness or irritation. Petal the cast edges as necessary.	These measures maintain cast and skin integrity and rapidly detect any complications.

Nursing Interventions

5. Do not put anything down into the cast, including powder or scratchers, unless specifically ordered by the doctor.
6. Assess the cast for any foul odor, warm spots, or drainage, which may indicate a wound infection or pressure sore under the cast. Report these signs to the doctor immediately.

Rationales

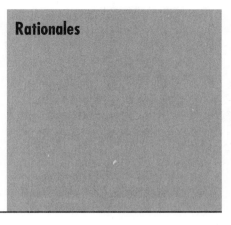

DISCHARGE PLANNING/CONTINUITY OF CARE
- Ensure patient is being cared for by physical therapy or occupational therapy according to treatment plan.
- Schedule follow-up doctor's appointments, if needed.
- Review medication regimen, including periodic blood work for those patients on warfarin.
- Ensure patient has necessary telephone numbers, e.g., the home care agency, therapist, and physician.

OTHER PLANS OF CARE TO REFERENCE
- Arthritis and Osteoarthritis
- Peripheral Vascular Disease
- Pain
- Skin Care

BIBLIOGRAPHY
American Academy of Orthopaedic Surgeons. (1993). *Live it safe.* Rosemont, IL: American Academy of Orthopaedic Surgeons.

Maher, A. B., Salmond, S. W., & Pellino, T. A. (1994). *Orthopaedic nursing.* Philadelphia, PA: W. B. Saunders.

National Association of Orthopaedic Nurses. (1992). *Guidelines for orthopaedic nursing.* Pitman, NJ: Anthony J. Janetti.

Salmond, S. W., Mooney, N. E., & Verdisco, L. A. (Eds.). (1991). *Core curriculum for orthopaedic nursing* (2nd ed.). Pitman, NJ: Anthony J. Janetti.

$\mathscr{A}$NTEPARTUM HOME CARE

Julie A. Loftus, RN, MSN

Antepartum nursing care is provided to pregnant women before the onset of labor. High-risk mothers-to-be may require home antepartum care due to complications, including placenta previa, preterm labor, preterm premature rupture of membranes, pregnancy-induced hypertension, and insulin-dependent diabetes. The nurse's role early in pregnancy (first trimester) includes hydrating patients with hyperemesis gravidarum. In the second and third trimesters, nurses focus on monitoring the mother and fetus, providing emotional support, and teaching techniques to minimize the risk of complications.

ETIOLOGIES
- Placenta previa
- Preterm labor
- Preterm premature rupture of membranes
- Pregnancy-induced hypertension
- Insulin-dependent diabetes
- Hyperemesis
- Uterine/vaginal infection
- History of preterm delivery
- History of uterine anomaly
- History of substance abuse/violence
- Teenage pregnancy
- Multipara

CLINICAL MANIFESTATIONS
- Increased uterine activity (more than 4 contractions in 1 h)
- Decreased fetal movement
- Headaches
- Blurred vision
- Edema (lower extremity, hand, facial)
- Increased vaginal discharge
- Foul vaginal odor/discharge
- Increased lower back pain (greater than norm)
- Vaginal bleeding
- Severe vomiting
- Dysuria (frequency, urgency, burning)

- Expressed feelings of inadequacy and/or guilt
- Frequent mood swings
- Lack of cooperation with medical regimen
- Expresses inability to rest because of lack of assistance

CLINICAL/DIAGNOSTIC FINDINGS
- Fever (>100.4)
- Elevated fetal heart rate (>160)
- Elevated fasting blood glucose (>110)
- Elevated urine protein/ketones (>2+)
- Elevated blood pressure (>140/90)
- Pelvic exam if ordered by physician (cervix dilated more than previous exam)
- Fundal height (appropriate for gestational age)
- Positive homan's sign
- Deep-tendon reflexes (brisk implies neurologic instability)

▶ NURSING DIAGNOSIS: *Knowledge Deficit*

Related To potential complications of high-risk pregnancy, care of high-risk mother/baby, diet/activity restrictions

Defining Characteristics
- Newly diagnosed as high risk
- Mother asks how to care for herself/fetus
- Lack of follow-through with diet instructions
- Lack of follow-through with activity restrictions
- Questions what to do if complications arise (e.g., vaginal bleeding, increased contractions)

Patient Outcomes
- Mother verbalizes rationale for activity restriction and proper diet.
- Mother verbalizes techniques for maintaining bedrest.
- Family participates in antepartum care regimen by assuming mother's tasks while she maintains on bedrest (measurable).
- Mother has emergency plan.

Nursing Interventions	Rationales
Assess mother/family knowledge level about antepartum care and possible complications.	Teaching strategy should be individualized to the patient's needs.

Nursing Interventions	Rationales
Provide individualized instructions to patient based on specific high-risk condition. Instruct on signs and symptoms to be reported to health care provider. For example, for mothers with placenta previa, report vaginal bleeding and decreased fetal movement. For pregnancy-induced hypertension, report sharp abdominal pain, vaginal bleeding, headache, blurred vision, and decreased fetal movement. For preterm labor, report increase in uterine activity (more than four contractions in 1 hour), rupture of membranes, fever, increase in sensation of baby "balling up," increase in usual vaginal discharge, and increase in lower back pain. For preterm premature rupture of membranes, report decreased fetal movement, fever, increase in amniotic fluid loss, foul smelling fluid, vaginal bleeding, and uterine contractions. For hyperemesis gravidarum, report headache, excessive vomiting, weight loss, and disorientation.	Recognizing and reporting complications early will minimize adverse effects.
Teach mother proper activity level given her diagnosis. Bedrest may mean bedrest with bathroom privileges or bedrest for a certain number of hours a day. Check physician's order.	Mothers with placenta previa, preterm labor, preterm premature rupture of membranes, or pregnancy-induced hypertension may require bedrest.
Discuss appropriate diversional activities. Individualize plan for the mother.	Diversional activities help mothers maintain bedrest.
Teach isometric exercises. Develop home exercise plan.	Bedrest may result in losses in muscular conditioning.
Teach mother to recognize normal fetal movement and uterine activity and distinguish from complications or abnormalities.	Fetal movement and uterine activity are subjective assessments. Mothers need to evaluate these assessments and know when to call nurse or physician.

Nursing Interventions	Rationales
Offer childbirth preparation video tapes. They are often available on loan from the public library or hospital patient education departments.	This provides distraction and helps prepare mother for labor and delivery.

▶ NURSING DIAGNOSIS: *Altered Role Performance*

Related To prenatal bedrest, uncertainty about pregnancy outcome, financial deficits

Defining Characteristics
- No one to help with woman's usual home care role (cooking, cleaning, child care, shopping, schooling)
- Mother taking time off from work, causing financial strain
- Mother verbalizing concern over inability to fulfill her previous roles
- Mother/father reporting stress in (marital) relationship
- Mother verbalizing lack of support systems/financial assistance
- Mother reporting social isolation

Patient Outcomes
- Mother verbalizes adequate resources to comply with antepartum bedrest or other restrictions.
- Support systems fulfill mother's previous role.
- Mother/family verbalizes that they are coping with antepartum care regimen.

Nursing Interventions	Rationales
Assess family's resources and plan for how they will cope with their new family roles.	Assists family in complying with medical regimen.
Refer to social services for financial assistance, respite, and child care services.	Social worker can access other nonnursing services.
Encourage mother/father/family to verbalize their feelings about their role changes. Have mother/family redefine their roles as a team effort.	Encourages family to be open and work together toward goal of healthy pregnancy outcome.
Remind the family that this change is timelimited. Recognize milestones in pregnancy: countdown to birth.	Helps family members cope with stress of role change.

Nursing Interventions	Rationales
Encourage the mother to accept help from others. Have mother give specific tasks to others who ask if they can help.	Family and friends may not know what will be most helpful to pregnant woman and family. Doing grocery shopping, providing transportation, and meal preparation are tangible tasks which may be designated to other family members.
Refer to support groups for high-risk mothers or teenage mothers.	High-risk mothers may have social support needs met through group activities; they may feel less social isolation through group contact.

▶ NURSING DIAGNOSIS: *High Risk for Fluid Volume Deficit*

Risk Factors
- Decreased fluid intake
- Living in warm climate without adequate cooling system
- Hyperemesis
- Premature rupture of membranes
- Pregnancy-induced hypertension
- Preterm labor
- Plasma protein loss
- Decreased urine output
- Inability to ingest and retain fluids

Patient Outcomes

Mother's urine
- Color is clear pale yellow
- Output is > 30 cc/h

Mother's skin
- Is warm and dry with good turgor

Mother
- Has no signs of generalized edema (headache, epigastric pain, dyspnea, nausea/vomiting)
- Has moist mucous membranes
- Has contractions < 4 per hour
- Has blood pressure 100–140/60-90
- Has orthostatic blood pressure < 20 mm Hg drop
- Denies dizziness when standing
- Has urine specific gravity < 1.040

Nursing Interventions	Rationales
Assess blood pressure, weight, contraction pattern, and signs and symptoms of dehydration (e.g., skin appearance and turgor, urine output and color, mucous membranes). Continue to assess fluid status throughout treatment plan.	Initial assessment is important to measure success of future interventions.
Monitor intake and output. Encourage intake appropriate for specific high-risk situation.	This monitors extent of fluid loss and assesses renal perfusion. It may not be possible to medicate women with hyperemesis by mouth. The patient may need intravenous (IV) hydration. Women with preterm labor may need 2–3 L fluids by mouth per 24 h.
If ordered by physician, begin and monitor IV infusion. Teach IV/heplock care (see Infusion Therapy chapter).	Mothers with severe hyperemesis may require IV fluid boluses or hyperalimentation (see Infusion Therapy chapter).
Assess lung sounds and respiratory rate.	Dyspnea and rales may indicate pulmonary edema, which may result if fluid moves from vascular space to interstitial space.
Weigh patient. Note weight loss or gain.	Weight loss may result with hyperemesis. Sudden weight gain (> 5 lb in 1 week) indicates fluid retention as fluid moves from vascular space to interstitial space.
Encourage bedrest as ordered; discuss benefits of left lateral position.	Left lateral position increases venous return and circulatory volume, improves uteroplacental perfusion and renal perfusion, and decreases vena caval pressure.

DISCHARGE PLANNING/CONTINUITY OF CARE
- Ensure that mother/family has plan for labor and delivery (e.g., site of care, physician, prenatal records, and emergency plan).
- Refer to parenting support groups and parenting classes.
- Refer to social services for Women, Infants, Children (WIC) or other financial assistance.
- Ensure mother has follow-up physician appointment.

BIBLIOGRAPHY

Goodwin, L. (1992). Home fetal assessment. *Journal of Perinatal and Neonatal Nursing, 5*(4), 33–45.

Grohar, J. (1994). Nursing protocols for antepartum home care. *Journal of Obstetric, Gynecologic, & Neonatal Nursing, 23*(8), 687–694.

Heaman, M., Robinson, M., Thompson, L., & Helewa, M. (1994). Patient satisfaction with an antepartum home-care program. *Journal of Obstetric, Gynecologic, & Neonatal Nursing, 23*(8), 707–713.

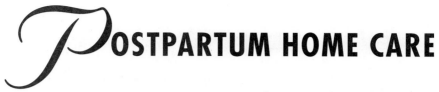

$\mathcal{P}$OSTPARTUM HOME CARE

Julie A. Loftus, RN, MSN

$\mathbf{P}$ostpartum home care is skilled nursing care provided to families following childbirth. The nurse's role in postpartum home care includes performing mother and newborn physical, psychosocial, and environmental assessments; breastfeeding assistance; blood draws; and referrals to community and medical resources as needed.

ETIOLOGIES
- Primiparas
- Mobile society (no family guidance network accessible)
- Early discharge/short hospital stay
- Lack of prenatal care and/or education
- Lack of support systems

CLINICAL MANIFESTATIONS (OF PROBLEMS)

Maternal
- boggy or soft uterus which does not respond to fundal massage
- blood clots (greater than size of a plum) passed per vagina
- uterine tenderness with palpation
- bright red, heavy flowing lochia rubra
- dysuria (frequency, urgency, burning)
- report of urinary incontinence since delivery
- episiotomy sutures not well approximated
- edema, ecchymosis, hematoma present on perineum or site of episiotomy repair
- purulent, foul-smelling lochial discharge
- poor hygiene
- engorged breasts

Infant
- wets less than six to eight diapers in 24 h
- bulging or depressed fontanels
- yellow sclera, skin
- green umbilical cord stump with drainage, foul smelling
- inconsolable crying
- poor hygiene

CLINICAL/DIAGNOSTIC FINDINGS

Maternal
- elevated blood pressure (> 140/90 mm Hg)
- fever (>100.4 F)
- increased pulse (>100 BPM)
- positive Homan's sign
- deep-tendon reflexes (brisk implies neurological instability)
- uterine fundal height above level of umbilicus
- distended bladder

Infant
- >10% weight loss from birth weight
- fever (>100.4 F)
- heart rate (>160 BPM)
- respiratory rate (>60 breaths/min)
- hypothermia: temperature < 97.7 F

▶ NURSING DIAGNOSIS: *Pain*

Related To mechanical trauma, episiotomy, perineal lacerations, hemorrhoids, engorged breasts, hormonal changes ("after-birth pains")

Defining Characteristics
- Reports pain
- Gait slow and stiff
- Reluctant to sit down
- Requests pain medication
- Reluctant to move bowels
- Two to 4 days postpartum
- Bottle-feeding infant

Patient Outcomes
Pain is reduced, as evidenced by:
- verbalizing decreased pain.
- ambulating with ease.
- being capable of caring for infant.

Nursing Interventions	Rationales
Assess degree and location of pain.	Provides nurse baseline information to measure outcome of further interventions.
Inspect perineum. Assess episiotomy or laceration repair for edema, hematoma, loss of approximation of sutures, and drainage from suture line. Assess hemorrhoids.	Excessive pain may indicate developing complications requiring further interventions.
Apply ice to hemorrhoids every 4 h for 15 min. Apply witch hazel compresses after pericare. Avoid direct pressure on hemorrhoids (use pillow). Avoid constipation.	Cold causes vasoconstriction, decreases edema, and provides local anesthesia. Witch hazel may decrease itching. Pressure on hemorrhoids may increase pain and increase size of hemorrhoid.
Encourage use of sitz bath or sitting in clean tub with 3–4 in. of warm water for 15 min three times per day.	Warm water soothes area, promotes vasodilation, increases circulation to area, and promotes healing.
Encourage use of topical antiseptic spray or pads and witch hazel compresses to perineum after pericare.	Produces local, cooling effect. Decreases pain.
Teach and/or review Kegel exercises.	Kegel exercises promote circulation, speed healing, and improve muscle tone.
For breast pain in nonnursing mother, encourage mother to wear tight-fitting bra or binder continuously until lactation ceases.	Weight of engorged breasts can be painful. Providing support decreases tension on breasts and decreases pain.
For nonnursing mothers, apply ice packs to axillary areas of breasts 20 min four times a day as needed.	Cold decreases inflammation and decreases pain.
For nonnursing mothers, instruct mother not to express milk or stimulate breasts.	Manually stimulating breasts causes release of oxytocin, which increases milk production. Producing more milk causes breasts to engorge.
Encourage mother to take pain medication as ordered.	This may relieve discomfort and allow her to care for self and infant.

▶ NURSING DIAGNOSIS: *Constipation*

Related To decreased muscle tone, effects of progesterone, and reluctance to put pressure on stitches

Defining Characteristics
- Reports no bowel movement since delivery
- Requests stool softener
- Reports reluctance to move bowels
- Reports hemorrhoid pain

Patient Outcomes
- Patient will return to predelivery elimination pattern, as evidenced by normal bowel movement.

Nursing Interventions	Rationales
Encourage early ambulation.	Ambulation promotes intestinal motility and improves muscle tone. Walking is a safe exercise in postpartum period.
Provide dietary information, including drinking six to eight glasses of water per day and eating high-fiber foods, including fruits, vegetables, and whole grains.	Water, fruits, vegetables, and whole grains soften and increase the volume of feces, leading to faster excretion.
Suggest over-the-counter stool softener.	Stool softeners lower surface tension of feces and permit water and fat to soften stool and facilitate elimination.

▶ NURSING DIAGNOSIS: *Knowledge Deficit—Newborn Care and Normal Growth and Development*

Related To inexperience with infant care and lack of role model

Defining Characteristics
- Questions about infant care
- Verbalizes lack of experience with infant care
- Verbalizes lack of confidence with infant care
- Inaccurately performs infant care skills

Patient Outcomes

Parents will:

- verbalize confidence with infant care.
- demonstrate appropriate behaviors necessary to safely care for infant's physical and emotional needs.
- verbalize rationale for appropriate caretaking activities.

Nursing Interventions	Rationales
Assess parent's knowledge of infant's physiological needs for nutrition, body temperature, sleep cycle, behavior state, and normal urinary and bowel outputs.	Establishes parent's knowledge base and helps nurse formulate teaching plan.
Perform infant physical assessment in the presence of parents. Explain findings to parents.	This assists parents in identifying normal variations in newborn and reassures them that infant is normal.
Demonstrate infant care techniques such as cleaning umbilical cord stump and diapering, feeding, and burping infant. Teach how to dress infant to reduce risk of hyperthermia and hypothermia. Teach circumcision care.	Provides role model for parents and encourages confidence in parents ability to perform infant care techniques. Provides opportunity for parents to ask questions.
In bottle-feeding infant, discuss proper preparation and storage of infant formula.	This ensures parents are providing nutrition in safe, appropriate manner.
Discuss potential dangers in bottle propping. (For breastfed infant, see Breastfeeding chapter).	Bottle propping can cause aspiration and airway occlusion if nipple is held against the back of throat. It also denies an opportunity for skin-to-skin contact and bonding between caretaker and infant.
Teach mother to position infant in crib on side with rolled towel or receiving blanket against back to keep infant in position or on back.	Reduces risk of sudden infant death syndrome.
Demonstrate taking axillary temperature and how to read thermometer. Discuss signs and symptoms of illness and when to call a health care provider.	Treating illness early improves outcomes. Axillary temperature is safe and accurate.

Nursing Interventions	Rationales
Encourage parents to make and keep appointments for follow-up with appropriate health care provider.	Encourages parents to continue involvement with health care system. Immunizations and monitoring for normal growth and development are essential in the first year of life.

▶ NURSING DIAGNOSIS: *High Risk for Infection*

Risk Factors
- Tissue trauma
- Break in skin integrity
- Decreased hemoglobin
- Prolonged rupture of membranes
- Poor hygiene in home
- Crowded living conditions

Patient Outcomes
Patient will:
- be afebrile.
- exhibit intact skin or wound without signs and symptoms of infection.
- produce negative cultures (if cultures are taken).

Nursing Interventions	Rationales
Assess vital signs.	Elevated temperature and rapid heart beat may indicate existing or developing infection.
Inspect perineum. Note any purulent drainage from episiotomy.	Purulent drainage indicates infection.
Instruct mother to change pads at least q4h, apply pad from front to back, and cleanse perineum with warm water after every void, cleaning from front to back. Use sitz bath/tub bath three times a day for 15 min. Make certain bath or tub is thoroughly cleansed prior to use to avoid contaminating open perineal wounds.	This helps prevent rectal contamination of vagina and urethra. Warmth promotes vasodilation and enhances healing.

Nursing Interventions	Rationales
Assess fundus and lochia. Review involution process and lochial progression.	Fundus should be firm without significant pain when massaged. Uterus descends approximately 1 cm below umbilicus per day. Failure to descend and/or contract ("boggy") may indicate infection. Foul-smelling and/or purulent lochia may indicate infection.
Encourage mother to empty bladder frequently and review signs and symptoms of a urinary tract infection (dysuria, frequency, urgency).	Urinary stasis and an overdistended bladder promotes bacterial growth. Inadequately emptying the bladder and urinary tract trauma during the birth process predispose mother to a urinary tract infection.

DISCHARGE PLANNING/CONTINUITY OF CARE
- Encourage mother to make and keep medical follow-up appointments for self and infant.
- Review emergency numbers and telephone referral sources.
- Refer family for social services as needed (WIC).
- Refer to community resources as needed (Department of Health).
- Refer to new mother support groups.

OTHER PLANS OF CARE TO REFERENCE
- Child Abuse/Neglect
- Violence against Women
- Parenting
- Failure to Thrive
- Breastfeeding

BIBLIOGRAPHY
Beck, C. T. (1994). Critique of the influence of postpartum visits on clinic attendance. *Nursing Scan in Research, 7*(1), 13.

Garcia, J., Renfrew, M., & Marchant, S. (1994). Postnatal homevisiting by midwives. *Midwifery, 19*(1), 40–43.

Kroll, D., & Dwyer, D. (1994). Postnatal care: Teamwork in the community. *Modern Midwife, 4*(10), 10–13.

Vines, S. W. (1994.) Effects of a community health nursing parent-baby (ad)venture program on depression and other selected maternal-child health outcomes. *Public Health Nursing, 11*(3), 188–194.

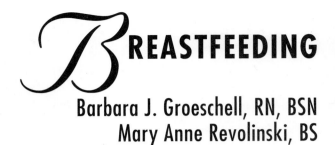

BREASTFEEDING

Barbara J. Groeschell, RN, BSN
Mary Anne Revolinski, BS

Breastfeeding is the best method of infant nutrition, and nurses should encourage and help mothers successfully diagnose effective, ineffective, and interrupted breastfeeding. In each case, the nurse has an opportunity to promote the breastfeeding relationship. With effective breastfeeding, the nurse should encourage the mother to continue, give her supportive information, and be able to answer any questions. With ineffective breastfeeding, it is crucial that the nurse identify the problem correctly and help the mother find a solution quickly. With interrupted breastfeeding (e.g., due to infant/mother separation or formula feeding), a nurse should be able to help a mother resume breastfeeding when that is the goal.

--- **Clinical Clip** ---

Breastfeeding
Advantages for baby

- Baby receives colostrum—baby's main defense against infection. Approximately half of a newborn's immunities come from colostrum. Colostrum has a laxative effect which helps baby pass meconium and is high in protein. Colostrum gradually changes to mature milk 10 days to 2 weeks after birth.
- Baby receives mother's milk, a superior infant food. It supplies all necessary nutrients in proper proportions. It digests easily because nutrients are easily absorbed and has a laxative effect so the baby is not constipated.
- It helps baby stay healthy and provides antibodies which protect against infection and illness. During sickness, it helps baby stay hydrated and speeds recovery. It also reduces the risk of allergies and reduces the risk of obesity later in life.
- General physical and emotional benefits. Promotes hand-eye coordination when baby is fed from both breasts. Promotes proper jaw, teeth, and speech development. Provides baby with emotional warmth—the building bonds of love.

Advantages for Mother

- Sucking stimulates hormones which contract the uterus after birth, thus reducing the risk of hemorrhaging.
- It helps mother return to prepregnancy weight faster (burns 500 calories a day).
- It helps mother get extra rest—night feedings are easier, less disruptive.
- Mother's body releases prolactin, or the "mother hormone," which helps her relax and makes mothering easier.
- It reduces the risk of breast cancer.
- It saves time and money.
- It makes going out with baby easier; the mother does not have to worry about food.
- It delays fertility if completely breastfeeding in most cases, i.e., no bottles, pacifiers, or solid food. However, when limiting or spacing family size is desired, alternative methods of protection should be considered.
- Close physical contact brings mother and baby closer together.
- There are physical differences in breastfeeding compared to bottle feeding which promote good feelings in the mother (e.g., baby's skin softer, bowel movements smell sweeter, spit-up does not stain clothing).
- Breastfeeding enables mother to comfort sick or unhappy baby, thus reducing her stress.

ETIOLOGIES

- Mother is well informed about the benefits of breastfeeding and how to get breastfeeding off to a good start.
- Mother is well informed about the benefits of breastfeeding but lacks basic information about starting breastfeeding.
- Mother has successfully breastfed previous children.

CLINICAL MANIFESTATIONS (PROBLEMS WITH BREASTFEEDING)

- Mother drowsy (from medication, complicated delivery); does not nurse baby immediately after delivery
- Feeds baby on a rigid schedule
- Bottles and/or pacifiers have been introduced
- Mother experiencing sore nipples
- Mother supplementing baby's diet (formula, water, juice, solids), and baby is refusing/fussy at breast
- Infant not gaining well, showing signs of dehydration, and/or sleepy/lethargic
- Mother concerned that baby is not getting enough—infant wants to nurse all the time

CLINICAL/DIAGNOSTIC FINDINGS (PROBLEMS WITH BREASTFEEDING)

- Baby is not gaining enough weight. Baby should regain birth weight (determined from lowest recorded weight) within 2–3 weeks of age, after which average weight gain is considered 4–8 oz/week.
- Infant is not well hydrated and wets less than five to six disposable or six to eight cloth diapers a day.

▶ NURSING DIAGNOSIS: *Effective Breastfeeding*

Related To baby thriving and doing well

Defining Characteristics

- Mother expresses desire to breastfeed but lacks knowledge.
- Mother has support system and can problem-solve if need arises.

Patient Outcomes

- Mother verbalizes and demonstrates correct techniques for breastfeeding.
- Breastfeeding begins and continues without difficulty.
- Mother verbalizes signs indicating infant's readiness to start solids.
- Mother has readily accessible support in case of problems.
- Mother states she is comfortable with normal breastfeeding patterns (i.e., breastfeeding "on demand").
- Mother does not use artificial nipples (i.e., bottle or pacifier).
- Baby is gaining weight and developing normally.

Nursing Interventions	Rationales
Assess mother's general knowledge and feeding techniques. Assess level of knowledge about proper positioning while breastfeeding, proper latch-on and sucking, and how to identify when baby is getting enough milk.	Patient teaching should be individualized according to patient needs. Assessing knowledge base helps identify patient needs.
Teach proper positioning. Mother should be comfortable and well supported while breastfeeding. Let her choose a comfortable nursing position. Mother should bring baby to breast and not lean into baby. Mother should support her nipple with four fingers underneath breast and thumb on top.	Mother is more relaxed when in comfortable position.
Teach proper latch-on techniques. Mother encourages her baby to open his or her mouth wide by tickling baby's lips with nipple, saying "open," and gently pulling down on baby's chin (see figure 31-1). Then quickly pull baby to breast and keeps infant close (see figure 31-2). The baby takes at least 1 in. of the areola into its mouth.	Proper latch-on will help avoid nipple trauma.
Teach proper sucking techniques. Baby is facing mother's breast so its head is not turned. Baby's chin and nose are touching breast (Figure 31-3). Baby's lips are flanged out and relaxed. (Mother can gently pull lips out if baby has sucked them in.) Baby's tongue is cupped underneath breast. (Check by pulling down on lower lip; tongue should be jutting forward as baby sucks.) Baby's ear and temple wiggle as it sucks. Baby swallows after every two to three sucks after mother's milk lets down for 5–10 min on each breast. Sucking will gradually decrease.	Proper positioning will decrease incidence of nipple trauma.

Nursing Interventions	Rationales
Teach mother how to remove baby from breast by first breaking suction by inserting her finger into baby's mouth.	This reduces nipple trauma.
Teach mother how to tell if baby is getting enough breast milk. Baby wets at least six to eight cloth (five to six disposable) diapers within a 24-h period. Urine is clear, not concentrated. (If a mother wants to check, have her pour ¼ cup of liquid in a dry diaper as a benchmark.) Baby has two to five bowel movements within a 24-h period during the first 6 weeks; it is normal for this to decrease after 6 weeks of age. Normal bowel movements are mustard colored and a loose, seedy consistency.	Normal urinary and bowel elimination patterns are evidence of adequate intake. Breastfed infants may have altered bowel consistency patterns, which are normal.
Teach mother how to care for herself while lactating: adequate diet, drinks to thirst, does not smoke or use drugs, gets enough rest, and does not overextend self.	Nutritious diet with good fluid intake and avoidance of drugs and alcohol promote optimal quality milk supply.
Encourage minimal elapsed time between birth and first feeding at breast.	Early breastfeeding promotes bonding and milk production and enhances uterine contraction/involution.
Encourage partner/family to support breastfeeding.	Support is an important element to success.
Encourage mother to breastfeed by discussing the benefits of breastfeeding.	Accurate information and support from health care providers are important elements to success.
Explain signs of readiness to start solids (usually around middle of first year): Baby needs to nurse more frequently, is sitting up, is interested in table food, and has teeth. Do not start solids before baby is ready.	Starting solids too early can shorten nursing time and can compromise nutrition by filling the baby up with carbohydrate instead of completely balanced mother's milk.

Nursing Interventions	Rationales
Inform mother about La Leche League International, a nonprofit breastfeeding organization.	As a support group and a resource for problem solving, La Leche League International can help contribute to a successful breastfeeding experience.

--- **Clinical Clip** ---

Proper Positions for Breastfeeding

Cradle Hold

Baby's stomach is pulled next to the mothers while the baby's ear, shoulder, and hip are in a straight line. A pillow can help support and bring the baby closer.

Football hold

The mother is sitting up with the baby clutched under the mother's arm. The baby's bottom is up against the couch with baby's feet pointing up. A pillow can help support the baby's back.

Side-lying

Both mother and baby are lying down, facing each other. The baby may be supported by pillows behind baby's back. The mother's head rests comfortably on her outstretched arm.

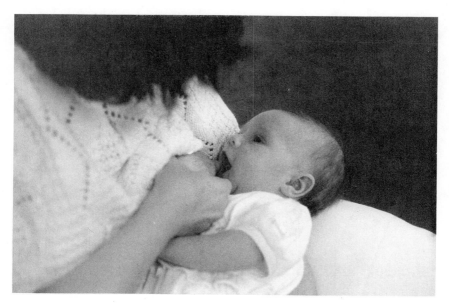

Figure 31-1.

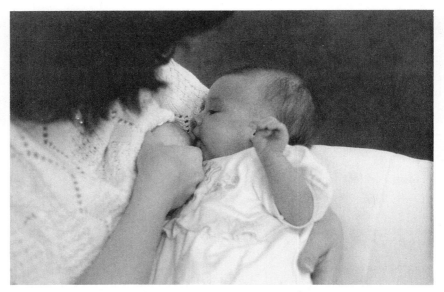

Figure 31-2.

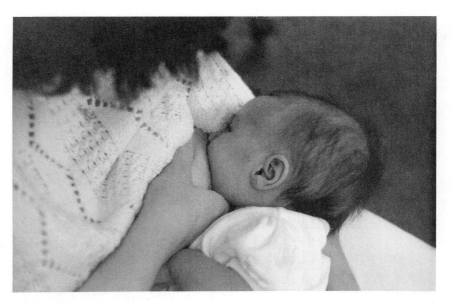

Figure 31-3. *Photos courtesy of La Leche League International.*

▶ NURSING DIAGNOSIS: *Ineffective Breastfeeding*

Related To mother's nipple soreness (irritated, red, cracked, or bleeding nipples)

Defining Characteristics
- Baby incorrectly positioned or latched on to breast
- Nipples constantly exposed to moisture
- Baby slipping from good position
- Sucking problems related to nipple confusion

Patient Outcomes
- Mother learns to correctly position baby at breast.
- Mother keeps nipples dry when not breastfeeding.
- Baby learns correct latch-on technique.
- Baby learns how to suck correctly at the breast.

Nursing Interventions	Rationales
Assess cause of nipple soreness by observing mother while breastfeeding and obtaining a detailed history.	Observation and a detailed history will indicate cause of soreness.
Teach mother proper positioning. It is sometimes helpful to have a doll handy to illustrate how to hold the baby. (See Effective Breastfeeding.)	A common cause of nipple soreness is improper positioning and latch on.
Teach the mother how to make sure baby latches on and sucks correctly.	Incorrect latch-on and sucking can cause nipple trauma.
Instruct mother about proper nipple care for sore nipples. Express some breast milk on sore nipples after nursing and let dry. Avoid creams, oils, and nipple shields.	Live antibodies in the milk will help heal any nipple lesions. Nipple shields may increase nipple trauma.
Keep nipples as dry as possible. Wear a nursing bra with the flaps down. Change wet nursing pads frequently.	Moisture can cause macerated tissue and promotes bacterial growth.
Nurse baby in a different position at each feeding.	Baby's mouth will put greatest pressure on different parts of nipple to give sore areas more time to heal.
Monitor nipple soreness for signs of healing and/or signs and symptoms of infection.	Nipple soreness may take several days to resolve. Evidence of infection will require further therapy and may rarely require temporary cessation of nursing.

Clinical Clip

Interrupted Breastfeeding

When breastfeeding has been interrupted (because of illness, mother/baby hospitalization, or the baby has been weaned from the breast), often breastfeeding can be resumed. This procedure is known as relactation. Its success will depend directly on the mother's motivation and the length of time the baby has been away from the breast. Relactation can be accomplished with the help of a good reference, such as *An Overview of Solutions to Breastfeeding and Sucking Problems* by Susan Meintz Maher, (1988), or contacting a local lactation consultant or a La Leche League leader.

▶ NURSING DIAGNOSIS: *Ineffective Breastfeeding*

Related To nipple confusion; i.e., baby has been given artificial nipples and can no longer suck effectively at the breast

Defining Characteristics
- Baby pushes nipple out of mouth and cries in frustration.
- Baby sucks at breast as if it were a bottle, causing sore nipples.
- Baby refuses and/or is fussy at the breast.

Patient Outcomes
- Mother stops using artificial nipples.
- Baby breastfeeds without difficulties.

Nursing Interventions	Rationales
Explain to mother the differences between sucking at the breast and bottle. Bottle feeding does not require the baby to open its mouth wide; thus, when breastfeeding, baby may only open its mouth partially, causing trauma to the nipple. Baby hardly needs to suck at the bottle because liquid drips out quite readily. In fact, baby learns to block too much liquid from bottle by pressing its tongue up to stop flow. This sucking action will push the	Information about nipple confusion will discourage casual use of artificial nipples.

Nursing Interventions	Rationales
mother's nipple out of baby's mouth when breastfeeding. Instead of flanging lips against breast, when sucking at a bottle, baby clamps down around smaller artificial nipple. This sucking technique will cause nipple pain and can delay mother's let-down reflex. With a bottle, baby is used to being met with an instant flood of liquid. At the breast, baby can easily become frustrated while waiting for milk to let down.	
Encourage mother to breastfeed every 2 h, paying special attention to good positioning and latch-on techniques.	This problem can usually be corrected over a 24-h period if mother avoids all artificial nipples.
Teach her alternative feeding methods if necessary (i.e. syringe, eye dropper, cup, or soft spoon) to use while persuading baby to take breast.	When intake is inadequate, a supplement can maintain hydration and caloric intake.
Instruct mother to express some milk before feeding to get milk flowing. This can be phased out once the baby is effectively sucking at breast.	Initiating a let-down prior to latch-on will encourage the baby, who is used to ready milk flow from bottle feeding.
Measure how much supplemental formula mother gives. If mother gives a lot of formula, caution her to reduce the amount slowly while she builds her milk supply. Do not give formula by bottle.	Mother's milk supply will increase with increased stimulation over a 24–48-h period.
Monitor baby's wet and dirty diapers to ensure that baby is getting enough breast milk.	Infant should have six to eight wet diapers daily and one to two stools.

▶ **NURSING DIAGNOSIS:** *Ineffective Breastfeeding*

Related To baby's slow weight gain

Defining Characteristics

- Baby is gaining less than 4–8 oz/week, losing weight, or exhibiting an inconsistent growth pattern.
- Mother is feeding on a rigid schedule.
- Mother only lets baby nurse for short periods of time.
- Baby only nurses from one breast at each feeding.
- Baby is improperly positioned at the breast.
- Baby receives supplements/artificial nipples.
- Baby is very sleepy and mother does not wake baby to nurse.

Patient Outcomes

- Baby's weight gain picks up to 4–8 oz/week.
- Mother verbalizes what caused slow weight gain and how to prevent its recurrence.

Nursing Interventions	Rationales
Assess baby's growth history. Include weight and growth parameters. Monitor weight as needed.	Baby's weight gain does not match normal growth patterns. Weight loss is normal for the first 3–4 days after birth. Normally, babies regain birth weight within 2–3 weeks after birth. Typical weight gain for the first 6 months after birth is 4–8 oz per week.
Instruct mother to nurse at least 10–12 times in a 24-h period.	Frequent feedings are needed to ensure growth and increase mother's milk supply.
Instruct mother to have baby nurse from each breast for 10–20 min.	This ensures that baby is getting the "hind milk," which is high in fat and calories. It also increases milk supply.
Show mother proper positioning and latch-on, necessary if baby is to get adequate nourishment.	Baby must grasp enough areolar tissue to empty and stimulate the milk ducts.
Instruct mother to wake a sleepy baby every 1½ h during the day and every three hours at night.	Babies should nurse 10–12 times per day.
Encourage mother to make nursing baby her priority for the next 24–48 h.	It takes 24–48 h to significantly increase her milk supply.

▶ NURSING DIAGNOSIS: *Ineffective Breastfeeding*

Related To infant wanting to constantly nurse

Defining Characteristics
- Mother feels baby wants to nurse all the time.
- Mother has bottle-fed previous children.
- Mother lacks knowledge of normal breastfeeding patterns.

Patient Outcomes
- Mother verbalizes how often and how long the average breastfed baby needs to nurse.
- Mother verbalizes how much breastfeeding meets baby's emotional needs.

Nursing Interventions	Rationales
Teach mother about normal nursing patterns. Baby should feed every 1 ½–3 h (from the start of one feeding to the start of the next feeding). Allow baby plenty of time at each breast.	Mothers often lack knowledge of normal breastfeeding patterns. Unlike formula, breast milk is readily digested, and frequent feedings are considered normal. Babies nurse for emotional as well as nutritional needs. Nonnutritive sucking allows the baby to be at the breast without fear of overfeeding. If nipples are sore, avoid nonnutritive sucking until nipples heal.
Encourage mother to let baby nurse on demand.	Stressing proper positioning and latch-on avoids nipple soreness.
Teach mother that breastfeeding meets baby's emotional needs.	Breastfeeding not only provides nourishment but also ensures plenty of necessary skin-to-skin contact. It also acts as a reminder of the womb and comforter for baby by hearing mother's voice, by smelling mother, and by hearing mother's heartbeat.

DISCHARGE PLANNING/CONTINUITY OF CARE
- Encourage mother to continue breastfeeding for as long as possible. The American Academy of Pediatrics recommends breastfeeding for at least 12 months.
- Refer to breast pump suppliers, if needed.

- Refer to La Leche League International, a nonprofit breastfeeding organization. Mothers interested in receiving breastfeeding support and/or attending monthly meetings can call 1-800-La Leche for the phone number of a local leader.
- Refer to lactation consultant.

REFERENCES/BIBLIOGRAPHY

Laurvers, J., & Waessner, C. (1983). *Counseling the nursing mother.* Wayne, NJ: Arrery Publishing Group.

Maher, S. M. (1988). *An overview of solutions to breastfeeding and sucking problems.* Franklin Park, IL: IBCLC, La Leche League Internations.

Mohrbacker, N., & Stock, J. (1991). *The breastfeeding answer book.* Franklin Park, IL: La Leche League International.

Cahill, M. A., Froehlich, E., Kerwin, M., Lennon, V., Tompson, M., Wagner, B., & White, M. (1991). *The womanly art of breastfeeding.* Franklin Park, IL: La Leche League International.

*U*RINARY INCONTINENCE

Susan Breakwell, RN, MS

Urinary incontinence (UI) is a symptom defined as the involuntary loss of urine of enough magnitude to be a problem. It is not a condition but a set of symptoms. Types of UI include:

- transient: involuntary loss of urine in which contributing factors are often reversible
- urge: involuntary loss of urine with a strong and often sudden sense of urgency to void
- stress: involuntary loss of urine occurring with activities that cause increased abdominal pressure, such as coughing, running, laughing, or sneezing
- overflow: involuntary loss of urine occurring when bladder is overdistended
- functional: involuntary loss of urine caused by chronic physical or cognitive impairment
- mixed: a combination of types of incontinence, generally urge and stress incontinence

Incontinence is commonly confused with toileting. Incontinence is an involuntary loss of urine while toileting refers to the activities related to using the bathroom or bedpan for elimination, including locating the bathroom, undressing, and positioning for voiding. Incontinence is a physical problem while toileting is a mobility problem.

Clinical Clip

The prevalence of incontinence varies; it goes as high as 25–30% for noninstitutionalized individuals over age 60 and 50% or more in the nursing home population (Urinary Incontinence Guideline Panel, 1992b). The physical, psychological, social, and financial impact of incontinence is extensive.

It is often underreported or hidden from health care providers or significant others even though many factors causing the incontinence can be ameliorated. Basic diagnostic testing and treatment has been underutilized, yet untreated incontinence is one of the most devastating problems an individual (especially an aged person) may face.

ETIOLOGIES

Transient incontinence
- infection
- fecal impaction
- weakness of supporting pelvic muscles
- atrophic urethritis/vaginitis
- excessive urine production
- medications, particularly diuretic and mind-altering drugs
- altered mental status, including confusion and depression
- limited mobility
- inadequate toileting facilities
- environmental factors

Urge incontinence
- involuntary detrusor contractions
- detrusor hyperactivity with impaired contractility of the bladder

Stress incontinence
- urethral hypermobility
- urethral sphincter weakness

Overflow incontinence
- obstruction of bladder outlet or urethra
- neurological conditions
- fecal impaction

Functional incontinence
- bladder cancer
- urethral and/or bladder anatomical abnormalities

CLINICAL MANIFESTATIONS
- Acknowledged history of incontinence
- Urinary frequency, urgency, burning sensation, polyuria
- Constipation, fecal impaction
- Odor
- Decreased attention to bladder cues
- Use of protective clothing, bedding
- Difficulty using bathroom without assistance
- Decreased fluid intake
- Vaginal atrophy, discharge, tenderness
- Social isolation, changes in socialization habits
- Restricted mobility
- Medication regimen
- Direct observation of urination for hesitancy, staining, altered urine stream

CLINICAL/DIAGNOSTIC FINDINGS

- Urinalysis/culture and sensitivity (C&S) reveals presence of infection [i.e., positive leukocytes, red blood cells (RBC's), bacteriuria] or other abnormalities
- Urine for cytology
- Voiding diary to serve as a baseline and help determine cause(s) and contributing factors to incontinence
- Stress testing for urine loss with coughing, sneezing
- Blood tests for abnormal blood urea nitrogen (BUN) or creatinine levels
- Measuring postvoided residual via abdominal assessment, catheterization, or pelvic ultrasound; inadequate emptying >200 cc residual
- Urodynamic tests (cystometry, cystometrogram, uroflowmetry)
- Urethral pressure profilometry (videourodynamics, electromyclography)
- Endoscopic cystourethroscopy

▶ NURSING DIAGNOSIS: *Altered Urinary Elimination*

Related To

- Infection
- Weak pelvic floor muscles
- Sphincter or bladder
- Enlarged prostate
- Constipation/fecal impaction
- Immobility
- Medications
- Dementia

Defining Characteristics

- Observed urine stains/soiled clothing/bedding
- Odor
- Observed episodes of urinary incontinence
- Affirmative patient response to open-ended question about incontinence (e.g., "Do you ever lose urine when you do not want to?" "Do you have any trouble with your bladder?")
- Demonstrated or reported difficulty with ADLs including self-dressing and self-toileting
- Observed absence of readily available and "user-friendly" toileting facilities

Patient Outcomes

Episodes of incontinence will stop or diminish in occurrence, as evidenced by:

- patient self-report (diary or verbal).
- decreased observable signs of incontinent episodes (i.e., bedding, clothing, odor).
- evidence of readily accessible toileting facilities.

Nursing Interventions	Rationales
Thorough physical, functional, and mental assessment.	Incontinence is a collection of symptoms which may need specifically targeted interventions.
Monitor and assess for fluid intake.	Adequate fluid intake (generally 2,000–3,000 mL/24 h) helps bladder to fill to normal capacity. Decreased fluid intake may exacerbate constipation, cystitis, and dehydration, leading to further incontinence.
Encourage/assure adequate intake of appropriate fluids.	Avoid caffeine, a bladder irritant. Inadequate hydration can lead to decreased attention to bladder cues and inadequate bladder filling, thus exacerbating incontinent episodes.
Maintain urine output or toileting record, including frequency, consistency, odor, volume, and color.	This provides additional information necessary to find and intervene in other underlying causes of incontinence.
Perform additional testing, including urinalysis, urine C&S, and blood work for BUN and creatinine levels.	Additional testing may be needed to adequately evaluate cause(s) of incontinence and establish specific treatments.

▶ NURSING DIAGNOSIS: *Self-Care Deficit, Toileting*

Related To difficulty accessing or using toilet facilities

Defining Characteristics
- Ineffective toileting skills with resulting episodes of UI

Patient Outcomes
Patient will:
- eliminate or minimize environmental roadblocks to effective continence program.
- verbalize/demonstrate use of effective toileting techniques to minimize UI.
- identify additional sources of help.

Nursing Interventions	Rationales
Assist patient and/or caregivers to establish a toileting schedule.	Patient may have altered cognitive functioning or decreased warning time. A regular schedule and regular cueing can diminish the effects of these problems on achieving continence.
Physical and verbal cueing may be needed.	Incontinent individuals may be more dependent in performing basic ADLs.
Minimize environmental roadblocks such as poor lighting, toilet of inappropriate height, cluttered pathway to bathroom, or poorly marked bathroom.	Eliminating factors which can increase the time between urge to urinate and getting properly positioned for urination in the bathroom can diminish the number of incontinent episodes.
Teach/monitor use of Kegel exercises when appropriate.	Techniques such as these can effectively decrease episodes of incontinence by strengthening pelvic floor muscles, thereby improving control over urination.
Teach behavioral techniques, including individualized positive reinforcers and consistent behavioral expectations, to appropriate patients and their caregivers.	Negative behavior patterns that may be contributing to continued incontinence can be gradually and positively modified using behavior modification techniques.
Provide information about additional sources of help for UI, including Help for Incontinent Persons (HIP), the Simon Foundation, and local incontinence clinics.	Additional resources can provide advocacy, support, and educational programs.
Offer emotional support and encouragement and allow patient/caregiver to ventilate.	There is social stigma related to incontinence. Individuals tend to believe that it is an inevitability of old age or that it cannot be treated. It may take several months to see significant improvement.
Teach good skin care and use of protective clothing or bedding (e.g., adult diapers, pads).	Skin needs to be clean and dry to prevent skin irritation, skin breakdown, and odor.

Nursing Interventions	Rationales
Coordinate findings and activities with the patient, caregivers, and other health care providers.	Communication and coordination with patient, caregivers, physicians, and other health care providers is crucial for effective patient care.

DISCHARGE PLANNING/CONTINUITY OF CARE

- Evaluate patient need for follow-up services after discharge from health care facility. Initiate referral to appropriate additional resources at least 2 days before discharge. Coordinating treatment with other health care providers for follow-through teaching and monitoring enhances patient outcomes.
- Refer patient for homemaker/home health aide services to assist with ADLs.
- Refer to specialist/incontinence clinic for necessary follow-up.
- Refer patient to support and self-help groups as needed.

REFERENCES/BIBLIOGRAPHY

Breakwell, S., & Walker, S. (1988). Differences in physical health, social interaction and personal adjustment between continent and incontinent homebound aged women. *Journal of Community Health Nursing, 5,* 19–31.

Cramer, D. (Ed.) (1993). Promoting continence: Strategies for success. *Perspectives in health promotion and aging.* Eldercare Institute on Health Promotion. Washington, DC: AARP.

Mitteness, L. S. (1992). Social aspects of urinary incontinence in the elderly. *AORN Journal, 5,* 731–737.

Newman, D. K. (1993). A guideline for the nation: Managing urinary incontinence. *Journal of Home Health Care Practice, 5,* 33–44.

Powers, I., & Williams, D. (1992). Urinary incontinence. Helping a patient regain control. *Nursing 92, 22,* 46–47.

Urinary Incontinence Guideline Panel. (1992a). *Urinary incontinence in adults: Clinical practice guideline.* AHCPR Publication 92-0038. Rockville, MD: Agency for Healthcare Policy and Research.

Urinary Incontinence Guideline Panel. (1992b). *Urinary incontinence in adults. Quick reference guide for clinicians.* AHCPR Publication 92-0041. Rockville, MD: Agency for Healthcare Policy and Research.

Warlemtom, R. (1992). Implementation of a urinary continence program. *Journal of Gerontological Nursing, 18,* 31–37.

CHRONIC RENAL FAILURE

Sally A. Steinhiser, RN, MSN

Chronic renal failure (CRF) is a functional diagnosis characterized by a persistent, progressive, and generally irreversible decline in glomerular filtration rate wherein there is little or no hope for significant improvement in kidney function. End-stage renal disease (ESRD) is the usual consequence of CRF, necessitating renal function replacement therapy, i.e., dialysis or renal transplantation. Most typically, this phenomenon develops slowly over the course of months and years, resulting from one- or multiple-disease processes or manifestations. In certain instances [e.g., rapidly progressive glomerulonephritis (RPGN) or associated diseases or diagnoses], the clinical course leading to this outcome is shorter, taking place or occurring over weeks to months.

The prognosis of a patient with ESRD depends primarily on the underlying cause of the CRF as well as the ability to prevent hyperkalemia, fluid overload, and congestive heart failure, all of which complicate renal failure.

The nurse's overall role is to identify complications, reinforce management plan and protocols, and provide emotional support.

ETIOLOGIES

Intrinsic renal disease
- glomerulonephritis (membranous, proliferative, membranoproliferative, crescentic, Berger's disease, congenital)
- interstitial (renal medullary) pylonephritis
- interstitial renal tubular (Fanconi's syndrome, analgesic abuse, heavy-metal intoxication)

Systemic disorders
- hypertensive (cardiovascular) renal disease (essential hypertension)
- diabetes mellitus
- collagen vascular disease (disseminated systemic lupus erythematosus (SLE), Wegener's granulomatosis)

Obstructive uropathy (e.g., hallmark—hydronephrosis)
- renal calculi
- prostatism
- congenital anomalies
- retroperitoneal fibrosis
- neoplasm
- urethral stricture
- bladder neck obstruction
- neurogenic bladder

Vascular disease
- arterial, arteriolar nephrosclerosis (hypertension, hypertensive cardiovascular renal disease, diabetes mellitus)
- renal vein thrombosis

CLINICAL MANIFESTATIONS
- Azotemia
- Uremia
- Edema
- Shortness of breath
- Pruritus
- Peripheral neuropathy (restless-leg syndrome)
- Nausea, vomiting
- Malnutrition, muscle wasting
- Fatigue
- Malaise
- Depression

CLINICAL/DIAGNOSTIC FINDINGS
- Elevated blood urea nitrogen (BUN) and creatinine
- Creatinine clearance reduced to <10%
- Serum electrolyte imbalance (hyperkalemia, hyper- or hypomagnesium, acidosis)
- Chronic anemia [reduced hemoglobin (Hgb) and hematocrit (Hct)]
- Renal Osteodystrophy (hypocalcemia, hyperphosphatemia, secondary hyperparathyroidism)
- Renal imaging and biopsy that confirm disease process

▶ NURSING DIAGNOSIS: *Knowledge Deficit*

Related To
- Disease process and potential complications
- Dietary modifications and restrictions, lifestyle changes
- Treatment procedures, supplies, and equipment (related to home dialysis patients)

Defining Characteristics
- Newly diagnosed
- Verbalizes lack of knowledge about disease process, potential complications, dietary modifications, lifestyle changes, treatment, and procedures

- Develops complications (i.e., fluid overload, hyperkalemia, hyperphosphatemia, hypocalcemia)
- Low score on verbal or written quizzing to assess knowledge base

Patient Outcomes

Patient will:

- describe disease process and identify possible complications.
- list signs and symptoms of most common and potentially life-threatening complication and limits after which medical help should and must be sought.
- identify dietary modifications and restrictions.
- avoid complications of which patient has control.
- achieve acceptable score on written quiz to assess knowledge base.
- successfully perform home peritoneal dialysis procedure (if applicable).
- completely manage home dialysis treatment and supplies (if applicable).

Nursing Interventions	Rationales
Assess current knowledge base and potential for understanding the disease process, possible complications, dietary modifications, lifestyle changes, medications, treatments, and procedures.	Teaching is individualized to match patient need, pace, and intellectual ability and capacity.
Establish relationship with multidisciplinary care team members at the ESRD facility.	Frequent, on-going and open communication between the nurse and the outpatient dialysis facility staff offers an additional source for input and participation and allows nurse to reinforce information consistently using the nursing process to maximize quality care interventions and minimize complications.
Reinforce patient teaching initiated by ESRD facility staff.	Generally, the ESRD facility medical, nursing, dietary, and social service staff provide ongoing patient education during the in-center dialysis treatments. Follow-up reinforcement and demonstrating how to apply concepts and activities in the home offer an opportunity for improved understanding and implementing care plans and goals.

Nursing Interventions	Rationales
Reinforce importance of dietary compliance, assuring understanding of nutritional needs and restrictions. Utilize creative teaching techniques, including written, verbal, and pictorial demonstrations to assist in patient comprehension.	Understanding dietary requirements and limitations will minimize complications related to dietary indiscretions.
Assure understanding of medication regimen and how to obtain prescribed drugs.	The dialysis patient medication regimen is complex and ever-changing. Ongoing review with demonstrations will increase probability of appropriate medication administration and minimize complications associated with the disease process.
Assure newly diagnosed patient referral to formal home dialysis training program, if appropriate and available.	Patients must successfully complete a comprehensive home dialysis teaching and training program provided by a Medicare-certified ESRD facility.
If the patient is on peritoneal dialysis, observe the patient performing the peritoneal dialysis fluid exchange procedure, assuring appropriate use of aseptic and sterile techniques and accurate medication administration. Consult the ESRD facility nursing staff, if appropriate.	Such observations can identify real and potential problems and complications with home patient therapy, including risk for infections or errors in medication administration.

▶ NURSING DIAGNOSIS: *Infection*

Related To dialysis access, break in aseptic technique, reduced immune response due to chronic illness

Defining Characteristics

Hemodialysis
- Fever, chills
- Tenderness, pain, inflammation, drainage at access site
- Leukocytosis
- Organism identification in specimen(s) obtained, e.g., site drainage, blood

Peritoneal Dialysis
- Fever, chills
- Abdominal tenderness, pain
- Drainage at catheter exit site
- Cloudy peritoneal dialysis fluid
- Leukocytosis
- Organism identification in specimen(s) obtained, e.g., site drainage, blood, peritoneal dialysis fluid

Patient Outcomes
Patient will:
- be asymptomatic.
- lack drainage at access site.
- have clear peritoneal dialysis fluid.
- have negative follow-up culture reports.

Nursing Interventions	Rationales
Assess for signs and symptoms of infection. Identifying a single or multiple defining characteristic warrants contacting the attending nephrologist immediately for medical assessment and intervention.	Suspecting or identifying a dialysis access infection is a critical situation, and initiating medical treatment is imperative and urgent. Therapies generally include the following: hemodialysis patients require parenteral antibiotics, which may be initially administered in an acute care center (e.g., Emergency Room) with subsequent infusions given in conjunction with the hemodialysis treatment. Peritoneal dialysis patients may begin self-administered intraperitoneal antibiotic therapy. Obtaining the requisite blood and additional specimen samples before initiating therapy ensures that organisms are properly identified and the most appropriate antibiotic regimen is selected.
Assess and evaluate the patient performing self-care procedures using dialysis access site care. Offer recommendations for improving technique. Consult the ESRD facility nursing staff, as appropriate.	An indwelling catheter provides a vulnerable site for bacterial growth and subsequent infection, leading to sepsis. Meticulous, methodical care and sterile technique must be used when providing catheter care

Nursing Interventions	Rationales
	(for either hemo or peritoneal dialysis access).
Assess patient's general hygiene and home (environmental) cleanliness and conditions, specifically observing for potential sources of contamination or infection. Encourage good hygienic techniques, addressing all general health care needs and concerns and especially emphasizing frequent hand washing, bathing, and oral and dental care.	Attention to excellent hygienic measures will minimize the risk and incidence of related infections.
Assess and evaluate the patient performing the peritoneal dialysis procedures. Identify any break in sterile technique. Provide recommendations for improvement, as appropriate. Notify ESRD facility nursing staff of observations and suggestions.	Continually entering into the peritoneal cavity enhances the risk for introducing pathogens, thus leading to infection. Absolute sterile technique must be used when performing peritoneal dialysis fluid exchanges.

▶ NURSING DIAGNOSIS: *Ineffective Coping*

Related To chronic illness, loss of control, time management, role changes, patient and family lifestyle changes

Defining Characteristics
- Mood and behavior extremes and swings
- Expressing anxiety, dysphoria, hopelessness, helplessness, nonaccepting, flat affect, depression, suicidal thoughts
- Noncompliance/rebellion
- Confrontational/argumentative
- Inflexible
- Indifference/withdrawal
- Self-destructive/suicidal gestures
- Indiscretions with treatment, medications, diet, and fluid management
- Inappropriately prioritizing health care and related problems and issues
- Dysfunctional (counterfunctional) family relations and behaviors

Patient Outcomes
Patient will:

- adhere to prescribed treatment regimen, including schedule, medications, diet, and fluid management.
- verbalize feeling of acceptance and empowerment over life.
- develop independence in modified lifestyle activities.
- enjoy participation in family and social events.

Nursing Interventions	Rationales
Explore and assess emotional response and adjustment to chronic illness, treatment regimens, role, family, and lifestyle changes. Allow patient maximal time to express feelings while observing associated behaviors. Be alert for subtle and obviously troubled and dysfunctional actions. Use nonjudgmental and therapeutic communication techniques.	Requisite adaptation to chronic illness, with associated vast and multiple changes, can be and frequently is overwhelming and devastating to patients and families. Feelings and emotions are sometimes difficult to verbalize and express and often will conflict with actual observed behaviors.
Identify ineffective coping characteristics or demonstrated regimen indiscretions. Discuss actions and subsequent consequences to assure appropriate knowledge base. Begin to explore and identify patient's rationale for behavior.	Often indiscretions in treatment regimens reflect rebellious behavior resulting from the patient's feeling a (real or imagined) loss of control. Allowing the patient as much control as possible and offering options in treatment regimen for patient selection can maximize the feeling of control. This can minimize these self-destructive and "acting-out" behaviors.
Assess patient time management, prioritizing, and categorizing skills. Assist with understanding, sorting, organizing, and arranging identified activities, needs, and concerns. Inform patient about the ramifications of their choices. Allow patient to make decisions; however, offer alternatives and compromises as appropriate.	This approach supports positive feelings of control and worthiness. In addition, it may help reestablish a "role" within the family unit and a feeling of contribution to the family lifestyle.

Nursing Interventions	Rationales
Assess for ongoing or severe extremes in coping actions and behaviors. Initiate additional support therapies, e.g., behavior modification techniques or psychological or psychiatric consult. Assure appropriate patient referral.	If successful adaptation does not occur as behaviors become more severe—and sometimes even life threatening—psychological consultation, support, or therapy is required.

DISCHARGE PLANNING/CONTINUITY OF CARE
- Assure availability of multidisciplinary care team for support and assistance in routine concerns and for emergent situations.
- Assure patient exercises good judgment in trouble-shooting and problem solving, and thereby understands limitations and is knowledgeable of how to call for assistance.
- Establish dialysis treatment schedule with ESRD facility.
- Identify follow-up therapy and clinical appointments.
- Assure availability of home care medication, supplies, and equipment.

OTHER PLANS OF CARE TO REFERENCE
- Medication Noncompliance
- Grief/Loss

BIBLIOGRAPHY
Czyrny, J. J. (1994). Rehabilitation of amputees with end-stage renal disease: functional outcome and cost. *American Journal of Physical Medicine and Rehabilitation, 73*(5), 353–357.

Oberley, E. T. (1994). Nursing interventions for rehabilitating renal patients. *Anna Journal, 21*(7), 407–411.

Oldrizzi, L. (1994). Nutrition and the kidney: How to manage patients with renal failure. *Nutrition in Clinical Practice, 9*(1), 3–10.

Shoop, K. L. (1994). Pruritis in end stage renal disease. *Anna Journal, 21*(2), 147–153.

$\mathcal{S}$KIN CARE

Jennifer A. Dore, RN, MSN, CETN

The skin is the largest organ system in the human body. It serves multiple functions, including protection, thermal regulation, and transmission of sensation. The skin is composed of three distinct layers: epidermis, dermis, and subcutaneous tissue.

The degree of damage to these tissue layers determines wound healing and the treatment plan. The wound is a partial-thickness injury when it is limited to the epidermis and the superficial dermal layer. Healing occurs with the inflammatory response and is followed by reepithelialization. A full-thickness injury extends through the dermis, involving the subcutaneous tissue and possibly deeper structures of fascia, muscle, or bone. Healing involves all three phases of wound repair: inflammation, proliferation, and maturation (see Table 34-1).

Many wounds encountered in the home care setting are considered chronic and exhibit prolonged or ineffective healing despite appropriate treatment. Managing these chronic wounds is a challenge due to the patient's underlying systemic disease. Therefore, nurses must assess for and prevent breakdown in the high-risk patient. Care is based on the wound etiology, underlying disease processes, and appropriate topical therapy.

ETIOLOGIES

Mechanical (external forces applied to skin)
- pressure greater than capillary closing pressure (25–32 mm Hg)
- friction
- shear forces

Chemical irritation/moisture
- feces
- urine
- intestinal secretions
- wound drainage

Vascular disease (see PVD chapter)
- venous stasis
- arterial insufficiency

Surgical wounds
- incisions
- percutaneous tubes (e.g., G-tubes, nephrostomy tubes)
- surgical drains (e.g., JP, penrose)

Infection (e.g., candida, herpes, impetigo)

Thermal/burn

CLINICAL MANIFESTATIONS
- Loss of one or more skin layers
- Presence of tubes, drains, or incisions
- Color change (erythema, cyanosis, pallor)
- Drainage
- Foul odor
- Warmth and swelling
- Pain at wound site

CLINICAL/DIAGNOSTIC FINDINGS
- Elevated temperature (>100.4 F)
- Positive cultures of wound, which indicates infection
- Low albumin/protein, which may predispose patient to skin breakdown
- Peripheral dopplers that show poor circulation [see also Peripheral Vascular Disease (PVD) chapter for additional vascular tests]

▶ NURSING DIAGNOSIS: *High Risk for Altered Skin Integrity*

Risk Factors
- Aging skin
- Malnutrition
- Chronic disease (e.g., diabetes, PVD, immunosuppression, hepatitis, chronic renal failure)
- Certain medications (e.g., corticosteroids)
- Immobility
- Loss of sensation
- Altered level of consciousness
- Incontinence

Patient Outcomes
- Patient's skin will remain intact.

Nursing Interventions	Rationales
Instruct patient to drink 6–8 glasses of fluid a day if medical condition permits. Lubricate skin with a lanolin or petrolatum-based moisturizer (Eucerin, Keri). Avoid massage over bony prominences.	Dry skin will rip and tear more easily. The aging process and corticosteroids reduce collagen in skin and make it more easily injured. Hydration and lubrication will reduce risk of injury. Massage may cause deep-tissue trauma.
Assess nutritional status and daily intake of food and fluids. If available, assess blood albumin and protein levels. If malnourished, instruct in good nutritional intake (see Nutrition chapter). Weigh patient weekly.	A decrease in subcutaneous tissue and muscle mass reduces padding between skin and underlying structures. This increases susceptibility to skin breakdown. Malnutrition increases risk of infection and skin breakdown. Weekly weights avoid measuring short-term fluid fluctuations.
Reinforce management of underlying chronic disease. (See chapters on diabetes, PVD, HIV, chronic renal failure.)	The skin's condition mirrors the patient's state of health.
For immobile patients, change position at least every 2 h.	Decreases pressure over bony prominences.
Provide pressure reduction devices, such as mattress overlays and chair cushions. Avoid donuts.	This redistributes the patient's weight over a larger surface area. Donuts cause venous congestion and edema; they decrease pressure in one area but increase pressure in surrounding areas.
Use elbow and heel protector devices. Use lift sheets rather than dragging patient up in bed.	This decreases shearing and friction forces.
If incontinent, assess why patient is incontinent. If possible, bowel/bladder train (see Incontinence and Spinal Cord Injury chapters).	The cause of bowel and bladder incontinence may be easily diagnosed and treated, thereby eliminating a risk factor for skin breakdown.
Use diapers only when necessary. Keep perineum clean and dry. Check and change diaper frequently. Apply moisture barrier products after cleansing following each incontinent episode. Use	Urine and stool are chemical irritants and moisture macerates the skin, leading to skin breakdown. Keeping skin clean, dry, and free of moisture will reduce the risk of skin breakdown.

Nursing Interventions	Rationales
cornstarch-based or antifungal powder in skin folds as needed.	

▶ **NURSING DIAGNOSIS:** *Altered Skin Integrity—Open Wounds*
Related To pressure, venous stasis, ischemic, and neuropathic ulcers

Defining Characteristics
• Partial- or full-thickness skin loss

Patient Outcomes
• Patient's skin integrity is restored in a comfortable and cost effective manner.

Nursing Interventions	Rationales
Assess etiology of wound. Manage underlying disease process, if possible (see PVD, Diabetes, Chronic Renal Failure, Hepatitis, Nutrition chapters).	An effective treatment plan is based upon the wound etiology.
Initiate all preventive measures discussed in first nursing diagnosis, as applicable.	An effective treatment plan will minimize effect of and treat underlying cause.
Assess open wound, including location, size, and depth in centimeters, presence of undermined areas and sinus tracks inside the wound, presence of exudate or odor, condition of tissue in wound bed (granulation/red, necrosis/black, slough/yellow), and condition of intact skin surrounding wound (inflammation, induration, maceration, tenderness).	Establishes baseline prior to initiating treatment and provides a comparison during treatment as an objective measurement of wound healing.
Identify clinical signs of wound infection (fever, increased exudate, odor, surrounding inflammation, or cellulitis). Obtain wound culture only if above signs are present.	All open wounds are colonized with bacteria, but not all are infected. Infection occurs when the bacterial load in the wound overwhelms the defense mechanisms of

Nursing Interventions	Rationales
Call physician for antibiotic order or emergency care.	the host. Infection prolongs the inflammatory phase of wound healing, interferes with the production of collagen, and causes additional tissue destruction.
Eliminate nonviable tissue (necrosis or slough). If a large amount of non-viable tissue is present, refer to physician for sharp debridement. Debridement is not appropriate in an ischemic ulcer with dry eschar unless signs of local wound infection are present. If a small amount of nonviable tissue is present, consider other forms of debridement: 1. mechanical, via wet-to-dry gauze dressings with normal saline; 2. autolytic, via moisture retentive dressings, including hydrocolloids, hydrogels, and transparent adhesive dressings (see table 34-2); and 3. chemical, via topical debriding enzymes (e.g., elase, collagenase, travase) (requires physician order).	Nonviable tissue provides an excellent medium for bacterial growth. Wet-to-dry dressings will facilitate removal of necrotic tissue but will also disrupt viable tissue in the wound bed. Discontinue wet-to-dry gauze when wound begins to granulate. Autolytic debridement via moisture-retentive dressings enhances the body's own natural debridement mechanisms by trapping white blood cells and enzymes under the dressing. This method is contraindicated in the infected wound or in the immuno-compromised patient who is not able to produce sufficient white cells to prevent infection.
Cleanse the wound with normal saline. In the infected or necrotic wound, irrigate with a 19-gauge needle and 35-cc syringe. In the clean, granulating wound, irrigate with a piston syringe or gently wipe with a saline-moistened gauze.	Wound irrigation with a 19-gauge needle and 35-cc syringe provides the appropriate pressure (8 psi) to remove foreign debris and bacteria. In the clean wound, gentle cleansing will protect new granulation tissue. Normal saline is the solution of choice. Antiseptic solutions are cytotoxic and can delay the wound-healing process.
Maintain a moist wound environment. Use damp-to-damp saline gauze dressings, hydrocolloids, transparent adhesive dressings, or hydrogels. The choice of dressing is dependent upon accurate wound assessment and individual patient usage considerations (see table 34-2).	A moist wound surface will promote wound healing by supporting autolysis and facilitating collagen synthesis and epidermal migration.

Nursing Interventions	Rationales
Lightly pack deep wounds and undermined areas and/or sinus tracks inside the wound with absorptive dressing products (e.g., gauze fluffs or ribbons or calcium alginates).	This prevents abscess formation or premature epithelization.
For venous stasis ulcers, provide compression therapy (ace wraps, support hose) following local ulcer care.	This promotes venous return, thereby decreasing edema.

▶ **NURSING DIAGNOSIS:** *Altered Skin Integrity—Tubes, Drains, and Surgical Wounds*

Related To surgical incisions, tubes, and drains

Defining Characteristics
• Closed incision
• Open incision
• Intact tube and drain sites
• Altered skin integrity at tube or drain insertion site

Patient Outcomes
Patient will exhibit:
• incision site healing without complications.
• tube and drain insertion sites that are free of skin breakdown and infection.

Nursing Interventions	Rationales
Assess incision, tube, or drain for healing, including wound approximation; presence/absence of drainage or odor; condition of skin surrounding incision, tube, or drain for inflammation or maceration; and presence of sutures or staples. Call physician for signs of infection.	Establishes a baseline prior to initiating treatment.
Assess appropriateness of dressing, if indicated. Use nonadherent	Protects wound from trauma or friction.

Nursing Interventions	Rationales
dressing (e.g., Telfa) if drainage is present from closed incision. Apply dressings around tubes and drains.	
If open incision, treat as an open wound. (See Altered Skin Integrity: Open Wounds.)	For healing to occur, the open incision must be free of infection and nonviable tissue and be packed with an appropriate dressing to maintain a moist surface and prevent premature closure.
For tubes, measure length of tube or drain. If tube or drain is dislodged, call physician.	This indicates tube movement.
Secure long tubes to skin without tension. Anchor tubes and drains to clothing.	This avoids pulling and tube dislodgement.
Have patient keep daily record of amount and type of tube or drain output. Should output increase suddenly, assess type and amount of drainage. For large amounts of bloody drainage, call physician or emergency services as indicated.	Increased output may indicate hemorrhages or infection.
Assess for leakage at the skin level; if present, call physician and apply skin barrier products.	Leakage at skin level may indicate blocked or misplaced tube or drain. Skin barrier products prevent skin breakdown from chemical irritation and moisture.
For amputations, use figure-eight dressing wraps.	This provides appropriate compression to minimize edema.

DISCHARGE PLANNING/CONTINUITY OF CARE
• Ensure patient has appropriate medications (antibiotics).
• Provide dressing supplies, if needed.
• Ensure patient has follow-up physician appointment.
• Refer to support groups, as needed.

Table 34-1 • Stages of Pressure Ulcers

Stage I: Nonblanchable erythema of intact skin; the heralding lesion of skin ulceration. Note: Reactive hyperemia can normally be expected to be present for one-half to three-fourths as long as the pressure-occluded blood flow to the area; it should not be confused with a stage I pressure ulcer.

Stage II: Partial-thickness skin loss involving epidermis and/or dermis. The ulcer is superficial and presents clinically as an abrasion, blister, or shallow crater.

Stage III: Full-thickness skin loss involving damage or necrosis of subcutaneous tissue that may extend down to, but not through, underlying fascia. The ulcer presents clinically as a deep crater with or without undermining of adjacent tissue.

Stage IV: Full-thickness skin loss with extensive destruction, tissue necrosis, or damage to muscle, bone, or supporting structures (e.g., tendon or joint capsule). Note: Undermining and sinus tracts may also be associated with stage IV pressure ulcers.

From panel for the Prediction and Prevention of Pressure Ulcers in Adults. Pressure Ulcers in Adults: Prediction and Prevention. Clinical Practice Guideline, Number 3. AHCPR Publication No. 92-0047. Rockville, MD: Agency for Health Care Policy and Research, Public Health Service, U.S. Department of Health and Human Services. May 1992.

Table 34-2 • Wound Care Products

Dressing Category	Clinical Characteristics	Primary Indications for Use	Examples
Moisture vapor/ permeable (MVP, or transparent adhesive dressings	Semipermeable: allows transmission of oxygen and water vapor	Wounds needing protection and a clean, moist surface	Tegaderm-3M
	Prevents entry of bacteria, protects against secondary infection	Threatened breakdown	OpSite-Smith & Nephew United
	Does *not* absorb drainage	Stages I and II wounds	Polyskin-Kendall
	Provides some protection against friction	May be used to facilitate autolysis of necrotic tissue	Bioclusive-J&J
	Provides for wound visualization		
Hydrocolloids	Occlusive: impermeable to oxygen	Wounds requiring minimal to moderate absorption, a moist wound surface, and protection	Duoderm, Duoderm CGF (Convatec)
	Supports autolytic debridement, especially for wounds with slough or a combination of necrosis and exudate	Stages I and II wounds	Duoderm Extra Thin (Convatec)
	Prevents secondary infection	Stage III wounds with minimal to moderate exudate and no dead space	Duoderm granules (Convatec)
	Provides limited to moderate absorption, depending on dressing formulation	May be used to facilitate autolysis of necrotic tissue	Duoderm paste (Convatec)
	Moldable: more likely to maintain a seal in difficult areas such as coccyx	Contraindicated in infected wounds or wounds with the potential for anaerobic infection	Comfeel paste (Coloplast)
	Available in wafer, paste, or powder form; also with special features (i.e., border, contour, extra thin)		Comfeel Ulcer Care-Dressing (Coloplast)
			Comfeel Pressure Relief Dressing (Coloplast)
			Tegasorb (3M)
			Restore (Hollister)
			Cutinova Hydro (Biersdorf)

Table 34-2 • *continued*

Dressing Category	Clinical Characteristics	Primary Indications for Use	Examples
Hydrogels	Supports autolytic debridement because of moisturizing effects Provides limited absorption of exudate Nonadherent surface provides a traumatic removal Available in amorphous and sheet form; must match appropriate form of hydrogel to the wound Amorphous form used in conjunction with moist gauze or other moisture-retentive dressing in full-thickness would; frequency of dressing change dependent on amount of exudate, usually once or twice a day. Sheet form is most appropriate for partial-thickness wounds. Sheet gels made primarily of water can macerate the surrounding skin, and so they must be cut to fit the lesion. Sheet gels must be monitored carefully and changed frequently enough to prevent dehydration of the dressing. Cover dressings selected based on amount of protection needed	Stages II, III, and IV wounds with minimal to moderate amounts of exudate (must match form of hydrogel to specific wound) May be used to support autolysis due to moisturizing effect	1. Amorphous forms: Biolex (Bard) Carrasyn—tube or spray bottle (Carrington) Intrasite (Smith & Nephew United) Normigel (Scott Healthcare) Hypergel (Scott Healthcare) Curasol (Healthpoint Medical) 2. Sheet forms: Vigilon (C.R. Bard) Nu-Gel (J&J)

Table 34-2 • *continued*

Dressing Category	Clinical Characteristics	Primary Indications for Use	Examples
Absorption Dressings	Supports autolytic debridement as long as moist wound surface maintained	Wounds with moderate to large amounts of exudate (stages III and IV)	1. Alginates: Algiderm (CONVATEC) Algosteril (J&J) Kaltostat (Calgon Vestal) Sorbsan (Dow Hickam)
	Absorbs large volumes of exudate, up to 20 times weight of each dressing	Wounds with sinus tracts**	
	Eliminated dead space	Wounds with a combination of necrosis and exudate	2. Copolymer starch dressing: Bard Absorption Dressing (C.R. Bard)
	Main Categories:		
	1. Alginates: Applied to the wound in *dry* form. They are appropriate only for exudative wounds. Available as standard size dressings as well as ropes/ribbons for *picking* sinus tracks/undermined areas. Frequency of change every 24–72 h depending on amount of exudate.		
	2. Copolymer starch dressings: Applied to the wounds in moist form, and so they may be used for wound with minimal exudate as well as for wounds with a large amount of exudate. They are usually changed daily; the wound is flushed and then lightly packed with the dressing.*		

**Note:* All dressings require a cover dressing. The cover dressing provides protection from environmental contaminants. The cover dressing should be selected based on wound location and amount of protection needed.

***Note:* Narrow sinus tracts are probably best managed with ribbon gauze packing.

OTHER PLANS OF CARE TO REFERENCE
- Peripheral Vascular Disease
- Nutrition
- Diabetes Mellitus
- Chronic Renal Failure
- Hepatitis
- Human Immunodeficiency Virus
- Intravenous Therapy
- Urinary Incontinence
- Spinal Cord Injury

BIBLIOGRAPHY

Banks, K., Jones, E. S., Law, M. S., & MacAvoy, S. (1993). An effective skin integrity program. *Journal of Nursing Staff Development, 9*(2), 93–96.

Bergman-Evans, B., Cuddigan, J., & Bergstrom, N. (1994). Clinical practice guidelines: Prediction and prevention of pressure ulcers. *Today's OR-Nurse, 16*(6), 33–40.

Friebel, L. M. (1993). The challenge of skin and wound care in the home setting. *Journal of Home Health Care Practice, 5*(3), 1.

Frantz, R. A. (1994). Clinical concerns: Management of dry skin. *Journal of Gerontological Nursing, 20*(9), 15–18.

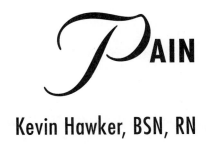

$\mathcal{P}$AIN

Kevin Hawker, BSN, RN

$\mathbf{P}$ain is a response to a noxious stimulus that arises from actual or potential tissue injury and elicits unpleasant sensory and psychic responses in the individual. Regardless of severity, pain is always subjective.

During the transition from the hospital to the home setting, pain and its effective management may often represent a patient's primary complaint and main concern. Research has determined that the primary cause of unresolved pain among patients is the failure of the health care team to adequately assess for and treat pain appropriately (Cleeland, 1991). Therefore, it is imperative that the nurse, in consultation with the physician, continually assess for and treat pain to ensure a pain-free convalescence.

ETIOLOGIES
- Acute pain: result of surgical or dental procedures, injury and trauma to the body, or an infectious process.
- Chronic pain: secondary to a disease process, overuse injuries, and repetitive-motion injuries.
- Cancer pain: acute, chronic, or intermittent manifestation of the disease process. Such pain usually has a precise cause that is related to tumor development or treatment interventions.
- Phantom pain (paraesthesia): experienced by the person who has had a limb amputated. Burning, stabbing, or throbbing sensations can be felt in the amputated (phantom) limb.

CLINICAL MANIFESTATIONS
- Tachycardia
- Elevated systolic blood pressure
- Tachypnea or shallow respirations
- Fatigue
- Sleep deprivation due to unresolved pain
- Increased energy expenditure to perform previously simple ADLs

- Loss of appetite
- Decreased motivation to prepare and consume meals
- Increased irritability, expressions of anger
- Social withdrawal, depression
- Decreased attention span, inability to concentrate

CLINICAL/DIAGNOSTIC FINDINGS

As pain is a subjective experience, there are no diagnostic procedures to assess the patient's condition. To objectify the pain experience, however, the nurse may employ pain-rating scales:
- Numerical: pain rated from 1, mild discomfort, to 10, severe pain.
- Visual analog: color gradient scale, with darker hues indicating low pain and brighter hues indicating intense pain.
- Faces scales: For children, a smiling face indicates comfort, while a frowning, tearful face indicates pain.

▶ NURSING DIAGNOSIS: *Pain*

Related To
- Infection, acute or chronic disease, injury
- Sequelae of surgical, diagnostic, or palliative interventions

Defining Characteristics
- Patient's subjective expression of discomfort or pain
- Vital signs outside of normal limits
- Activity intolerance

Patient Outcomes
The patient will exhibit mediation or complete alleviation of the pain syndrome, as evidenced by:
- subjective reporting that pain has resolved or diminished to a tolerable level.
- vital signs returning to patient's baseline parameters.
- ability to resume ADLs relative to the patient's diagnosis or condition.

Nursing Interventions	Rationales
Perform physical assessment and monitor vital signs during initial and subsequent nursing visits.	This provides a baseline and determines ongoing status of patient's condition.
Query patient to determine presence of pain.	This allows for timely and effective analgesic intervention.

Nursing Interventions	Rationales
Assess patient's ability to perform ADLs.	Decline or increase in patient's activities, sleeping, and eating is often an indicator of the efficacy of the analgesic regimen.
Instruct patient in proper administration of prescribed analgesics. Help patient/family to plan for securing an adequate supply of pain medication.	Incorrect administration may decrease drug's efficacy. Planning ahead will ensure that patient has medication when needed.
Advise patient to adhere to scheduled dosing of analgesics. Employ medication reminder techniques such as "days of the week" pill boxes or color-coded medication vials to facilitate schedule compliance.	Continuous scheduled dosing of analgesics provides more consistent pain relief than "as-needed" regimens.
Monitor patient for drug side effects (euphoria, oversedation, nausea, constipation, pruritus).	Interventions to lessen drug side effects enhance patient's feelings of well-being and encourage medication compliance.
Monitor patient's response to analgesic regimen. In consultation with primary physician, adjust analgesic dosages as pain escalates or subsides.	Titrating medications allows for effective analgesia or prevents unwanted side effects for the patient.
As an adjunct to the analgesic regimen, assist the patient with non-pharmacological pain interventions such as guided imagery, relaxation, and distraction techniques.	Patient-directed techniques to relieve pain enhance the patient's sense of autonomy and control over his or her condition, enabling active participation in pain alleviation.

▶ NURSING DIAGNOSIS: *Anxiety*

Related To pain

Defining Characteristics
- Feelings of nervousness, fear, helplessness
- Emotional lability, withdrawal, heightened sensitivity to criticism
- Memory lapses, decreased attention span, inability to concentrate

Patient Outcomes
Patient will report:
- that his or her anxiety related to the pain experience has lessened.

- a resumption of normal physical and cognitive functioning.

The caregiver and family members will participate in alleviating stressors that heighten the sense of anxiety in the patient.

Nursing Interventions	Rationales
Assess patient's level of anxiety (mild, moderate, severe, panic).	Assessment will determine specific intervention and therapeutic approach to employ with patient.
Provide reassurance to the patient.	This establishes nurse as a focal point of trust for positive interaction with patient.
Determine what specific element of the pain experience provokes anxiety for the patient.	Having patient's verbalize their sense of anxiety assists both the patients and the nurse in identifying its cause.
Provide anticipatory guidance for the patient and family.	Teaching about the pain experience before it occurs provides information, allows a sense of control, and alleviates unfounded assumptions.
Assess family members' responses during episodes when the patient is experiencing pain and intervene accordingly.	Negative or inappropriate responses may heighten anxiety for patients and alienate them from the family nucleus. Positive responses should be encouraged to enhance a sense of shared coping.
Assess patient's cognitive and affective domains on an ongoing basis.	As the patient's anxiety lessens, cognitive functioning should become more acute and affective behavior more appropriate.
Refer patient and family members to community support groups, chaplin, social events, if appropriate.	Support systems help decrease anxiety.
Refer to home health aide, if appropriate.	Assisting with ADLs on a daily basis can decrease anxiety and stress.

DISCHARGE PLANNING/CONTINUITY OF CARE

- If the patient's condition is stable, but he or she still requires long-term analgesics, ensure that a specific pain-management regimen is in place.

- Provide patient with a 24-hour contact person (physician or nurse) for consultation if pain should unexpectedly occur.
- If the condition or diagnosis warrants, discuss with patient, family, and physician the appropriateness of hospice care.

REFERENCES/BIBLIOGRAPHY

Cleeland, C. S. (1991). Analgesic trials to clinical practice: When and how does it happen? In M. B. Max, R. D. Portenoy, & E. M. Laska (Eds.) *The Design of Analgesic Clinical Trials*. New York: Raven.

Kelly, J., & Payne, R. (1991). Cancer pain syndromes. *Neurologic Clinics of North America, 9,* 937–953.

Max, M. B. (1990). Improving outcomes of analgesic treatment, Is education enough? *Annals of Internal Medicine, 113,* 885–889.

Shannon, M., & Berde, C. B. (1989). Pharmacologic management of pain in children and adolescents. *Pediatric Clinics of North America, 26,* 855–873.

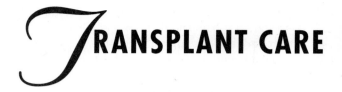RANSPLANT CARE

Kathleen Klauseger, MSN

Transplanting major organs—such as the heart, lungs, and kidneys—has become more commonplace in the last decade. Shorter postoperative stays and increased technological capabilities in the home setting have resulted in developing a population of patients with highly specialized needs. This chapter will address common postoperative needs and possible major complications of heart, lung, and kidney transplant patients.

ETIOLOGIES
- Heart: cardiomyopathies, anomalies, coronary artery disease
- Lung: hereditary and congenital diseases, chronic obstructive pulmonary disease (COPD), malignancy
- Kidney: end-stage renal disease, hypertension, glomerulonephritis

CLINICAL MANIFESTATIONS
Normal posttransplant (include normal physical findings)
- heart: tachycardia (100–110 bpm), no chest pain with angina secondary to deinnervated heart
- lung: breath sounds normal, breathing pattern should return to normal by hospital discharge (patients may need to be reminded not to use accessory muscles)
- kidney: outpouching of transplanted kidney which feels like a fist; may have numbness or swelling of leg on transplanted side, normal urinary patterns

Infection posttransplant (most common abnormal findings for all transplants)
- elevated temperature
- elevated white blood cell (WBC) count
- abnormal chest x-ray
- redness of wounds
- burning on urination

Rejection posttransplant (most common abnormal findings)
- heart: elevated temperature, shortness of breath (SOB), edema, weight gain, cough, elevated WBC count
- lung: tired, SOB, weight gain, cough and sputum production, 15% reduction in home spirometry readings
- kidney: tenderness at graft site, decreased urine output, sudden increase in weight, peripheral edema

CLINICAL/DIAGNOSTIC FINDINGS

Normal posttransplant
- heart: heart biopsy at regular intervals, cultures for fever >38°C, chest x-ray for persistent cough, routine laboratory work cyclosporin levels, CBC, and SMAC at regular intervals
- lung: lung biopsy 1 month postoperatively and as needed; cultures for fever >38°C; routine laboratory work includes cyclosporin levels, CBC, and SMAC at regular intervals; bronchoscopy as needed
- kidney: biopsy performed only when rejection is suspected; CBC, cyclosporin levels, creatinine, and SMAC at regular levels

▶ NURSING DIAGNOSIS: *High Risk for Infection*

Risk Factors
- Immunosuppressive medications

Patient Outcomes
Patient will verbally identify:
- immunosuppressive precautions and therapy.
- preventive activities related to immunosuppression.

Nursing Interventions	Rationales
Instruct and monitor for signs and symptoms of infection or infectious process, such as urinary tract, respiratory, or local infection. Take daily temperature. Instruct in good hand-washing technique. Screen visitors with communicable diseases. Avoid fresh flowers, live plants, pet care, or cleaning of litter boxes and cages.	Immunosuppression will suppress the natural inflammatory response. Low-grade fevers can represent significant infection. Avoiding known and possible sources of infectious agents reduces risk of infection.
Instruct in self-administration of medication. Include specific adverse effects and consequences of altering medication schedule.	Familiarity with medication and adverse reactions is critical in preventing infection.

Nursing Interventions	Rationales
Instruct in preventive self-care skills such as monitoring blood pressure, weight gain, behavior changes, gastrointestinal (GI) intolerances, wound healing, and good skin and mouth care. Reinforce life-long follow-up with transplant team.	Immunosuppressive therapy can cause many severe adverse reactions. Recognizing these reactions is critical for medical management.

▶ NURSING DIAGNOSIS: *Impaired Tissue Integrity*

Related To rejection

Defining Characteristics

Heart
- acute rejection (seen within 3–6 months posttransplant): SOB, weight gain, change in vital signs, lethargy
- chronic rejection (onset 3–6 months posttransplant): same as for acute rejection plus increasing abdominal girth

Lung
- acute rejection: fever, increased sputum production, cough, SOB, change in activity tolerance
- chronic rejection: decreasing activity tolerance, SOB with oxygen requirements, change in vital signs, lethargy

Kidney
- acute rejection: signs/symptoms of infection, hematuria, generalized edema, pain/tenderness over transplanted kidney
- chronic rejection: fluid retention, weight gain, rising blood pressure, malaise, lethargy, anorexia, edema of legs on side of transplanted kidney

Patient Outcomes
- The patient will verbally identify signs and symptoms of acute and chronic rejection episodes.

Nursing Interventions	Rationales
Monitor patient of signs and symptoms of rejection (specific to transplanted organ).	Recognizing impending periods of rejection is imperative in successful treatment.

Nursing Interventions	Rationales
Administer organ-specific antirejection medications and treatments; monitor laboratory and x-ray results as ordered.	Treating rejection is essential if transplanted organ is to be salvaged.
Instruct patient in signs and symptoms of rejection.	The patient must self-monitor for rejection their entire life.

DISCHARGE PLANNING/CONTINUITY OF CARE
- The patient should be able to verbally demonstrate self-care abilities in the following areas: medication administration, preventive activities, and importance of life-long follow-up with the health care and transplant teams.

BIBLIOGRAPHY
Lake, K., & Kilkenny, J. (1992). The pharmacokinetics and pharmacodynamics of immunosuppressive agents. *Critical Care Nursing Clinics of North America, 4*(2), 205–221.

Lekander, B. (1988). Preventing complications for heart and lung transplant recipient. *Dimensions of Critical Care Nursing, 7*(1), 18–27.

Perez, R. (1993). Managing nutrition problems in transplant patients. *Nutrition in Clinical Practice, 8*(1), 28–32.

Schaefer, M., & Williams, L. (1991). Nursing implications of immunosuppression in transplantation. *Nursing Clinics of North America, 26*(2), 291–314.

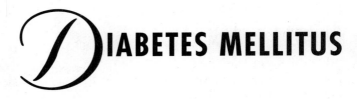

DIABETES MELLITUS

Cynthia Fryhling Corbett, MN, RN

Diabetes mellitus is a heterogeneous group of hyperglycemic disorders characterized by glucose intolerance as a result of abnormal insulin secretion or resistance to insulin in peripheral tissue. This causes alterations in carbohydrate, protein, and lipid metabolism. The two most common forms of this syndrome are type I, insulin-dependent diabetes mellitus (IDDM), and type II, non-insulin-dependent diabetes mellitus (NIDDM). Insulin-dependent diabetes mellitus is characterized by grossly inadequate, often absent, insulin production which quickly leads to ketoacidosis if untreated. In contrast, NIDDM is generally the result of insulin resistance by hepatic or peripheral tissue rather than a lack of insulin production.

Diabetes mellitus affects virtually every organ system in the body, and managing diabetes affects nearly every facet of a diabetic's life. Therefore, assisting patients and families to manage diabetes mellitus requires comprehensive and individualized care planning.

ETIOLOGIES
- Insulin-dependent diabetes mellitus (type I): Exact causes are unknown, but the main theories are:
  - a genetic, immunological abnormality involving certain human leukocyte antigens (HLAs) on chromosome 6
  - beta islet cell damage due to viral illness or chemical toxicity
  - environmental stimuli, such as stress, triggering the onset of IDDM in those who are genetically or otherwise predisposed to the disease
- Non-insulin-dependent diabetes mellitus (type II): Exact causes are unknown, but associated factors are:
  - genetic predisposition
  - environmental and lifestyle factors such as obesity and stress

CLINICAL MANIFESTATIONS

Insulin-dependent diabetes mellitus
- hyperglycemia, prone to ketoacidosis
- weight loss
- polyuria
- polydipsia
- glycosuria, ketonuria, increased urinary nitrogen
- hyperlipidemia
- rapid onset
- patient generally younger than age 30
- sensitive to exogenous insulin

Non-insulin-dependent diabetes mellitus
- hyperglycemia without ketoacidosis
- obese, and may have had recent weight loss or weight gain due to the onset of diabetes; gestational diabetes may occur during pregnancy
- polyuria
- polydipsia
- gradual onset
- patient generally older than age 40
- resistant to exogenous insulin

CLINICAL/DIAGNOSTIC FINDINGS
- Fasting blood glucose >140 mg/dL on at least two testings
- Sustained elevated oral glucose tolerance test ($\geq$ 200 mg/dL) on two samples taken post–glucose administration

▶ NURSING DIAGNOSIS: *Knowledge Deficit*

Related To self-management of diabetes mellitus

Defining Characteristics
- Subjective statements by the patient and/or significant others indicating a lack of knowledge or incorrect information
- Sustained hyperglycemia evidenced by mean blood glucose readings or glycosylated hemoglobin levels
- Frequent episodes of hypoglycemia
- New diagnosis of diabetes mellitus

Patient Outcomes
Patient:
- verbalizes understanding of appropriate self-care behaviors related to diet, exercise, medication use, and glucose monitoring.
- verbalizes signs and symptoms of hypoglycemia and action to take in event of hypoglycemia.

- verbalizes signs and symptoms of hyperglycemia and action to take in event of hyperglycemia.
- verbalizes understanding of potential complications associated with diabetes and health maintenance behaviors to prevent such complications.
- has mean blood glucose levels of approximately 180 mg/dL.
- has glycosylated hemoglobin levels of 10 or less.
- experiences infrequent episodes of hypoglycemia.
- demonstrates appropriate meal planning.
- demonstrates appropriate medication use and storage of medications.
- demonstrates appropriate glucose monitoring.
- participates in regular exercise program.
- demonstrates appropriate integumentary and foot care.
- has regularly scheduled appointments with primary care provider.
- has annual eye examination.
- verbalizes diabetic management plan for "sick days."
- wears pendant or bracelet identifying diabetic status.

Nursing Interventions	Rationales
Instruct on appropriate American Diabetic Association (ADA) diet that is tailored to patient's food preferences and ethnic/religious practices.	An ADA diet is designed to provide optimum nutritional intake, including selections from all four food groups and less simple carbohydrate foods. Tailoring the diet to the patient's preferences increases the patient's ability to understand and adhere to the diet.
Instruct the patient on how to interpret food labels so they can follow the ADA diet.	Understanding food labels will facilitate selecting and preparing food.
Instruct the patient that more frequent, smaller meals/snacks may prevent extreme blood glucose levels.	Frequent, smaller meals with snacks prevent wide blood sugar fluctuations, which usually result from a high caloric intake followed by long periods of no caloric intake.
Instruct the patient to always have a bedtime snack.	The long interval between the evening meal and the morning meal is a high-risk time period for hypoglycemia. This is especially dangerous because the patient may not be awake to notice the onset of hypoglycemic signs and symptoms.

Nursing Interventions	Rationales
Instruct the patient about the relationship between glucose transport and exercise and the importance of regular exercise in the management of diabetes. However, advise the patient to have a thorough physical exam prior to beginning an exercise program.	Aerobic exercise enables glucose transport across cell membranes without insulin. The systemic benefits of exercise (e.g., cardiovascular, musculoskeletal) can help prevent complications associated with diabetes. Exercise may be especially beneficial for type II diabetics who are attempting to lose weight. A thorough history and physical prior to initiating an exercise program is recommended for the patient's safety.
Instruct patient about medication use, including proper preparation and storage, administration, dose, and potential side effects. For those requiring insulin, instruct about insulin storage, insulin preparation, administration (including mixing different types of insulin and site rotation), peak action of insulin, and needle disposal.	Knowledge of medication use, actions, potential side effects, and appropriate storage and handling fosters patient safety and prevents adverse reactions.
Instruct the patient that blood glucose levels fluctuate throughout the day. Together, set goals for target fasting and preprandial, postprandial, and bedtime blood glucose levels.	Knowledge that blood glucose levels fluctuate will help the patient realistically evaluate glucose control. Mutual goal setting allows patients to participate in their care and may promote feelings of control over the disease process.
Instruct on importance of regular blood glucose monitoring. For patients using a blood glucose monitor instruct on the care and use (including trouble-shooting) of the monitor and how to obtain additional supplies.	Patients may need to monitor their blood sugar depending on how well they control their blood glucose and take care of themselves. However, all patients should regularly see their primary care provider, community health nurse, or health departments/centers so they can be monitored and evaluated. Health care practitioners provide reinforcement for those maintaining good control and provide information

Nursing Interventions	Rationales
	and an opportunity to learn for those with less than optimal blood glucose levels.
Instruct the patient about the signs and symptoms of hypoglycemia and hyperglycemia and the actions to take to counteract these reactions.	Detecting adverse reactions early and returning blood glucose to more normal levels can prevent serious complications, such as insulin shock and ketoacidosis.
Instruct the patient about the potential complications of diabetes mellitus and accepted methods for preventing these complications, including good blood glucose control, regular exercise, good hygiene and foot care, and regular physical and eye exams with a primary care provider.	The degree of blood glucose control is thought to play a factor in the rate at which complications develop. Knowledge of the many and varied complications may motivate patients to strive toward good blood glucose control. Vascular changes associated with diabetes mellitus predispose diabetics to eye disease, cardiovascular complications, and skin breakdown, making diabetic self-care activities and regular check-ups essential.
Instruct the patient and significant others on medication use, fluid and food selections, and blood glucose and urine monitoring during times when the patient is sick. Instruct the patient to notify his or her primary care physician when an illness that disrupts eating patterns lasts more than 3 days.	While illness may decrease the patient's caloric intake and exercise/activity, the stress of illness may elevate blood glucose levels. Therefore, in general, instruct patients to take some/all of their normal medication, drink juices, or other *caloric* beverages if solid foods are not tolerated. Also monitor blood glucose levels closely, preferably with a glucose monitor. Both IDDM and NIDDM are at risk for ketoacidosis during illness. Therefore, test urine for ketones prior to each insulin dose, for those requiring insulin, and daily for diabetics who do not require insulin.
Instruct the patient on the importance of obtaining and wearing a bracelet or necklace that identifies	In the event of diabetic ketoacidosis, insulin shock, or other medical emergency, such information can

Nursing Interventions	Rationales
him or her as a diabetic. In addition, patients should be instructed to carry diabetic identification, names and doses of current medications, and the name of their primary care provider in purse/wallet.	facilitate diagnosis and treatment of the patient's condition.
Instruct the patient to carry hard candy or other type of high-glucose snack when away from home. Patients who require insulin to control their blood glucose should also be advised to carry a glucagon kit. Instruct the patient's significant other on how to use the glucagon kit.	Foods high in glucose should be available to the patient at all times to counteract hypoglycemia. Those requiring insulin are most at risk for severe hypoglycemia, resulting in loss of consciousness. When loss of consciousness occurs, administer glucagon.

▶ NURSING DIAGNOSIS: *Ineffective Individual or Family Coping*

Related To management of diabetes mellitus

Defining Characteristics
- Subjective statements by the patient or family indicating an inability to cope with the demands of diabetes and other life stressors or daily hassles
- Signs and symptoms of depression or emotional instability (patient or one or more family members)
- Hostility or isolation among family members
- Incidence of violence or abuse
- Poor glycemic control
- Use of detrimental coping mechanisms such as overeating, alcohol, or chemical substances
- Problems at school or work

Patient Outcomes
Patient and/or family members exhibit decreased stress and improved coping abilities, as evidenced by:
- improved blood glucose control.
- decreased signs of depression and evidence of emotional stability.
- improved relationships among family members.
- demonstration of adaptive coping mechanisms such as use of problem-solving skills, effective communication, and physical exercise.
- involvement in support groups and/or spiritual and mental health or family counseling.

- no signs of violence, neglect, or abuse.
- resumption of normal school/work patterns.

Nursing Interventions	Rationales
Use therapeutic communication skills to allow patient/family to verbalize feelings and problems in a supportive, nonthreatening environment; to explore realistic choices; and to provide decision-making support.	Therapeutic communication helps them identify sources of stress and methods of coping.
Contract with patient/family to facilitate behaviors that will promote glucose control, decrease hostility or social isolation, and improve coping skills and self-esteem. (Refer to Contracting chapter for more information.)	Contracting provides a method to involve the patient/family in the care-planning process, promotes more positive behaviors, and specifies measures that promote patient/family safety.
Refer them to support groups or a diabetic camp (children and adolescents), a mental health professional, and/or a spiritual counselor.	Support groups and/or a diabetic camp provide the patient with peer support that may be unattainable from health care professionals. Patients/families may also need a mental health professional or pastoral counselor to work through problems that inhibit effective coping.
Provide crisis intervention and refer to appropriate social service agencies in cases of abuse or neglect.	This ensures patient and family safety.

▶ NURSING DIAGNOSIS: *High Risk for Impaired Skin Integrity*

Risk Factors
- Microvascular changes
- Peripheral neuropathy
- Long history of diabetes
- History of poorly controlled diabetes
- Poor hygiene practices
- Other complications of diabetes, such as cardiovascular disease, retinopathy, or decreased renal function
- Decreased mobility

Patient Outcomes

Patient:

- demonstrates appropriate hygiene and foot care.
- wears well-fitting slippers and shoes at all times.
- does not display skin breakdown.
- identifies early signs and symptoms of impending skin breakdown.
- verbalizes that signs and symptoms of skin breakdown need to be reported to primary care provider *immediately*.

Nursing Interventions	Rationales
Instruct the patient about the reason(s) that he or she is at high risk for skin breakdown.	Understanding the rationale may help motivate the patient to participate in behaviors that prevent skin breakdown.
Together, develop a realistic plan to increase the patient's activity level.	Increased activity facilitates circulation and can prevent pressure sores for people with mobility limitations. Mutual goal planning facilitates patient participation.
Instruct the patient about the importance of appropriate hygiene practices, including examining their feet daily, providing nail care, and wearing well-fitting shoes/slippers, even when indoors. Refer the patient to a home health aide or homemaker if he or she requires assistance with hygiene. Refer to a podiatrist as needed for more difficult nail care. Demonstrate and have patient return-demonstrate foot inspection procedure and nail care. Evaluate how well the patient's shoes and slippers fit.	Preventing lower extremity skin breakdown is a priority in maintaining the patient's mobility, independence, and overall quality of life and in reducing health care costs associated with diabetes. Patients must take an active part in preventing complications since it is dependent on basic self-care behaviors. Patients may need assistance with hygiene, depending on their overall health status. Patients who are unable to provide their own foot care due to visual or mobility deficits or if in need of complicated foot or nail care (e.g., ingrown nails, neglect of nails for long periods of time) may need podiatry care.
Instruct the patient about early signs and symptoms of skin breakdown (pain, reddened areas). Also stress the need to notify the primary care provider immediately should any of these signs and symptoms occur.	If treated in the early stages, more severe breakdown and related morbidity can be prevented.

DISCHARGE PLANNING/CONTINUITY OF CARE

Ensure that the patient\family has the following resources in place for ongoing care needs:

- A primary care provider who is familiar with the patient's health history and with whom the patient has regularly scheduled follow-up appointments
- A pharmacy for medication and other diabetic supplies
- Names and numbers of diabetic support groups, diabetic camps, and counseling services

---

Clinical Clip

It is estimated that there are nearly 14 million diabetics in the United States, but only half have been diagnosed with diabetes. Approximately 90% have type II diabetes and 10% have type I diabetes. The prevalence of diabetes increases with age. Hence the number of people with diabetes will continue to grow as the U.S. population ages.

OTHER PLANS OF CARE TO REFERENCE

- Contracting
- Skin Care

BIBLIOGRAPHY

Anderson, R. M. (1991). The challenge of translating scientific knowledge into improved diabetes care in the 1990s. *Diabetes Care, 14,* 418–421.

Daly, J. M. (1993). *NIC interventions linked to NANDA diagnoses.* Iowa City, IA: University of Iowa.

Fain, J. A. (1993). National trends in diabetes: An epidemiologic perspective. *Nursing Clinics of North America, 28,* 1–7.

Helms, R. B. (1992). Implications of population growth on prevalence of diabetes: A look at the future. *Diabetes Care, 15*(Suppl. 1), 6–9.

Lebovitz, H. E., DeFronzo, R. A., Genuth, A., Kreisberg, R. A., Pfeifer, M. A., & Tamborlane, W. V. (Eds.). (1991). *Therapy for diabetes mellitus and related disorders.* Alexandria, VA: American Diabetes Association.

McCloskey, J. C., & Bulechek, G. M. (Eds.). (1992). *Nursing interventions classifications (NIC).* St. Louis: Mosby Year-Book.

Rubin, R. R., & Peyrot, M. (1992). Psychosocial problems and interventions in diabetes: A review of the literature. *Diabetes Care, 15,* 1640–1657.

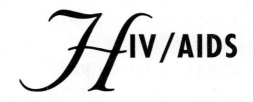
HIV/AIDS

Scott L. V. Chinburg, RN, MSN

Acquired immuno deficiency syndrome (AIDS) represents the later stages of a disease associated with infection by human immunodeficiency virus (HIV). It represents the results of the progressive deterioration of the immune system's ability to resist opportunistic infections and neoplasms. Progression from HIV infection to AIDS may be as long as 10–15 years (Fauci, 1993). During this period, people with HIV infection may lead healthy and productive lives, although they remain potentially infectious to others.

Managing HIV infection as a chronic condition in the community setting plays a vital role in delaying disease progression and in maintaining quality of life (O'Brien, 1993). Additionally, because HIV infection is associated with deteriorating multiple body systems, maintaining nutritional status is of utmost importance because this deters muscle wasting, opportunistic infections, and morbidity/mortality (Kotler, 1992).

Clinical Clip

The Changing Face of AIDS

The HIV epidemic in the United States is increasingly affecting women, communities of color, and children. In 1988, the average American with AIDS was a gay, white male in his early 30's. By the year 2000, it is estimated that the average American with AIDS will be African-American or Hispanic, female, and under 25 years of age (Cleve, 1993).

ETIOLOGIES
- Exposure to HIV through contact with contaminated bodily fluids (blood, semen, and vaginal secretions)
- Exposure to HIV through contact with contaminated parenteral drug use equipment (needles)

- Exposure to HIV via maternal-fetal transmission (in utero, peripartum, and breastfeeding)

CLINICAL MANIFESTATIONS

Fatigue
- loss of motivation unrelated to activity or sleep patterns
- acute viral syndrome (fever, fatigue, and myalgia); occurs in approximately 75% of individuals 7–10 days following exposure to HIV

Weight loss
- very common in mid to late stages of HIV disease
- severe malnutrition associated with increased rate of opportunistic infections and shorter survival

Self-concept
- loss of control
- preexisting negative self-concept
- spiritual distress
- changes in body image
- fear of sexual dysfunction

Social isolation
- social stigmatization
- loss of ability to work
- changes in lifestyle/culture/primary group
- depression/antisocial behavior
- impaired communication (HIV-related dementia/progressive multifocal leukoplakia)

CLINICAL/DIAGNOSTIC FINDINGS

Serology testing for HIV
- positive enzyme-linked immunosorbent assay (ELISA) for HIV antibody production (within 6 months of exposure)
- confirmed by Western blot assay
- gradual decline in number and percent of CD4 lymphocytes (approximately $50/mm^3$ per year after exposure)

Testing for HIV-related diseases
- *Pneumocystis carinii* pneumonia (PCP) by bronchoscopy and cytological stain
- candidiasis (esophageal, recurrent vaginal) by physical examination
- cytomegalovirus (CMV) by retinal exam for eye involvement or endoscopy for gastrointestinal (GI) involvement
- *Mycobacterium avium* complex (MAC) by acid fast bacillus (AFB) culture
- *Mycobacterium tuberculosis* (TB) by purified protein derivative (PPD)
- Kaposi's sarcoma by pathology report
- non-Hodgkin's lymphoma by pathology report
- Papanicolau (pap) smear q 6 months for early detection of cervical dysplasia

Screening for complications due to HIV infection

- complete blood count (CBC) with differential for thrombocytopenia, neutropenia, or anemia
- chemistry profile for elevated renal tests (BUN/Cr), elevated liver function tests [aspartate amino transferase (AST), alanine transferase (ALT), lactic dehydrogenase (LDH), Alk phosphatase], poor nutrition (low albumin, low globulin, high triglycerides), and electrolyte imbalance (low potassium, low CO_2, high sodium)
- rapid plasma reagent (RPR) elevated ratio to indicate untreated syphilis

▶ NURSING DIAGNOSIS: *Fatigue*

Related To
- HIV infection
- side effects of antiretroviral and/or other medications

Defining Characteristics
- Physical deterioration, nutritional compromise, and/or muscle wasting
- Psychosocial concerns/depression

Patient Outcomes
Patient will exhibit increased energy levels, as evidenced by:
- improving performance of activities of daily living (ADLs).
- seeking psychosocial support resources.
- modifying medication regimen.

Nursing Interventions	Rationales
Assess ability to perform ADLs.	Establishes level of need for education/assistance and provides baseline to monitor progression.
Instruct in energy-saving techniques.	This maximizes efficiency of work to perform ADLs.
Instruct caregiver in assisting with ADLs.	Lessens anxiety regarding personal contact with patient and reinforces supportive role.
Assess psychosocial needs of patient and family system.	Identifies needs commonly not discussed openly due to stigmatization and/or denial.
Encourage patient and family to discuss feelings and needs.	Reinforces open communication in family system.
Refer as needed for professional therapy, peer-based support groups, and/or pastoral provider.	Utilizes community resources for psychosocial support.

Nursing Interventions	Rationales
Assess medications for potential side effects and interactions.	Fatigue is a common side effect of medications used to treat HIV and/or opportunistic infections.
Instruct regarding potential side effects/interactions of medications and possible modifications to lessen symptoms.	Patients frequently tolerate alternative antiretroviral therapies with less fatigue.
Monitor for signs and symptoms of opportunistic infections.	Fatigue is often an initial symptom of an opportunistic infection.

▶ **NURSING DIAGNOSIS:** *Altered Nutrition—Less Than Body Requirements*

Related To HIV infection

Defining Characteristics
- Ten percent or greater unintentional loss of usual body weight
- Loss of muscle mass with increased fat stores with same, usual body weight

Risk Factors
- Anorexia
- Dysphagia
- Nausea
- Opportunistic infections
- Malabsorption syndromes and/or chronic diarrhea
- Inadequate food availability/inability to prepare food
- Medication side effects
- Fatigue
- Neurological complications (e.g., weakness leading to inability to prepare food)

Patient Outcome
Patient will recover and maintain optimal body weight.

Nursing Interventions	Rationales
Assess current and optimal body weight.	Establishes level of need for nutritional education and intervention.

Nursing Interventions	Rationales
Assess patient's educational needs regarding basic nutrition and nutritional support in HIV infection.	Establishes level of need for patient instruction.
Instruct about proper nutrition and appropriate diet as indicated.	Reinforces importance of nutrition support in overall management of illness.
Assess risk factors associated with altered nutrition.	Clarifies multifactorial etiology and intervention plan.
Instruct regarding compensatory diet modifications, supplements, and potential medication side effects.	Reinforces means to recover and maintain optimal body weight.
Assess availability of food and ability to prepare food.	Identifies socioeconomic and personal assistance needs regarding nutritional support.
Refer as needed to registered dietitian, community-based resources (e.g., Meals on Wheels), and suppliers of nutritional supplements.	Utilizes community resources for nutritional support.
Continue to monitor changing nutritional needs associated with new risk factors.	Maintains appropriate level of nutritional support with progression of disease.

DISCHARGE PLANNING/CONTINUITY OF CARE

- Reinforce need for regular follow-up visit to primary health care clinic and/or physician (see Table 38-1).
- Refer patient to home care/hospice agencies as needed.
- Ensure that patient can perform appropriate home management and ADLs.
- Refer patient to nutritional counseling, social work counseling, case management services, community resources, support groups, and substance abuse programs as needed.
- Refer patient to AIDS/HIV clinical trials available in your institution and/or area.

Table 38-1 • CD4 Count as Clinical Marker of Progression of HIV Disease and Its Indication for Medical Management (Sande et al., 1993)

CD4 > 500/mm^3 and asymptomatic	Follow q 6 months with CD4 testing q 6 months.
CD4 200–500/mm^3 and asymptomatic	Instruct regarding potential benefits and risks of initiating antiretroviral therapy.
CD4 200–500/mm^3 and symptomatic	Encourage antiretroviral therapy. Monitor side effects, compliance, and new symptoms.
CD4 < 200/mm^3 (diagnosis of AIDS regardless of symptomatology)	Reinforce importance of antiretroviral therapy, encouraging alternatives if AZT is not tolerated. Instruct regarding need for prophylaxis against PCP, monitoring of antiretroviral therapies and CD4 counts, nutritional support, and early intervention and medical management of opportunistic infections and/or neoplasms if and when they occur. Most opportunistic infections and neoplasms associated with HIV infection generally occur in patients with CD4 < 200.

OTHER PLANS OF CARE TO REFERENCE

- Social Isolation
- Grief/Loss
- Altered Mental Status
- Human Sexuality
- Death/Dying
- Substance Abuse
- Medication Noncompliance
- Infusion Therapy
- Contracting
- Patient's Rights and Self-Determination
- Caregiver Burden

REFERENCES/BIBLIOGRAPHY

Castro, K., Ward, J., Slutsker, L., Buehler, J. Jaffe, H., & Berkelman, R. (1992). 1993 Revised classification system for HIV infection and expanded surveillance case definition for AIDS among adolescents and adults. *Morbidity and Mortality Weekly Report, 41*(RR-17), 1–19.

Cleve, J. (1993). Facing change: The changing face of AIDS in America. *Lifetimes II, 3*(3), 5.

Fauci, A. (1993). Multifactorial nature of human immunodeficiency virus disease: Implications for therapy. *Science, 262,* 1011–1018.

Jewett, J., & Hecht, F. (1993). Preventive health care for adults with HIV infection. *Journal of the American Medical Association, 269*(9), 1144–1153.

Kotler, D. (1992). Causes and consequences of malnutrition in HIV/AIDS. *PAACNOTES, 1,* 5–8.

O'Brien, M. (1993). Physical and psychosocial nursing care for patients with HIV infection. *Nursing Clinics of North America, 28*(2), 303–333.

Sande, M., Carpenter, C., Cobbs, D., Holmes, K., & Sanford, J. (1993). Antiretroviral therapy for adult HIV-infected patients. *Journal of the American Medical Association, 270*(21), 2583–2589.

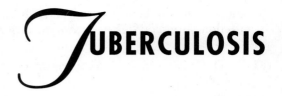

$\mathcal{T}$UBERCULOSIS

Barbara G. Konestabo, RN, MSN

Tuberculosis (TB) is an inflammatory, chronic bacterial infection caused by *Mycobacterium tuberculosis*, which commonly affects the lungs, although other organs may be involved. The major mode of transmission is via droplet nuclei suspended in the air when individuals with pulmonary TB cough, sneeze, talk, or sing. Extrapulmonary transmission routes (e.g., ingestion, invasion of skin, or mucous membranes) are well documented but pose a very limited risk compared to the aerial route.

ETIOLOGIES
- Inhaled tubercle bacillus *M. tuberculosis* (only 5–10% of all newly infected persons develop progressive primary TB when host response is inadequate or the mass of infection inocula is too great)
- High-risk lifestyles (substance abuse, alcohol abuse, crowding, poor ventilation, smoking, poor nutritional intake)
- High-risk groups (malnourished, elderly, young, chronically ill, immunodeficient persons)
- Individuals with noninfectious primary TB who have a high-risk lifestyle or who are in a high-risk group also at risk for secondary TB

CLINICAL MANIFESTATIONS
- May be asymptomatic
- Generalized weakness, fatigue
- Anorexia
- Weight loss, dehydration
- Low-grade fever
- Drenching night sweats
- Shortness of breath, usually with activity
- Chronic cough progressing to mucopurulent, possible hemoptysis, in later stages

- Chest pain that may be vague or sharp and stabbing and pleuritic in origin
- Patient often appearing chronically ill

CLINICAL/DIAGNOSTIC FINDINGS
- Tachycardia, blood pressure (B/P) changes, increased respirations, especially with activity
- Auscultation of lungs: may be normal or may reveal diminished breath sounds and/or adventitious breath sounds
- Sputum smear and culture for definitive diagnosis
- Histological examination or by culture in extrapulmonary disease in urine, body fluids, and tissue
- Positive PPD Tuberculin test: provides presumptive evidence of exposure but does not distinguish between active and past exposure
- Chest x-ray for further confirmation: shows abnormalities, often including fibrocavity apical disease, nodules, and pneumonic infiltrates
- Needle biopsy of pleura: usually reveals TB granulomas

▶ NURSING DIAGNOSIS: *Ineffective Breathing Pattern*
Related To inflammatory, infectious process

Defining Characteristics
- Respiratory rhythm, rate, and depth changes
- Productive or nonproductive cough, possible hemoptysis
- Shortness of breath, may have pain with respiration
- Possible diminished breath sounds, adventitious sounds
- Possible areas of thoracic dullness detectable on percussion

Patient Outcomes
Patient will:
- maintain desired activity level with adaptations as needed to ensure effective respiratory functioning to gradually resume usual lifestyle.
- show a reduction in cough.
- show a resolution of fever.
- maintain adequate course of chemotherapy.
- have decreased bacilli on smear or culture (eventually sputum free of bacilli).
- have a chest radiograph reflecting healing to healed lung areas.

Nursing Interventions	Rationales
Perform physical assessment and history. Pay particular attention to home safety, heating, and ventilation. Take into account where patients spend the most time and where household members and frequent visitors spend time.	Both general and specialized assessments are key to understanding patient's physical and environmental baseline and to developing a realistic plan of treatment.
Perform thorough respiratory assessment at initial visits and subsequent visits. Analyze breath sounds according to pitch, intensity, quality, and relative duration of inspiratory and expiratory phases (compare to baseline at each visit). Monitor for absent or decreased breath sounds and adventitious breath sounds. Perform systematic thorax percussion (abnormalities may be appreciated only in the presence of extensive disease).	This provides baseline and ongoing objective comparative data to assess severity of disease and the amount of healing over time.
Monitor temperature and respirations for depth, frequency, and work of breathing and pulse for rate increase and quality (especially with activity). Instruct how to take temperature and how to count respirations and pulse; instruct to record information in the a.m and p.m. Review entries at every visit.	Recording objective baseline and ongoing data assists nurses and patients/caregivers to safely plan daily activities toward gradual recovery.
Instruct and reinforce during each visit that patients will require more sleep and will need to pace activities with rest periods throughout the day to maintain vital signs within safe parameters.	Infectious disease is a major stressor to the body. For effective healing, patients/caregivers should appreciate the importance of regulating activities based on subjective and objective signs and symptoms. Patient's/caregiver's day-to-day participation and adherence to this concept is essential to patient recovery.
Obtain baseline description of cough and sputum (e.g., color, amount, frequency, odor,	Cough should decrease as patient's condition improves. Sputum specimens are necessary in ascertaining

Nursing Interventions	Rationales
hemoptysis) and monitor for changes. Instruct how to splint to avoid stress to chest wall. Instruct how to safely collect early morning sputum specimen for laboratory analysis.	the effectiveness of chemotherapy, monitoring drug treatment response over time, and identifying possible drug-resistant organisms or patient noncompliance.
Instruct to report new or unusual signs/symptoms. Instruct when to call nurse/physician and when to call for emergency assistance (e.g., chest pain, unrelenting shortness of breath, hemorrhaging).	A trusting environment and open communication between health care team members and patients/caregivers helps to identify the most effective treatment plan and appropriate modifications to maximize the quality of care. Even though few medical emergencies are anticipated with TB home care patients, nurses and patients/caregivers must be prepared to deal with them.
Monitor results of serial sputum testing and x-ray studies. Explain findings and progress. Answer questions and promote therapeutic discussion.	Patient's/caregiver's understanding and appreciation of laboratory testing promotes trust and their participation and compliance in the treatment plan.

▶ **NURSING DIAGNOSIS:** *Altered Nutrition—Less Than Body Requirements*

Related To
- Increased nutritional requirements secondary to the febrile, infectious illness
- Anorexia as a symptom of the disease

Defining Characteristics
- Reported inadequate food intake less than recommended daily allowance
- Reported lack of interest or altered taste for food and/or motivation, ability, or resources to maintain regular, nutritious meals
- Weakness, fatigue, mental irritability, or confusion
- Possible weight loss below ideal for height and frame
- Possible decreased serum albumin
- Possible dehydration, as evidenced by poor skin turgor, dry mucous membranes, and elevated blood urea nitrogen (BUN)

Patient Outcomes

- Patients/caregivers demonstrate verbal and behavioral understanding, as evidenced by ongoing compliance with nutritious, regular eating patterns.
- Optimal nutritional status is validated by objective and subjective data (no further weight loss with gradual weight gain, laboratory values within normal limits (WNL), improving appetite), regular eating habits, and increasing energy levels and endurance.

Nursing Interventions	Rationales
Perform a nutritional assessment, including patient's food and fluid preferences. Identify who buys groceries, prepares meals, and maintains the kitchen. Assess how many meals patients typically eat a day and at what times and assess if patients are currently following a special diet [e.g., American Dietetic Association (ADA), no added salt (NAS), low fat/cholesterol].	Obtaining a dietary baseline and developing individualized diet plans will make the diet both acceptable and achievable. Successful diets also must incorporate dietary preferences and restrictions.
Assess elimination patterns and determine if the current illness has altered these activities (e.g., diarrhea, constipation, change in voiding pattern). Incorporate appropriate foods and fluids in the diet plan and stress that improving diet and fluid intake will help alleviate elimination problems.	Patients/caregivers learning about and improving dietary and fluid intake will promote better elimination, which may improve patient's sense of well-being and may increase appetite.
Instruct about basic nutrition, including using food variety and food groups at every meal. Provide guidelines for choosing a healthy diet and stress the importance of regular meals. Ask patients/caregivers to keep a food diary so that the nurse can assess understanding and compliance. Allow patients/caregivers some control in selecting foods and in choosing meal times. Encourage supplements and frequent small meals.	Improving patient's/caregiver's knowledge of a healthy diet is vital to full recovery. Achieving understanding through education, coaching, and support promotes cooperation and improves long-term dietary compliance.

Nursing Interventions	Rationales
Coordinate social worker and/or home health aide/homemaker referrals as needed.	Resources may be available to supplement finances for patients on limited incomes so that more food and healthier foods can be purchased on a regular basis. A home health aide or homemaker can assist patients with limited informal support networks to grocery shop, to plan and to prepare meals, and to reinforce regular, healthy meals.
Encourage good oral hygiene, including cleaning partials and dentures. Suggest patients brush their teeth or at least rinse their mouths before and after meals. Encourage drinking fluids (unless contraindicated).	The infection and frequent coughing may coat the oral cavity and teeth, decreasing the sense of taste or smell and the desire for food. Frequently cleaning and rinsing the mouth and increasing fluid intake will enhance oral hygiene and improve appetite.
Obtain baseline weight at initial visit and at subsequent visits. Instruct in taking weight and explain the relationship of satisfactory weight and good health. Relate importance of dietary intake to returning to preillness weight.	Regular weight monitoring will alert nurse to a change in patient condition. A gain or loss may be due to dietary intake, hydration status, or infectious disease process.

▶ **NURSING DIAGNOSIS:** *Knowledge Deficit*

Related To
- Lack of information about efforts to prevent the transmission of disease and to protect susceptible persons from infection
- Inadequate information about activities to effectively comply with medical regimen, long-term chemotherapy, and follow-up

Defining Characteristics
- Lack of information
- Actions that indicate a lack of information and/or ability to comply (or have a history of noncompliance) with therapeutic regimen and follow-up

- High-risk patients who require more comprehensive assistance and coordination for safe management of disease at home (e.g., elderly, altered-cell-mediated immunity, prolonged corticosteroid therapy, alcoholism, malnutrition, diabetes, neoplasia, renal dialysis)

Patient Outcomes

- Patients/caregivers verbalize adequate knowledge of causes of disease, transmission, susceptibility, presentation of disease, and signs/symptoms of complications.
- Patients/caregivers are able to comply with all aspects of treatment plan and improve clinically by following through with lifestyle adaptations, complying with medication regimen, and cooperating with health care team.

Nursing Interventions	Rationales
At initial visit, assess abilities to sustain activities of daily living, motivation for learning, and access to informal support systems.	To ensure greater cooperation and success, treatment plans should be individualized and based on such factors as patient ability, resources, motivation, teaching/readiness/ learning style, age, past experience, and disease burden.
Creatively apply teaching/learning theory to the level of the patient/ caregiver. Include disease process, transmission, susceptibility, and signs and symptoms of complications. Begin at initial visit and continue throughout episode of care.	Teaching is geared to the level of the learner. Without this consideration, learning and compliance will be less effective.
Instruct patients/caregivers in proper medication administration during the first visit and continue with teaching and monitoring for compliance at every visit. Alert patients/caregivers to report potential hypersensitivities or adverse drug reactions to nurse/physician. Advise patients not to smoke or drink alcohol. Caution patients to use nonprescription drugs only with physician's permission. Stress at every visit that successful treatment requires several months of consistent, uninterrupted medication.	All TB medications must be taken as prescribed. Compliance with long-term chemotherapy is critical to arrest the disease. Incomplete or inadequate drug treatment not only delays recovery, but also encourages multiple-drug-resistant (MDR) strains of TB with a potential increase in morbidity and mortality. First line anti-TB drugs include isoniazid (INH), rifampin, pyrazinamide ethambutol, and streptomycin. Combination therapy for TB cure is critical to help prevent the emergence of resistant organisms, to

Nursing Interventions	Rationales
	lower concentrations of compounds that have toxic potential, to treat polymicrobial infections, and to provide a broad spectrum of coverage for immunodeficient patients. Patients with drug-resistant TB may require second-line drugs such as cycloserine, ciprofloxacin,ethionamide, and aminosalicylic acid (PAS).
Instruct patient contacts (if not already screened in the previous 3 months) to obtain skin testing, possible follow-up chest x-ray, and drug treatment according to the Centers for Disease Control (CDC) and American Thoracic Society guidelines.	Case source investigation with community follow-through is critical in controlling TB transmission. Tuberculosis is still an avoidable, curable disease. Curing infectious cases in early stages helps prevent further transmission to others.
Teach that persons visiting the home may need to take precautions. These precautions include instructing patients how to contain coughs and sneezes and how to dispose of infectious expectoration. If needed, instruct in respiratory isolation procedures, suggest a private well-ventilated room with a door that can be kept closed, and discuss using masks, gloves, thorough hand-washing techniques, and proper handling and disposal of waterproof bags for articles contaminated with respiratory secretions. Stress that hand washing is essential to prevent cross-infection. Gloves are worn when touching infective material.	Usually infectiousness decreases within 2-3 weeks after initiating TB drug therapy. However, failure to take medications as prescribed and the ever-increasing presence of drug-resistant diseases will impede patient's recovery and increase the risk for transmission. Guidelines for home care patients and agency personnel should be written for the infectious and the potentially infectious patient.
Health care personnel should wear respiratory protection while visiting the patients' homes. Perform cough-inducing procedures in a well-ventilated room and away from other family members. If	The U. S. CDC recommends the use of particulate respirators (PR) by health care personnel when providers must share space with suspected or confirmed infectious TB patient. The PR mask must be

Nursing Interventions

immunocompromised persons or young children are living in the same household as an infectious or potentially infectious patient, alternative living arrangements should be considered until the patient has a negative sputum smear.

Rationales

individually fitted for all personnel. A disposable PR that is designed to provide a tight fit and adequate protection through efficient air filtration is still under investigation at the time of this printing. The U.S. CDC, OSHA, and the National Institute of Occpational Safety and Health (NIOSH) are presently evaluating for an acceptable level of respiratory performance for a proposed industry standard.

DISCHARGE PLANNING/CONTINUITY OF CARE

- Stress to patient/caregiver the importance of completing chemotherapy to ensure effective drug treatment for cure of infection.
- Instruct patient/caregiver to keep all appointments with physician or public health department for follow-up and for further diagnostic studies.
- Reinforce that patient/caregiver should report any unusual signs/symptoms or complications immediately to physician or public health department.
- Provide additional information as indicated to patient/caregiver for social services or other community resources for further education and support.

— Clinical Clip —

Tuberculosis cases are rising and major outbreaks of multi-drug resistant (MDR) strains of TB are developing because patients are not completing their treatment. Drug-resistant strains of TB grow when drug treatment is incomplete or inadequate. These difficult-to-treat strains are now resistant to isoniazid and rifampin and are more difficult and expensive to treat. Under normal circumstances, with proper management, the cure rate for TB is over 90%, as compared to MDR TB, which is 50–80% fatal. Human immunodeficiency virus (HIV) infected TB carriers and poorly managed TB control programs that treat infectious patients but do not ensure cure spread MDR strains. Also, patients with MDR TB can pass the disease onto susceptible persons, who will then be MDR from the outset. A growing trend with the best documented succes rate is by administering directly observed therapy which involves the use of healthcare workers bringing the medication, two to three times a week, directly to the patients. This strategy has been particularly successful in populations, that in the past, were poorly compliant and had limited recovery rates.

BIBLIOGRAPHY

Centers for Disease Control. (1990). *Guidelines for preventing the transmission of tuberculosis in health-care settings, with special focus on HIV-related issues (Morbidity and Mortality Weekly Report,* Vol. 39, No. RR-17). Atlanta, GA: U.S. Department of Health and Human Services.

Comstock, G. W. (1994). Tuberculosis: Is the past once again prologue? *American Journal of Public Health, 84*(11), 1729–1731.

Lancaster, E. (1993). Tuberculosis comeback: Impact on long-term facilities. *Journal of Gerontological Nursing, 19*(7), 16–21.

TB: A global emergency. (1993). *World Health, 4* (July/Aug.).

Walsh, K. (1994). Guidelines for the prevention and control of tuberculosis in the elderly. *Nurse Practitioner: American Journal of Primary Health Care, 19*(11), 79–84.

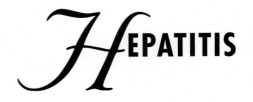

HEPATITIS

Dorothy Fraser, MSN, FNP

Hepatitis is an inflammation of the liver that can be caused by bacterial or viral infections, parasitic infestation, alcohol and drug toxicity, toxins, and other infectious etiologies such as infectious mononucleosis. The course of the disease can be acute or chronic. Acute infections are usually self-limiting and are localized to the liver or associated with systemic disease. Chronic hepatitis is characterized as lasting for 6 months or longer and may lead to cirrhosis of the liver.

ETIOLOGIES

- Hepatitis A (or infectious hepatitis): Hepatitis A virus is most commonly spread by the fecal/oral route (15–40 days incubation) and is associated with close contact, overcrowded conditions, and institutional settings.
- Hepatitis B (or serum hepatitis): Hepatitis B virus (HBV) is spread by parenteral route by contact with blood, contaminated needles, or sexual contact (50–160 days incubation) and is occasionally spread by fecal/oral route. Individuals can have the disease or be a carrier. Carriers are individuals who remain infectious and demonstrate the presence of the HBV surface antigen at least twice in a 6 month period.
- Hepatitis C (or non-A, non-B hepatitis): Hepatitis C virus is spread parenterally and is the cause of 90% of posttransfusion hepatitis cases.
- Hepatitis D: Hepatitis D virus is spread the same way as hepatitis B. It occurs as a coinfection with hepatitis B or is occasionally superimposed on an individual who is a carrier of the HBV.
- Toxic hepatitis is caused by toxic effects of alcohol, drugs, and environmental toxins such as carbon tetrachloride on liver cells. Also drugs—such as acetaminophen in large doses, isoniazid, and various antibiotics—cause liver cell necrosis.

CLINICAL MANIFESTATIONS
Preicteric prodromal stage
- nausea and vomiting
- low-grade fever/chills
- dyspepsia
- anorexia: may be the most important symptom noted during this stage
- arthralgias
- malaise/fatigue
- right upper quadrant (RUQ) tenderness
- aversion to the smell of smoke and to the taste of cigarettes

Icteric phase (some individuals do not develop icteric phase)
- increasing tenderness of liver in RUQ
- jaundice
- dark amber urine
- pruritus
- erythematous macular papular rash
- splenomegaly
- anterior cervical lymphadenopathy

CLINICAL/DIAGNOSTIC FINDINGS
- Blood work
  - complete blood count (CBC) shows granulocytopenia, lymphocytosis, and a mild anemia.
  - elevated total bilirubin indicates severity of disease.
  - serum aminotransferase—ACT (SGOT), ALT (SGPT)—usually rises before the onset of jaundice and will remain elevated for several weeks with a gradual decline as the patient improves.
  - alkaline phosphatase rises early in the disease, will usually remain elevated throughout the disease, and is often the last enzyme to return to normal
  - prothrombin time may be prolonged.
  - serum albumin decreases in later stages of the disease.
- Urinalysis: shows elevated bilirubin levels
- Immunological findings for specific types of hepatitis
  - antibodies to hepatitis A (Anti-HA) are in the serum. Found within 4 weeks of infection and can remain present for over 10 years.
  - hepatitis B surface antigen (HBsAG) is in the blood. Found 1–2 weeks before onset of the symptoms and is usually not present 2 months after symptoms have cleared. Can indicate a chronic carrier state if it is in the serum for 3 months after symptoms have cleared.
  - antibodies to hepatitis B surface antigen (Anti-HBs) are in the serum. Demonstrates prior infection or immunization to hepatitis B.
  - antibodies to Hepatitis C (Anti-HC) are in the serum. Found 4–32 weeks after the appearance of symptoms.

▶ NURSING DIAGNOSIS: *Fluid Volume Deficit*

Related To
- Increased fluid volume loss secondary to nausea/vomiting
- Decreased fluid intake due to anorexia

Defining Characteristics
- Decreased skin turgor
- Increased specific gravity of urine
- Decreased blood pressure
- Increased pulse rate
- Postural changes in blood pressure and pulse
- Elevated hemoglobin (Hgb) and hematocrit (Hct) due to hemoconcentration
- Elevated serum sodium
- Increased thirst
- Decreased urine output

Patient Outcomes
Fluid volume is adequate, as evidenced by:
- blood pressure and pulse returning to patient baseline.
- normal skin turgor.
- urine specific gravity between 1.015 and 1.025.
- absence of postural changes in blood pressure and pulse.
- moist mucous membranes.
- normal serum sodium.
- elevated blood urea nitrogen (BUN).

Nursing Interventions	Rationales
Monitor temperature, blood pressure, pulse, and postural changes in vitals.	Hypovolemia is characterized by a decrease in blood pressure and increase in pulse rate. A drop of blood pressure of 10–15 mm Hg and an increase of 10–20 beats in pulse rate with a change in position reflect a hypovolemic state and are indicators of both circulating volume and perfusion status.
Instruct patient to monitor and record intake and output and weigh themselves daily. Draw and monitor BUN and creatinine and obtain urine samples to monitor specific gravity.	Anorexia, nausea, and vomiting all can cause decreased intake with fluid volume loss. Decreasing urine output with increasing urine specific gravity and increasing BUN are all evidence of fluid volume deficit.

Nursing Interventions	Rationales
Assess for peripheral indicators of fluid balance, i.e., skin turgor, status of mucous membranes, and thirst.	These are signs of hypovolemia and dehydration.
Monitor Hgb, Hct, albumin, and prothrombin time drawn in the home or at the physician's office. Assess for evidence of bleeding tendency, such as bruising and bleeding.	Albumin will reflect protein status needed for repairing damaged liver, maintaining normal fluid volume status, and preventing edema. Clotting factor formation can decrease, which increases the risk of hemorrhage and adds to the fluid volume deficits.
Offer clear liquids in small amounts with more frequent intervals.	Anorexia and aversion to smells and food make fluid replacement at home difficult.

▶ NURSING DIAGNOSIS: *Altered Nutrition—Less Than Body Requirements*

Related To
- Insufficient intake to meet increased metabolic needs secondary to nausea, vomiting, anorexia, and aversion to food
- Abnormal metabolism of foods with decreased energy sources secondary to inflammation of the liver and decreased metabolic efficiency

Defining Characteristics
- Reported aversion to food
- Weight loss
- Fatigue
- Abdominal pain
- Decreased serum albumin

Patient Outcomes
Patient will exhibit:
- gradual weight gain.
- normalization of serum albumin, Hgb, and Hct.
- gradual increase in activity tolerance.

Nursing Interventions	Rationales
Monitor dietary intake of calories and food intake by encouraging the patient or family to maintain a food diary.	Decreased caloric intake secondary to nausea and vomiting can lead to a malnourished state that decreases the body's ability to heal. Accurate

Nursing Interventions	Rationales
	intake information helps identify correct interventions to meet caloric needs.
Encourage small, frequent meals with intake of fat, protein, and carbohydrate proportional to individual patient needs.	Large servings in the presence of anorexia can decrease appetite even more. Individual patients will have very individualized needs depending upon the stage and severity of the disease. Fat intolerance may be present. Individuals with a marked decrease in liver function may need to restrict protein intake. A dietary consult may be valuable. Adding high-calorie foods in small frequent servings can maintain individualized caloric needs.
Monitor serum albumin, Hgb, and Hct levels drawn by nurse or at physician's office.	Malnutrition and liver disease are associated with a decrease in serum albumin secondary to a decrease in protein synthesis. Low serum albumin is also associated with edema. Decreased nutritional intake can lead to anemia from folic acid or iron deficiency.
Identify patient's beverage and food preferences and plan with patient and family to obtain and prepare these foods.	Providing patients with their favorite foods will encourage them to eat. Small frequent meals will decrease nausea and increase nutritional intake.

▶ NURSING DIAGNOSIS: *Activity Intolerance*

Related To
- Decreased gluconeogenesis secondary to liver dysfunction
- Anorexia causing fatigue and weakness

Defining Characteristics
- Verbal reports of fatigue or weakness
- Decreased exercise tolerance
- Decreased muscle strength

Patient Outcomes

Patient will:
- have decreased reports of fatigue and weakness.
- have increased muscle strength.
- gradually increase exercise intervals without fatigue.

Nursing Interventions	Rationales
Promote periods of rest associated with periods of activity.	Prolonged rest can decrease muscle strength and endurance. Increasing activity before liver inflammation subsides can increase liver function tests and worsen the disease. It is important to teach patients and family the importance of gradually increasing exercise.
Monitor liver enzyme levels drawn by nurse or at physician's office. Watch for signs and symptoms of increased fatigue and exhaustion.	Premature increase in activity can increase enzyme levels. Fatigue is frequently an indicator of too rapid escalation of activity.
Prior to beginning exercise program, discuss exercise regimen with patient and physician.	Communication between nurse, patient, and physician is vital to maximize healthy outcomes and treatment success.

▶ NURSING DIAGNOSIS: *High Risk for Infection*

Risk Factors
- Immunosuppression
- Granulocytopenia
- Malnutrition

Patient Outcomes

Patient will:
- be free of secondary infection.
- verbalize the principles of disease transmission.
- make lifestyle changes needed to prevent disease transmission.

Nursing Interventions	Rationales
Explain to patient and family the method of disease transmission, the importance of hand washing, and how to isolate urine, stool, and blood.	Most cases of hepatitis are treated on an outpatient basis. Individuals who live in close contact are at high risk for disease transmission. Proper handling of infected body waste can lower the risk of cross-infection.
Limit visitors and minimize exposure to individuals with respiratory infections.	Patients are at high risk for developing secondary infections due to immunosuppression. Prevention is essential.

DISCHARGE PLANNING/CONTINUITY OF CARE
- Refer family members to health care provider for early signs and symptoms of hepatitis.
- Refer patient to health care provider or public health clinic to determine possibility of carrier status at the end of 3 months.
- Refer to community health clinics, private health care provider, or school health clinics to learn more about preventive health practices, such as safe sex and how to avoid exposure to other communicable diseases.
- Refer to drug rehabilitation program, if appropriate.
- Refer to social services for crowded living conditions, poor hygiene, or inadequate finances. These increase the risk of reexposure.

BIBLIOGRAPHY
Beneson, A. S. (Ed.). (1990). *Control of communicable disease in man*, (15th ed.). Washington, DC: American Public Health Association.

Gilchrist, E. (1991). Hepatitis B: It will never happen to me. *Today's OR Nurse, 13*, 15–18.

Jackson, M., & Rymer, T. (1994). Viral hepatitis: Anatomy of a diagnosis. *American Journal of Nursing, 94*(1), 43–48.

Poss, J. E. (1989). Hepatitis D virus infection. *Nurse Practitioner, 14*, 14–15.

Health
Behaviors

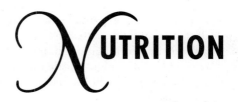

NUTRITION

Pamela K. Roark, BSN, MA, MSN

Nutrition is the study of processes by which living organisms receive and utilize nutrients from food for maintaining tissue function and growth. Nutrition can be viewed along a continuum, with the malnourished population—including undernourished and obese—at one end and those with optimal nutrition at the opposite end. In the middle of this continuum—where most of the population is found—are those who exhibit some healthy behaviors but have not reached optimal nutrition. In addition, certain diseases, such as cardiovascular disease, diabetes, and renal disease, require special diets that must be followed to obtain optimal nutritional status. To adopt these healthy behaviors, patients need appropriate information, motivation, and supportive environments. Nursing care should focus on treating the malnourished and teaching and reinforcing health-promoting, optimal nutritious diets.

ETIOLOGIES

Undernutrition/underweight
- inadequate intake of calories
- malabsorption of the intake (due to swallowing and structural abnormalities)
- lack of access to wholesome, nutritious food supply (availability, cost, convenience)
- cultural and/or religious influences on food choices and eating habits
- misconceptions, lack of adequate nutrition information
- noncompliance with diet
- anxiety/depression
- psychological body image disturbance (anorexia or bulimia)

Overnutrition/overweight
- dysfunctional eating patterns

- imbalance between intake and activity level (increased intake and decreased activity patterns)
- cultural and/or religious influences on food choices and eating habits (eating high-fat, high-calorie meals)
- lack of access to wholesome, nutritious food supply (availability, cost, convenience)
- misconceptions, lack of adequate nutrition information
- noncompliance with diet
- anxiety/depression

CLINICAL MANIFESTATIONS

Undernutrition/underweight
- loss of body weight with adequate food intake
- food intake less than recommended daily allowances
- general appearance listless, apathetic, cachectic
- flaccid, poor muscle tone, "wasted" appearance
- anorexia, indigestion, constipation or diarrhea
- easily fatigued, no energy
- skin rough, dry, scaly, pale
- sore, inflamed buccal cavity
- hyperactive bowel sounds
- pale conjunctival and mucous membranes

Overnutrition/overweight
- food intake more than recommended daily allowances
- pairs food with other activities
- majority of food intake at end of day
- eating in response to external clues such as time of day or social situation
- eating in response to internal clues other than hunger, such as stress, anxiety, depression
- rotund appearance
- lack of energy, easily fatigued

CLINICAL/DIAGNOSTIC FINDINGS

Undernutrition/underweight
- weight 10% or more under ideal
- decreased serum protein level (adult normal range 6.0–8.2 g/dL)
- decreased serum albumin level (adult normal range 3.5–5.0 g/dL)
- increased transferrin levels (adult normal range 250–450 ug/dL)
- anthropometric measures below standards

Overnutrition/overweight
- weight 10% or more over ideal
- anthropometric measure above standards

▶ NURSING DIAGNOSIS: *Altered Nutrition—Less Than Body Requirements*

Related To inability to ingest or digest food or absorb nutrients because of biological, chemical, psychological, or economic factors

Defining Characteristics
• Body weight 10% or more under ideal
• Food intake less than recommended daily allowance

Patient Outcomes
Nutritional status is adequate, as evidenced by:
• weight within normal range for height and age.
• a diet that contains the recommended daily food allowances.
• no signs and symptoms of malnutrition.

Nursing Interventions	Rationales
Determine if weight loss or gain is intentional.	Etiology of altered nutritional status will affect nursing approach. Psychiatric causes need to be treated differently than lacking knowledge or "will power."
Assess and monitor caloric and nutrient intake. Use a self-report diary to assist in assessing actual intake.	Provider can use information to calculate the patient's nutritional intake and compare it with recommended allowances.
Weigh patient at regular intervals (weekly) with the same scale.	This will detect changes that may indicate improved or deteriorating nutritional status.
Assess ability to chew and swallow. If problems with chewing, refer to speech therapist or dentist.	Inability to properly chew and/or swallow food is a contributing factor to malnutrition and additional workup and referral are required.
Monitor for changes in physical assessment findings.	Changes in assessment observations indicate improved, unchanged, or worsening condition.
Monitor laboratory values.	Abnormal levels of albumin, serum total protein, and transferrin indicate continued nutritional deficiencies.

Nursing Interventions	Rationales
Determine cultural and religious influences on food selection. Encourage patient to incorporate these foods in the diet plan.	Incorporating these foods, as appropriate, into the diet plan will promote compliance.
Assess socioeconomic factors such as food availability, economic issues, and social/family supports. Refer to appropriate community resources, such as a local food pantry and Meals on Wheels. If appropriate, refer to social worker.	Community resources can help to ensure that the patient has access to nutritious food in order to achieve or maintain desired weight.
Determine time of day when patient's appetite is greatest and plan highest caloric meal for that time.	This is the most likely time that patient will take in the proper amount of food.
Encourage eating by offering small amounts of food at one time.	Smaller meals facilitate gastric emptying and promote an overall larger food intake.
Encourage moderate exercise.	This stimulates appetite and prevents complications from sedentary lifestyle.
Provide frequent, positive reinforcement of patient self-care activities that promote a healthy, nutritious lifestyle.	Positive feedback promotes self-care activities.
Reassess anthropometric measures at established goal date.	This allows for comparison with baseline measurements taken prior to nursing intervention. (Note standards have not been established for the elderly over 75 years of age.)
Assist patient/family to prepare meal plans and grocery lists.	The more involved the patient/family is in planning, the greater the probability of compliance with diet and recommended daily allowances.

▶ **NURSING DIAGNOSIS: *Altered Nutrition—More Than Body Requirements***

Related To excessive intake in relation to metabolic needs

Defining Characteristics
- Body weight 10% or more over ideal
- Imbalance between diet and activity levels (increased intake and decreased activity)
- Dysfunctional eating patterns

Patient/Family Outcomes
Patient will:
- exhibit progressive weight loss toward desired goal within established length of time.
- consume a balanced nutritional diet that facilitates weight reduction.
- follow a regular exercise plan (see also Exercise chapter).
- identify and modify dysfunctional eating behaviors.

Nursing Interventions	Rationales
Assess and monitor caloric/nutrient intake and eating patterns. Use a self-report diary to assist in assessing what, when, and where patient eats.	Identifies nutritional intake and dysfunctional eating patterns.
Assist patient to identify motivation for eating and associated internal and external cues to eating. Discuss behavior modification needed to correct dysfunctional eating patterns.	Patients identifying and understanding dysfunctional eating patterns will positively affect their ability or willingness to modify intake.
Assess patient's activity level and compare with dietary intake.	Increased intake and decreased activity is the primary cause of overweight/obesity.
Determine patient's desire and motivation to reduce weight.	This will assist in developing personalized short- and long-term goals for weight loss. However, without desire or motivation, the patient may be unwilling to modify nutritional intake regardless of nursing interventions and education.
Recommend a diet plan. If, indicated, refer to dietician or nutritionist for recommended diet.	A nutritious, calorie-reduced diet will assist in achieving long-range weight loss goals.
Weigh patient or have patient record weight at regular intervals (weekly) with the same scale.	Provides a visible means of assessing progress toward reaching weight loss goal; more frequent weights may reflect temporary

Nursing Interventions	Rationales
	weight gains and cause patient to become discouraged.
Assist patient in selecting an exercise plan that he or she will enjoy.	Promotes compliance for adhering to exercise plan.
Teach stress reduction techniques such as progressive relaxation, quiet time, and time management.	Reduces eating associated with stress and facilitates behavior modification.
Determine cultural and religious influences on food selection. Identify foods high in fats and refined sugars and encourage patient to reduce or eliminate these foods in diet. Encourage using those low in fats and refined sugars.	Because of cultural background and religious preferences, patient may not know the nutritional content of these foods and their effect on weight management.
Encourage patient to grocery shop with a list and soon after eating.	This enhances compliance to recommended diet and reduces impulsive food buying.
Provide positive reinforcement for consistent progress toward weight loss goals. Encourage patient to develop internal reward system for when goals are accomplished.	This promotes positive behavior changes and enhances patient's sense of control.
Identify available community resources such as support groups (TOPS, Overeaters Anonymous, Weight Watchers) and community weight control programs.	Provides long range support for continued success with weight loss and weight maintenance.

▶ NURSING DIAGNOSIS: *Knowledge Deficit*

Related To lack of nutritional information or misinformation about newly prescribed diet

Defining Characteristics
- Patient/family verbalizes lack of understanding regarding recommended diet and nutritional requirements.
- Patient/family exhibits poor selection of foods to meet nutritional requirements.

Patient Outcomes
Patient/family will:

- state the recommended daily food allowances.
- verbalize understanding of his or her own prescribed diets.
- verbalize understanding of Federal Drug Administration (FDA) food labels.
- design and implement a personalized nutritional improvement plan.
- describe how to contact and access community support services.

Nursing Interventions	Rationales
Assess patient/family current level of understanding of prescribed diet.	Individualized teaching plan avoids needless repetition and improves learning.
Design teaching plan specific to patient/family needs and educational level.	This is best suited to meet the needs of the patient/family and improve understanding.
Provide dietary instructions that are written at the appropriate educational level and in the patient's/family's primary language.	These are a valuable resource for the patient/family that is readily available at all times. These instructions must be understandable for patient to use them.
Provide both verbal and written information on purpose of the diet, diet requirements and food preparation, weighing and measuring food, signs and symptoms of malnutrition, recommended exercise plan, and benefits of optimal nutritional status.	This aids in reinforcing information and is a resource for long-term planning.
Inform patient of possible drug/food interactions as appropriate.	Patient must be able to identify these when making food choices to avoid adverse reaction.
Instruct patient how to accommodate his or her food preferences into the prescribed diet.	Promotes compliance with prescribed diet.
Instruct patient how to plan appropriate meals. Provide written meal plans using food pyramid concept.	Knowledge of menu planning and food preparation enhances compliance with prescribed diet.
Instruct patient/family how to read food labels and select appropriate foods in compliance with prescribed diet.	Patient/family should be able to identify the nutrient content of foods to select appropriate food items that are in compliance with recommended dietary plan.

Nursing Interventions	Rationales
Encourage verbalization of concerns and anxiety about willingness and ability to adhere to prescribed diet.	Assists in reducing fear and anxiety and provides a means for identifying possible resources.
Provide forms for recording dietary intake and weight and instruct on how to keep a food diary.	Provides a valuable resource for the patient and family to chart progress. Is also a valuable document for health care providers in assessing nutritional intake and eating patterns during follow-up.
Provide literature and forms for planning a food budget.	This provides a planned strategy for how and when to purchase recommended food items.
Refer to dietician, particularly when starting a new diet.	Dieticians can initiate a teaching plan for a new diet therapy.

DISCHARGE PLANNING/CONTINUITY OF CARE

- Refer to local continuing support services, including food pantries, Meals on Wheels, and community health services.
- Ensure patient has follow-up appointment with physician.
- Refer to dietician for follow-up advise and information.

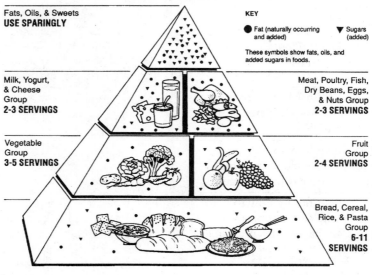

Food Guide Pyramid
A Guide to Daily Food Choices

Fats, Oils, & Sweets
USE SPARINGLY

KEY

● Fat (naturally occurring and added)   ▼ Sugars (added)

These symbols show fats, oils, and added sugars in foods.

Milk, Yogurt, & Cheese Group
2-3 SERVINGS

Meat, Poultry, Fish, Dry Beans, Eggs, & Nuts Group
2-3 SERVINGS

Vegetable Group
3-5 SERVINGS

Fruit Group
2-4 SERVINGS

Bread, Cereal, Rice, & Pasta Group
6-11 SERVINGS

Figure 41-1.

BIBLIOGRAPHY

Cerrato, P. L. (1993). Deciphering the new food labels. *RN, 56*(8), 57–58.

Herron, D. G. (1991). Strategies for promoting a healthy dietary intake. *Nursing Clinics of North America, 26,*(4), 875–884.

Treseler, K. M. (1998). *Clinical laboratory and diagnostic tests: Significance and nursing implications* (2nd ed.). Norwalk, CT: Appleton & Lange.

U.S. Department of Agriculture and Health and Human Services. (1990). *Nutrition and your health: Dietary guidelines for Americans,* (3rd ed.). Washington, DC: U. S. Government Printing Office.

SLEEP AND REST PATTERNS

Pamela K. Roark, BSN, MA, MSN

Adequate sleep is essential for health and well-being. Sleep is a basic human need and is defined as a recurrent, altered state of consciousness that occurs for sustained periods, restoring energy and well-being. Everyone requires different amounts and qualities of sleep and rest. It is generally thought that 6–8 h of sleep each night is necessary. However, the best advice for patients is to obtain an average amount of sleep that is needed to avoid fatigue. Identifying disturbances in sleep and rest patterns is an important goal for preventive and restorative nursing care.

ETIOLOGIES
- Emotional stress
- Nonfunctional sleep habits
- Use of drugs or alcohol
- Environmental factors such as noise, light, and temperature
- Physical illness
- Pain or discomfort

CLINICAL MANIFESTATIONS
- Difficulty falling asleep
- Not feeling well rested
- Awakening earlier/later than desired
- Interrupted sleep
- Complaints of fatigue
- Changes in behavior and performance
- Increasing irritability, restlessness, disorientation, or lethargy
- Physical signs such as hand tremor, ptosis of eyelid, expressionless face, dark circles under eyes, frequent yawning, or changes in posture

CLINICAL/DIAGNOSTIC FINDINGS
None

▶ **NURSING DIAGNOSIS:** *Sleep Pattern Disturbance*

Related To difficulty falling and remaining asleep, life events, and stress

Defining Characteristics
- Difficulty falling asleep, taking up to an hour or more to go to sleep
- Interrupted sleep, awakens two to three times nightly with difficulty falling back to sleep
- Complaints of not feeling well rested

Patient Outcomes
Patient will:
- fall asleep within 30 min of going to bed.
- awaken less during the night.
- verbalize feeling refreshed and less fatigued during the day.
- verbalize plan to implement beneficial bedtime routine.

Nursing Interventions	Rationales
Assess for factors that are interfering with sleep.	Physiological, psychological, and environmental factors can alter the quantity and quality of sleep.
Assess for signs/symptoms of sleep disorders, such as long-term insomnia, sleep apnea, narcolepsy, and severe sleep deprivation. Refer patient to a physician who deals with sleep disorders.	Significant sleep disorders may need further workup in a sleep laboratory.
Assess patient's normal sleep pattern.	Knowing a patient's normal sleep pattern will assist the nurse in developing a sleep plan.
Instruct patient and/or bed partner to keep a sleep-wake log for 1–2 weeks. Review log with patient.	This log can help to identify the factors that are interfering with sleep and distinguish beneficial habits from detrimental ones.
Assist patient in developing plan to restrict caffeine or alcohol from diet in the evening and to avoid large meals late at night.	Caffeine and alcohol act as stimulants and disrupt sleep patterns. The digestive process may interfere with normal sleep patterns.

Nursing Interventions	Rationales
Assist patient in developing an effective bedtime ritual. Determine those habits that are beneficial for the individual patient. Drink a glass of milk before retiring if not contraindicated.	Following a bedtime ritual that includes going to bed at the same time each night enhances the patient's ability to fall asleep. L-Tryptophan in milk is believed to induce sleep.
Instruct patient to perform relaxation techniques as part of the bedtime ritual. These may include a soothing bath, meditation, or progressive relaxation.	Relaxation will help induce sleep and decrease stress and anxiety.
Assess bedtime environment. Identify factors that can be reduced or controlled such as noise, light, and amount of ventilation.	Loud noises and light can prevent and interfere with sleep.
Determine if sleep disturbance is related to a situational crisis or emotional problem. Refer for psychiatric evaluation.	Identifing underlying causes of sleep disturbance help determine if referrals to additional health care providers are necessary.
Encourage adequate physical exercise during the day.	Moderate fatigue from enjoyable work or exercise will enhance restful sleep.
Identify medications being taken and their effect on sleep.	Medications being taken for sleep often cause more problems than benefits and should be avoided. Numerous other drugs cause sleep pattern disturbance, such as diuretics, stimulants, digoxin, beta blockers, valium, and narcotics.
Refer patient to community services and support groups that deal with stress management.	Patient will receive long-term benefits from support groups.

DISCHARGE PLANNING/CONTINUITY OF CARE

- Refer to local community health services and support groups.

Clinical Clip

Johnson (1991) suggests that, instead of reaching for the bottle of sleeping pills, progressive relaxation may be the answer to ensure a good night's sleep. Johnson selected 55 noninstitutionalized women 65 years of age or older to participate in an 8-day sleep laboratory study. Results suggested that progressive relaxation is an effective intervention. The women fell asleep more readily, woke up less frequently during the night, and slept more soundly. Limitations of the study included prior medication use and health status of the subjects. However, progressive relaxation is an intervention that the nurse can easily learn and teach.

REFERENCES/BIBLIOGRAPHY

Glick, O. J. (1992). Interventions related to activity and movement. *The Nursing Clinics of North America, 27*(2), 541–568.

Johnson, J. (1991). Progressive relaxation and the sleep of older noninstitutionalized women. *Applied Nursing Research, 4*(4), 165–170.

Miller, C. A. (1993). Interventions for sleep pattern disturbances. *Geriatric Nursing, 14*(5), 235–236.

Spenceley, S. M. (1993). Sleep inquiry: A look with fresh eyes. Image: *Journal of Nursing Scholarship, 25*(3), 249–256.

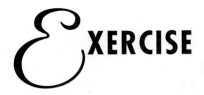

$\mathcal{E}$XERCISE

Pamela K. Roark, BSN, MA, MSN

Exercise is an important component of a healthy lifestyle. Regular exercise, combined with a proper diet, promotes health and well-being. There are a number of physiological and psychological benefits of regular exercise and fitness. These include improved muscle strength, aerobic capacity, immune response, and psychological well-being. Regular exercise can also reduce the risk of cardiovascular disease and cancer. Exercise is a health promotion activity that requires minimal or no financial investment. Everyone can exercise! However, despite the current "fitness craze," the majority of Americans lead sedentary lifestyles. Studies have shown that only 20 percent of Americans are physically active.

Nurses are in key positions to reinforce the positive benefits of exercise for all of our patients, both young and old. All individuals should exercise based on their physical condition and abilities. Exercising appropriately will increase energy levels, making daily tasks easier, and increase self-esteem and self-confidence.

Clinical Clip

Activity Intolerance

Inadequate or inappropriate exercise causes or places the patient at risk for activity intolerance. This also places the patient at risk for medical complications—for example, a heart attack for a cardiac patient. Activity intolerance is a state in which an individual is at risk of experiencing or is experiencing an insufficient physiological or psychological energy to endure or complete required or desired daily activities. There are several clinical conditions that might affect the patient's activity tolerance. These include anemias, cardiovascular disease, pulmonary disease, metabolic disorders, and musculoskeletal disorders.

ETIOLOGIES
- Sedentary lifestyle
- Lack of knowledge regarding proper exercise

CLINICAL MANIFESTATIONS
- Verbalizes complaint of fatigue or weakness
- Unable to perform desired activities
- Complaint of dizziness, dyspnea, diaphoresis with increased activity

CLINICAL/DIAGNOSTIC FINDINGS
- Abnormally elevated pulse rate, respiratory rate, and blood pressure in response to activity

▶ NURSING DIAGNOSIS: *Activity Intolerance*

Related To sedentary lifestyle

Defining Characteristics
- Exhibits physical symptoms of fatigue, such as shortness of breath or vertigo, or weakness upon minimal activity
- Verbalizes minimal or lack of regular exercises
- Misconceptions, lack of exercise/fitness information
- Lack of understanding regarding health benefits and physiological effects of exercise
- Lack of knowledge regarding adequate and appropriate exercise activities

Patient Outcomes
Patient will:
- experience diminished fatigue and weakness with daily activities.
- participate in regular exercise program.
- verbalize increased sense of health and well-being.
- have a pulse rate less than the recommended maximum heart rate (220 minus person's age) and that returns to baseline within 5–7 min.

Nursing Interventions	Rationales
Assess patient's health history and physical status.	It is necessary to determine if patient has any health problems that would contraindicate participation in a regular exercise program.
Assess patient's current activity level. Have patient self-report a normal week's exercise activities.	Establishes baseline for planning.

Nursing Interventions	Rationales
Assess range of motion and determine muscular strength. This can be done by having patient perform sit-ups and push-ups for 1 min. Determine how far patient can walk or jog before becoming fatigued.	
Evaluate patient's beliefs regarding physical exercise. Reinforce accurate information and dispel myths.	Incorrect information may discourage patient from either starting an exercise program or maintaining one.
Assist patient in developing personal short- and long-term goals for desired activities.	Encourages adherence to exercise plan. Meeting short-term goals promotes a sense of accomplishment and is a method to motivate positive behavior.
Encourage family involvement in planning and maintaining the exercise program.	Family involvement provides positive reinforcement for the program.
Instruct patient about exercise plan, including type, intensity, duration, and frequency of each activity.	A specific, written plan that is individualized to the patient maximizes the benefits and reduces risks for the patient.
Assist patient to prepare and maintain a graph or log to chart his or her progress.	This provides visual feedback of progress and serves as an incentive to adhere to exercise program.
Monitor vital signs before, immediately after, and 5–7 min after activity. Alter type or intensity of exercise in response to vital signs. Modify type or decrease exercise intensity in response to vital signs. Instruct patient on how to palpate carotid pulse for 1 min to determine heart rate.	Pulse, respiratory rate, and blood pressure should return to baseline within 5–7 min after exercise.
Instruct patient about signs and symptoms that warrant stopping or modifying the exercise. These include undue fatigue, chest pain, shortness of breath, dizziness, and/or muscle or joint pain.	If the patient is beginning an exercise program after being sedentary, closely monitor the patient for the above signs and symptoms to reduce cardiovascular and musculoskeletal injuries.

Nursing Interventions	Rationales
Instruct and demonstrate proper warm-up and cool-down exercises.	Warm-up and cool-down exercises improve circulation and decrease risk of injuries.
Instruct patient on importance of a well-balanced diet and adequate hydration (6–8 glasses per day).	Increased activity level will increase metabolic and fluid requirements. (See Nutrition chapter.)
Assist patient to identify incentives and barriers for adhering to exercise plan.	This improves the patient's motivation and can identify ways in which to decrease barriers.
Provide positive reinforcement for patient's efforts.	Positive reinforcement increases self-esteem as well as the probability exercise program will continue.
Identify available community services that offer exercise programs and support groups, i.e., community centers, park district recreation programs, and adult education offerings.	Provides location for and support in exercise.

▶ **NURSING DIAGNOSIS:** *High Risk for Injury*

Risk Factors

- History of chronic illness
- Recent hospitalizations or surgeries
- Cardiac medications
- Obesity
- Musculoskeletal disease or injury

Patient Outcomes

Patient will:
- experience diminished fatigue and weakness with daily activities.
- increase endurance and flexibility.
- participate in regular exercise program.
- verbalize increased sense of health and well-being.
- demonstrate exercise activities using proper body mechanics and safety measures.

Nursing Interventions	Rationales
Perform an initial assessment which includes a thorough health history and physical exam.	There is a need to identify contraindications to participate in a regular exercise program. Examples

Nursing Interventions	Rationales
	of contraindications are: cardiovascular disease, shortness of breath, dizziness, pulmonary disease, renal disease, musculoskeletal problems, and certain medications.
Arrange for a physician consultation prior to initiating an exercise program.	Physician consent should be obtained prior to engaging in a regular exercise program. Closer monitoring may be required.
Refer to physical therapy (PT), occupational therapy (OT), and/or cardiac/pulmonary rehabilitation programs.	Patients with special needs will benefit from the expertise of specialists in this field. Exercise programs provided through these resources also offer the patient a unique opportunity to meet and develop support systems with other patients that have the same problems and concerns. This will enhance compliance.
Develop an individual exercise plan that is tailored to the patient's specific capabilities, goals, and resources. The exercise plan should contain a combination of dynamic and flexibility exercises. Examples of dynamic exercises are walking, cycling, and swimming. Flexibility exercises involve stretching movements that enhance range of motion.	These patients have special needs due to their health status. Their exercise plan must maximize the benefits and minimize the risk of each exercise. Static exercises are often contraindicated.
Instruct patient about exercise plan, including type, intensity, duration, and frequency. Demonstrate how to properly perform prescribed exercises using proper body mechanics.	Increased knowledge and understanding will enhance motivation and compliance.
Instruct patient about signs and symptoms that warrant stopping or modifying the exercise. These include undue fatigue, chest pain, shortness of breath, dizziness, headache, and/or muscle or joint pain. Patients should seek advise	Identifying warning signs early will reduce risk factors associated with exercise in this patient population.

Nursing Interventions	Rationales
from their health care provider if these symptoms occur.	
Assess patient's perception of exertion level during exercise to determine optimal training intensity. Decrease intensity if perceived exertion is "hard."	Target heart rate measurements may not be appropriate for this patient population, especially those that take medications to depress or accelerate their heart rate.
Assess patient's fears and concerns regarding exercise.	Patients with health problems are often concerned of beginning exercise programs and are fearful that it may exacerbate their health problems. Talking about these feelings will assist the patient in working through these fears and in identifying the benefits of this safe exercise plan and how to reduce the risks.

DISCHARGE PLANNING/CONTINUITY OF CARE

Continue community services, PT, OT, and cardiac/pulmonary rehabilitation programs. If possible, encourage patient to join formal exercise group or program or plan exercise activities with others.

BIBLIOGRAPHY

Edmunds, M. W. (1991). Strategies for promoting physical fitness. *Nursing Clinics of North America, 26*(4), 855–866.

Field, L. K., & Steinhardt, M. A. (1992). The relationship of internally directed behavior to self-reinforcement, self-esteem, and expectancy values for exercise. *American Journal of Health Promotion, 7*(1), 21–27.

Moore, S. R. (1989). Walking for health: A nurse-managed activity. *Journal of Gerontological Nursing, 15*(7), 26–28.

Topp, R. (1991). Development of an exercise program for older adults: Preexercise testing, exercise prescription and program maintenance. *Nurse Practitioner, 16*(10), 16–28.

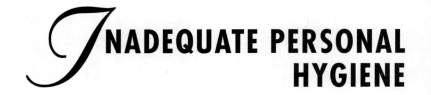

*I*NADEQUATE PERSONAL HYGIENE

Pamela K. Roark, BSN, MA, MSN

Personal hygiene is personal care of the skin, teeth, oral and nasal cavities, eyes, ears, and perineal and genital regions. Many view personal hygiene as a private matter, influenced by cultural, social, familial, and personal factors. Adequate hygiene promotes health and prevents disease, and poor personal hygiene is a risk factor for disease transmission. The nurse's overall role is to educate the patient and provide supports.

ETIOLOGIES
- Unwillingness to perform adequate hygiene
- Intolerance to activity
- Pain
- Neuromuscular impairment
- Musculoskeletal impairment
- Severe depression

CLINICAL MANIFESTATIONS
- Disheveled appearance
- Visible dirt on skin and nails
- Strong body odor
- Inflamed oral mucosa, discolored teeth, halitosis

CLINICAL/DIAGNOSTIC FINDINGS
- Lice
- Scabies

▶ **NURSING DIAGNOSIS:** *Inadequate Personal Hygiene*

Related To perceived need to perform hygiene activities for oneself

Defining Characteristics
- Disheveled appearance
- Visible dirt on skin and nails
- Strong body odor
- Inflamed oral mucosa, discolored teeth, halitosis

Patient Outcomes
Personal hygiene is adequate, as evidenced by:
- intact, clean skin, nails, hair, oral and nasal mucosa, eyes, ears, genital and perineal regions.
- being free of body odor.
- verbalizing and demonstrating adequate hygiene measures.
- establishing realistic self-care activities to be achieved.

Nursing Interventions	Rationales
Assess patient's feelings and beliefs regarding self-care hygiene activities.	Hygiene practices are a very personal matter. Identifying and discussing the patient's feelings will build a trusting, caring relationship.
Assess patient's ability to independently perform self-care hygiene activities.	Limitations or barriers must be evaluated and addressed to develop a realistic personal hygiene plan.
Assess status of oral cavity. Refer to dentist if necessary.	The oral cavity is often overlooked during patient assessment and provides valuable clues to the patient's overall health and hygiene practices.
Assist patient in developing a schedule to perform personal hygiene.	Developing a written plan and schedule will assist patient and family in establishing a repetitive hygiene routine.
Assess resources that are needed for adequate hygiene measures, including soap, water, toothbrush, and towels. Refer patient to local resources such as food pantries and community assistance offices if he or she cannot afford these items.	Adequate personal hygiene requires equipment.

Nursing Interventions	Rationales
Provide positive reinforcement for each self-care accomplishment.	This enhances self-esteem and increases motivation.
Arrange referral(s) to physical therapy (PT), occupational therapy (OT), and home health aide if appropriate.	These community resources may be needed to assist the patient who is unable to perform these self-care activities.
Refer to social worker if financial difficulty exists.	The social worker will assist the patient in obtaining financial assistance, if needed.

▶ **NURSING DIAGNOSIS:** *Knowledge Deficit*

Related To lack of information or misinformation regarding personal hygiene measures

Defining Characteristics
- Lack of understanding regarding recommended personal hygiene activities

Patient/Family Outcomes
Patient/family will:
- verbalize understanding of how to perform the recommended personal hygiene measures.
- explain and discuss importance of establishing a consistent routine of basic personal hygiene activities.
- list resources that can be utilized if supplies or more information is needed.

Nursing Interventions	Rationales
Observe patient performing personal hygiene practices such as bathing, grooming, and brushing teeth.	Nursing assessment based on direct observation of patient's personal hygiene habits will be key in developing an effective teaching plan.
Assess patient's current level of knowledge and understanding of hygiene practices.	The teaching plan must be personalized based on patient's knowledge and understanding to best meet his or her needs.

Nursing Interventions	Rationales
Instruct patient on benefits of adequate personal hygiene and risks of inadequate hygiene.	Personal hygiene activities are self-directed and self-motivated. Understanding the benefits and risks increases the probability the patient will adhere to the plan.
Instruct patient on proper hygiene practices, including care of the skin, eyes, ears, and perineal and genital regions.	Adequately understanding proper care will enhance compliance.
Demonstrate proper hygiene practices.	A demonstration will reinforce didactic instruction and increase learning.
Instruct patient on proper oral hygiene measures.	Dental health is a vital part of oral health. Poor oral hygiene practices will result in caries and periodontal disease.
Instruct patient on proper care of dentures (if applicable).	Dentures must also be kept clean to prevent bacterial and fungal organisms from accumulating.
Demonstrate proper teeth brushing and gum care.	A demonstration will reinforce didactic instruction and increase learning.
Provide written materials for patient and family regarding purpose and instruction of proper personal hygiene practices.	Patient and family can refer to these written materials as needed.

DISCHARGE PLANNING/CONTINUITY OF CARE
• Refer to or continue community services, PT, OT, and home health aide, if needed. Arrange scheduled follow-up with dental professionals as necessary.

BIBLIOGRAPHY
Winkley, G. P., Brown, J. O., & Stone, T. (1993). Interventions to improve oral care: The nursing assistant's role. *Journal of Gerontological Nursing, 19*(11), 47–48.

$\mathcal{S}$UBSTANCE ABUSE

Karen Egenes, RN, EdD

$\mathcal{S}$ubstance abuse/dependence exists when at least three of the following are present:

1. Ingesting a substance more frequently or in larger quantities than planned
2. Unsuccessfully attempting to stop or decrease substance use despite a desire to do so
3. Expending excessive time in procuring and in using substances and recovering from their use
4. Having an impaired ability to function at work and in social situations due to substance use or withdrawal
5. Reducing or ceasing other important life activities because of substance abuse/dependence
6. Continuing substance use despite physical, psychological, social, or occupational problems related to its use
7. Developing a tolerance for the substance

Continued substance abuse/dependence leads to serious physiological and psychological impairments. Family members, friends, or co-workers might notice these changes but attempt to "protect" the patient by making excuses for inappropriate patient behaviors. Slowly, the substance abuse/dependence adversely affects family and associate relationships.

Health care professionals often have first contact with the substance abuser when he or she seeks treatment for related health problems, including gastric ulcers, cirrhosis, or hepatitis. Usually the patient denies any problem with substance abuse/dependence and does not initiate treatment for abusive behavior. The patient often manipulates others by overusing denial, rationalizing, and blaming defense mechanisms.

The community health nurse can participate in combatting substance abuse/dependence by promoting mental health in families, identifying early stages of the addiction process, and referring patients for treatment. Nurse-initiated referrals to community resources also can help meet family needs for food, housing, and financial assistance.

ETIOLOGIES
- Biological: Patient is genetically predisposed to chemical dependence and is unable to cease its use.
- Psychological: Patient is regressed and fixated at the oral level of psychosexual development. The patient is highly dependent, with poor impulse control and low self-esteem.
- Sociocultural: Social conditions and contexts help to create and sustain substance abuse/dependence. Psychosocial stressors or deviant sub-cultures encourage a substance-dependent lifestyle.
- Family systems: Patient is the product of an enmeshed, overprotective family that lacks emotional warmth. Family members assume codependent roles in and attempt to control the patient's behavior, or "enabler" roles that help perpetuate the patient's substance abuse/dependence.

CLINICAL MANIFESTATIONS

Physical problems
- impaired speech, motor, and mental abilities
- cachexia and tremors due to vitamin deficiencies
- tremors/seizures, memory loss, neuritis, and sleep disturbances: indicate central nervous system dysfunction and irritability
- elevated temperature and lesions on mucous membranes: indicate low resistance to infection

Dysfunctional behavior patterns
- manipulation: exploits others to meet personal needs
- impulsivity: acts on whims; reckless, potentially self-injurious behavior
- dysfunctional anger: irritable and aggressive with explosive behavior
- avoidance: pattern of emotional distancing of self from others; poor parenting skills, marital relationship
- grandiosity: sense of uniqueness, superiority
- denial of addiction and problems caused by it
- low self-esteem

CLINICAL/DIAGNOSTIC FINDINGS
- Drug screen identifies drugs being used, including morphine, Percodan, and Quaalude.
- Blood alcohol level of 0.10 and above is considered "legally drunk" in most states.
- The addiction severity index (ASD) is an assessment tool that yields a "problem severity profile" and indicates areas of patient treatment needs.
- Liver function tests (SGOT and SGPT) might be elevated, reflecting liver damage.
- Elevated serum amylase indicates pancreatic damage.
- Hypokalemia and hypomagnesemia.

- Decreased hemoglobin reflects problems of iron deficiency anemia or gastrointestinal (GI) bleeding.
- White blood cell count might be increased if infection is present or decreased if immunosuppressed.

▶ NURSING DIAGNOSIS: *Powerlessness*

Related To dependent lifestyle and helplessness

Defining Characteristics
- Psychological craving for substance abused
- Ineffective attempts at recovery
- Statement of inability to discontinue substance abuse

Patient Outcomes
Patient will:
- identify factors that can be controlled by self.
- verbalize self-control alone will not lead to cessation of substance abuse.
- verbalize need for treatment.
- participate in treatment program.
- maintain sobriety and substance-free lifestyle.

Nursing Interventions	Rationales
Discuss patient's need for help in caring, nonjudgmental way.	A caring, nonmoralistic, nonjudgmental approach decreases patient defensiveness.
Discuss ways in which substance abuse/dependence has interfered with patient's life, work, and interpersonal relationships.	Awareness can help to decrease patient denial.
Inform patient about treatment options and self-help groups.	Knowledge of options promotes patient involvement in the treatment process.
Refer patient to a treatment program and help patient make first appointment.	Making the first appointment is often the most difficult for the patient.

▶ NURSING DIAGNOSIS: *Altered Nutrition—Less Than Body Requirements*

Related To:
- Replacing dietary intake with substance ingestion
- Chemicals interfering with nutrient absorption and metabolism

Defining Characteristics
- Reporting inadequate dietary intake
- Weight 10–20% or more below ideal for height and frame
- Poor muscle tone and skin turgor

Patient Outcomes
Patient will increase oral intake, as evidenced by:
- gaining 2 or more pounds per week.
- discussing relationship between substance abuse and malnutrition.
- discussing a well balanced diet.

Nursing Interventions	Rationales
Explain to patient the relationship between substance abuse and malnutrition and teach the components of a well-balanced diet.	This corrects patient knowledge deficits and provides needed information.
Help patient to plan a diet high in protein and carbohydrates.	Protein rebuilds nutritional status and elevates serum albumin, B vitamins promote central nervous system functioning, and carbohydrates decrease the craving for the abused substance. Enlisting patient collaboration in planning increases the probability that patient will follow plan.
Monitor patient's adherence to medication regimen, i.e., vitamins (especially thiamine) to replace losses and antacids to reduce gastric irritation.	Medications correct deficiencies and facilitate physical healing.
Weigh patient weekly and record.	Monitors patient progress.

▶ NURSING DIAGNOSIS: *High Risk for Violence—Self-Directed or Directed at Others*

Risk Factors
- History of overt aggressive acts
- Increase in stressors within a short period of time
- Perceived threats to self-esteem
- Dysfunctional coping mechanisms
- Rage reaction in response to frustration

Patient Outcomes

Patient will:
- abstain from violence toward others.
- verbalize causes of behavior and precipitating factors.
- describe alternative methods for appropriately expressing anger and frustration.

Nursing Interventions	Rationales
Assess patient history for violent or self-destructive behaviors related to substance abuse.	A history of previous violent behaviors is the best predictor of violent behavior. Being aware of the possibility of recurrent violence is the first step in preventing further episodes.
Encourage patient to verbally express feelings of anger and frustration.	Encouraging verbalization of feelings teaches the patient an effective and appropriate method of coping.
Assist patient to identify situations that provoke anger.	Awareness might help the patient consciously attempt alternative and appropriate methods of coping.
Discuss using physical activity as a means for appropriately expressing anger.	Gross motor activities can decrease aggressive drives.

▶ NURSING DIAGNOSIS: *Ineffective Denial*

Related To negative self-concept, anger, frustration, powerlessness, and sense of failure

Defining Characteristics
- Denying substance abuse, which is problematic or destructive to patient and significant others
- Refusing to seek treatment or assistance for problems related to substance abuse
- Blaming others for substance abuse
- Displaying impaired adaptive behavior and problem-solving skills

Patient Outcomes

Patient will:
- admit problems caused by substance abuse.
- seek treatment for substance abuse problem.
- verbalize relationship of substance abuse to current situation.

- use effective problem-solving and coping skills.
- maintain sobriety (or alert, optimum functioning) through abstinence from alcohol and/or drugs.

Nursing Interventions	Rationales
In an accepting, nonjudgmental manner, discuss with patient the problem of substance abuse and its consequences.	A nonjudgmental approach conveys to the patient the nurse's ability and willingness to understand the patient's situation without instilling guilt.
When patient uses denial, redirect interaction by saying, "I'm interested in hearing about your part in this."	Redirecting the patient's statements might decrease overusing denial. The nurse must especially avoid premature or ill-timed confrontation that increases patient defensiveness.
Help patient examine response to stressors at home, at work, and in social situations.	Helps the patient become aware of sources of stress and dysfunctional methods of coping used in the past. Helps the patient identify other methods of coping with stress.
Provide information about substance abuse and its deleterious effects on one's physical, psychological, and social functioning abilities.	Increased knowledge about the deleterious effects of substance abuse might encourage the patient to decide to abstain from substance use.
Teach the patient new coping skills such as relaxation techniques, assertiveness skills, and problem solving.	The opportunity to learn and practice new coping skills will reduce the patient's tendency to revert to dysfunctional coping methods.
Refer the patient to a self-help group such as Alcoholics Anonymous or Narcotic Anonymous.	Self-help groups help the patient relinquish excessive use of denial and learn alternative, functional coping strategies.
Refer patient's family members to appropriate self-help groups such as Alanon, Alateen, Codependents Anonymous, or Adult Children of Alcoholics.	Self-help groups help family members to recognize and change their dysfunctional responses (enabling, codependency, etc.) to the substance abuser. Family members require insight and support to assist the substance abuser in changing behaviors and to maintain their own emotional well-being.

Nursing Interventions	Rationales
Praise the patient and family members for acknowledging the substance abuse problem and for using more functional methods of coping.	Positive reinforcement builds self-esteem and encourages continued therapy.

▶ NURSING DIAGNOSIS: *Diversional Activity Deficit*

Related To cessation of substance abuse and loss of companions in substance abuse subculture

Defining Characteristics
- Statements of boredom/depression from lack of activity/interests
- Expressing feeling different from others
- Difficulty interacting with others in social situations

Patient Outcomes
Patient will:
- identify cause of boredom.
- verbalize willingness to be involved with others not involved in substance abuse.
- participate in diversional activities not connected to substance abuse subculture.
- structure leisure time with activities promoting sobriety.

Nursing Interventions	Rationales
Assist patient to find activities of interest that provide personal satisfaction.	Replaces time previously used in substance abuse activities with rewarding, satisfying activities.
Encourage interactions between patient and other persons in recovery from substance abuse.	Provides the patient with support and instills hope for continued sobriety.
Encourage patient to avoid previous companions who remain members of the substance abuse subculture.	This helps remove patient from potential sources of temptation.
Discuss with patient ways to find new friends not associated with the substance abuse subculture.	This provides support and encourages chemical-free lifestyle.
Praise patient for attempts to become involved in diversional activities supportive of sobriety.	Positive reinforcement builds self-esteem and encourages continued abstinence.

────────────────── **Clinical Clip** ──────────────────

Twelve-Step Self-Help Programs

Alcoholics Anonymous (AA) and Narcotic Anonymous (NA) are not specifically treatment programs but, rather, programs of recovery. They are international fellowships of men and women who meet together to attain and maintain sobriety. The groups are nonprofessional, self-supporting, nondenominational, and apolitical. Groups meet in halls, hospitals, churches, and schools almost every night of the week. Meetings are open to anyone who desires to stop taking drugs or alcohol.

Both AA and NA are based on the principle "Once an alcoholic/addict, always and alcoholic/addict." They believe total abstinence is essential to recovery. Through a series of 12 steps, members admit they are powerless over chemical substances, express belief in "a power greater than man," turn their problems over to "God as understood" by them, admit to and make amends for harm to others, and carry the message to other victims of substance abuse.

Through AA and NA, patients learn to correct negative attitudes and behaviors. As members become substance free, they are asked to "sponsor" or act as a supportive contact for other substance abusers. Regularly attending meetings and supporting other members are essential to the recovery process.

Note: Twelve-step programs are also effective with eating disorders and compulsive behaviors.

DISCHARGE PLANNING/CONTINUITY OF CARE
- Refer patient to self-help group (Alcoholics Anonymous or Narcotic Anonymous) and encourage continued participation.
- Refer patient's family members to appropriate self-help groups such as Alanon, Alateen, Naranon, Codependents Anonymous, or Adult Children of Alcoholics.
- Review and reinforce realistic plan for maintaining sobriety.
- Reinforce setting daily, short-term, attainable goals (i.e., sobriety "one day at a time").
- Refer patient to vocational counseling or social services as indicated.

OTHER PLANS OF CARE TO REFERENCE
- Social Isolation
- Parenting
- Neglect/Abuse: Child
- Nutrition

- Neglect/Abuse: Adult/Elderly
- Violence Against Women
- Communicable Diseases
- Exercise

BIBLIOGRAPHY

Barton, J. A. (1991). Parental adaptation to adolescent drug use: An ethnographic study of role formulation in response to courtesy stigma. *Public Health Nursing, 8*(1), 39–45.

Brent, N. J. (1992). Chemical use: Taking care of oneself. *Home Healthcare Nurse, 10*(1), 8–9.

Sheehan, A. (1992). Nurses respond to substance abuse. *International Nursing Review, 39*(5), 141–144.

Sullivan, E. J., & Handley, S. S. (1993). Alcohol and drug abuse. *Annual Review of Nursing Research, 11*, 281–297.

Wilson, H., & Kneisl, C. (1992). *Psychiatric nursing* (4th ed.). Redwood City, CA: Addison-Wesley.

MEDICATION COMPLIANCE/ NONCOMPLIANCE

Dana E. Clark, BSN, MBA

Medication compliance refers to patients taking prescribed medication at the correct dose, time, and route of administration. Noncompliance with prescription medication has been referred to as primary when the prescription is not filled and secondary when it is filled but subsequently not taken correctly because of either errors of omission or commission, schedule misconceptions or schedule noncompliance (Saunders, 1987). Compliance should be used in the context of failure to follow a regimen regardless of the reason.

The problem of medication noncompliance is frequently encountered by home care nurses and poses a continuous challenge in daily practice. Estimates on the rate of noncompliance vary. Poor compliance has been shown to cause inadequate disease control among patients with hypertension, epilepsy, childhood asthma, affective disorder, and other health problems. Reports indicate patients are frequently rehospitalized secondary to medication-related reasons. Therefore, the nurse's role is to encourage and assist the patient to maintain medication compliance.

The nurse's overall role is to assess for and to identify noncompliance and to provide education and assistive devices to assist the patient to be more informed and compliant.

Clinical Clip

In one study, 28.2% of elderly patients admitted to an acute-care hospital were drug related, 11.4 percent due to noncompliance, and 16.8 percent due to adverse drug reactions (Kluckowski, 1992). In addition to being detrimental for the patient, rehospitalizing patients also increases the cost of health care.

ETIOLOGIES/RISK FACTORS

It is important to understand the factors that contribute to noncompliance. Once these are identified, a plan can be put in place to help solve the problem. The factors that contribute to noncompliance are:
- Taking medications for prolonged periods of time for chronic disease management
- Financial difficulties
- Lack of understanding regarding medication regimen
- Poor cognitive function/poor literacy
- Complexity of regimen and presence of multiple medications
- Presence of undesirable side effects
- Emotional problems/refusal to control health
- Absence of support from family/friends
- Environmental difficulties (lack of delivery services, use of multiple pharmacies)
- Fear of administration/dislikes route of administration
- Vision/dexterity problems (packaging, dosage)
- Patient's beliefs or lack of belief about their susceptibility to illness and presence of special folk beliefs
- Lack of acceptance of medical diagnosis
- Patient's relationship with the physician/health care provider
- Misunderstanding about the purpose of the drug and the goal of drug therapy

CLINICAL MANIFESTATIONS
- Errors in drug administration (dosage, timing, crushing)
- Errors in drug use (wrong drug)
- Unsupervised use of nonprescription medications
- Noncompliance with prescribed regimens
- Medication sharing between family and friends
- Taking medications no longer prescribed
- Recurrent hospitalizations
- Incorrect pill count
- Anticipated actions of medication not occurring
- Excessive/unusual side effects

CLINICAL/DIAGNOSTIC FINDINGS
- Nontherapeutic blood levels of specific medications

▶ NURSING DIAGNOSIS: *Medication Noncompliance*

Related To forgetfulness, lack of understanding, fear

Defining Characteristics
- Recurrent hospitalizations
- Incorrect pill count

- Anticipated actions of medication not occurring
- Excessive/unusual side effects
- Patient states that they do not understand how to take the medications
- Patient states fear in taking medications

Patient Outcomes

- Patient will demonstrate adequate compliance with medication regimen, as evidenced by:
  - –therapeutic blood levels of specific medications.
  - –correct pill count.
  - –improved patient health and well-being.
- Patient will demonstrate adequate knowledge regarding medication regimen and ability to recite drug name, actions, reason for medication, dosage, side effects, contraindicated medication and substances, and the use of over-the-counter medications.

Nursing Interventions	Rationales
Obtain a complete and thorough drug history, including prescription drugs, alcohol, caffeine, nicotine, and home remedies. Record the name, dosage, and frequency of administration.	Assists in evaluating the patient's medication regimen. Nonprescription drugs can interact or cause additive adverse effects with prescription drugs.
Ask to see all the patient's medications or look in the medicine cabinet for old or expired drugs and duplicate therapy.	Often the patient visits more than one prescribing physician, resulting in duplicate drug therapy. Patients may keep old prescription bottles and confuse them with the current medication regimen.
Thoroughly assess the possible reasons why the patient is not following through with the prescribed regimen.	This provides the basis for determining how to creatively solve the problem. Blindly attempting to increase compliance without considering the reasons for altered compliance can lead to major problems. This starts with ignoring the patient's free will and the fact that the patient's analysis and actions may be correct and the prescriber's wrong.
Assess compliance by periodically counting the number of pills left in a prescription bottle to determine if the correct number of pills are missing.	This helps to confirm suspicions of poor cognitive functioning or forgetfulness on the part of the patient.

Nursing Interventions	Rationales
Assess if financial difficulties are affecting compliance. Notify the physician if this is the case.	The physician may be willing to switch to a similar medication that costs less. The patient may be eligible for state prescription plan programs and elderly discounted prescription plans.
Assess for visual/dexterity problems.	Many forms of packaging are difficult to open. Prefilling devices can be used for insulin administration.
Continually assess and question the patient about the presence of side effects. Notify the physician if present.	If side effects are present, they can hinder compliance. Perhaps the medication can be adjusted, changed, or discontinued.
Evaluate how well the patient/caregiver knows the purpose of each medication. Instruct on the drug name, its actions, reason for medication, dosage, side effects, contraindicated medications and substances, and use of over-the-counter medications. Leave written drug information for later referral. Ask the patient/caregiver to post the written drug schedule on the refrigerator or another frequently accessed area.	Knowledge about the medications and written reminders improve medication compliance.
Information should be presented clearly; simplify the medication regimen as much as possible.	Each time a regimen is simplified, compliance improves. Most patients are much more likely to comply with a once- or twice-daily dosage schedule than those given three or more times daily.
Provide both brand and generic names of the drug for the patient/caregiver.	Generic medications may be used instead of brand names, causing confusion for some patients.
Tailor medication times to a patient's individual routine or daily schedule.	Through tailoring, the patient's everyday life will not be drastically altered and the patient will feel in control of the medication schedule. A feeling of control may increase compliance.

Nursing Interventions	Rationales
Instruct the patient/caregiver to keep a record of all drugs the patient is receiving—prescription and nonprescription—and show it to all the physicians.	Often the patient visits more than one prescribing physician, resulting in duplicate drug therapy.
Provide educational information explaining the patient's disease process.	Knowledge of the disease process will help the patient understand the importance of taking the medications properly.
Encourage patients to use one pharmacy only.	Study results indicate increased drug reactions with patients using two or more pharmacies (Kluckowski, 1992).
Ask a clinical pharmacist to review medication regimens for drug interactions, potential side effects, and ways to maximize medication benefits.	A clinical pharmacist associated with a home health care agency can review medication regimens for drug interactions and potential side effects, provide in-service education, and serve as a liaison between the home care nurse and the physician. Clinical pharmacists can help nurses ensure that patients receive maximum benefits from their medication therapy.
Use over-the-counter medication organizers which are available in pharmacies.	The organizers can improve medication compliance for the cognitively limited patient.
Use other solutions such as "picture schedule," instruction/reminder sheets, calendar blister packs, and egg cartons (Kluckowski, 1992).	The organizers can improve medication compliance for the cognitively limited patient.
Involve a family member, caregiver, or other responsible party if the patient is unable or unwilling to follow through with the administration of a particular medication. This is not ideal; however, if all other alternatives have been explored, it may be necessary.	

DISCHARGE PLANNING/CONTINUITY OF CARE

- Patients are often discharged on a medication regimen different from what they had prior to rehospitalization as a result of dosage adjustment or the addition of new medications. Even if patients are instructed about their new medications prior to discharge, they may not fully understand the instructions and retention may be poor. The role of the home health care nurse becomes extremely important in counseling the patient and caregiver about the proper medication administration.
- Set up periodic visits to physician to ensure medication regimen is therapeutic. Encourage patient to question and clarify any confusing aspects of the medication treatment plan.
- If applicable, involve a family member, caregiver, or other responsible person to identify signs and symptoms of possible medication noncompliance postdischarge.
- Refer to physical or occupational therapy for dexterity problems in administering medications (e.g., insulin injections).
- Refer to social services for financial problems in purchasing medications.
- Refer to local stores to purchase medication assistance tools, if necessary.

REFERENCES/BIBLIOGRAPHY

Cornish, J. L. (1992). Color coding patient medications. *Caring Magazine,* Nov., 46–51.

Fineman, B., & DeFelice, C. A Study of medication compliance. *Home Healthcare Nurse, 10*(5), 26–29.

Forman, L. (1993). Medications: Reasons and interventions for noncompliance. *Journal of Psychosocial Nursing & Mental Health Services, 31*(10), 23–25.

Kluckowski, J. C. (1992). Solving medication noncompliance in home care. *Caring Magazine,* Nov., 34–41.

McPherson, M. L. (1990). Medicating home health patients. *Caring Magazine,* Jan., 38–40.

Mullen, R. A. (1993). Noncompliance: The homecare provider's critical role. *Computertalk for Homecare Providers, 1,* 19.

Saunders, C. E. (1987). Patient compliance in filling prescriptions after discharge from the emergency department. *American Journal of Emergency Medicine 5,* 283–286.

Stein, J. E., Keefner, K. R., & Haddad, A. M. (1992). The emergence of the home care pharmacist. *Caring Magazine,* Nov., 4–9.

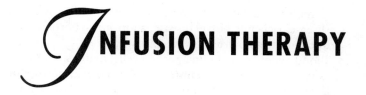

$\mathcal{J}$NFUSION THERAPY

Jackie Kareb, MS, RN

Infusion therapy involves the use of medications, fluids, or nutrients that are administered intravenously or subcutaneously to treat a variety of acute and chronic conditions. Infusion therapy has become an accepted and frequently used treatment modality in the home setting because of cost concerns to decrease hospital lengths of stay and because of patients' desires to receive care in a familiar setting.

A variety of new devices and technology allows patients and caregivers to provide safe health care in the home that is compatible with normal daily routines. These devices and technology include implantable intravenous ports, peripherally inserted central catheter (PICC) and portable or ambulatory infusion pumps. Pharmaceutical technology has followed this trend, with the creation of products that can be more easily administered in the home setting. Examples include nutrition mixtures that combine hyperalimentation formulas with lipids in one bag and antibiotics that can be administered as infrequently as once daily.

ETIOLOGIES/USES
- *Fluid hydration* therapy is generally of short duration to correct acute fluid loss occurring with hyperemesis, high-output syndromes, and decreased intake. Occasionally, long-term hydration therapy may be used to replace chronic losses.
- *Antibiotics/antiviral* treatment of infective processes may be short term (1–2 weeks) or long term (3–6 weeks or longer). Disease processes treated at home include endocarditis; opportunistic infections associated with acquired immunodeficiency syndrome (AIDS) and other immunosuppressive states; and soft tissue, bone-joint, respiratory, and genitourinary infections.
- *Parenteral nutrition* therapy is indicated when the gastrointestinal tract is unable to adequately absorb and process nutrients or in depletion states that require intensive refeeding. Common disease processes that require

parenteral nutrition include gastric neoplasm with obstruction, Crohn's disease, ischemic bowel disease, short-gut syndromes, acute pancreatitis, and cytomegalovirus (CMV) gastritis.

- Blood products including packed cells, platlets, and various factors are administered to restore normal hematological status.
- *Chemotherapy* can be infused at home when risk from extravasation and side effects are minimal and can be safely managed.
- *Antirejection therapies* to treat acute and chronic rejection of transplanted organs can be managed at home when patients are medically stable and can tolerate such agents. Commonly used agents include OK-T3, At Gam, Gamma Guard, and various steroids.
- *Cardiac inotropic* therapy manages chronic, end-stage disease and patients awaiting heart transplant.
- *Continuous subcutaneous heparin therapy* has been used for patients requiring anticoagulants during pregnancy when warfarin agents are contraindicated.

Clinical Clip

Clinical Factors in Patient Selection

1. The patient is medically stable.
2. Etiology for the presenting problem is clearly defined.
3. Venous access can be maintained in the home.
4. The product can be safely administered in the home.
5. The patient's general medical condition can be adequately and routinely evaluated while in the home setting.
6. The managing physician is comfortable with home infusion therapy.
7. A responsible adult is available to be with the patient when indicated. In the absence of another adult, consider whether the patient can responsibly and competently manage and trouble-shoot the infusion.
8. The patient has access to a telephone in the event of an emergency or equipment malfunction.

CLINICAL MANIFESTATIONS

Complications related to the venous access device

- Infection may be manifested by temperature elevation and pain, erythema, or drainage at the catheter exit site.
- Mechanical phlebitis.

- Occlusion from clotted blood or precipitates formed by the mixing of incompatible agents within the intravenous (IV) catheter. Occlusion may impede ability to obtain a blood return as well as infuse prescribed products.
- Displacement of IV catheter manifested by absence of blood return, pain, or discomfort along the route of the catheter. Displaced peripherally placed catheters will result in infiltration of intravenous fluids into surrounding tissues.

Extravasation
- Leakage of vesicant or irritant agents into surrounding tissues that are capable of causing pain, necrosis, and/or sloughing off of tissue.

Fluid/electrolyte imbalances
- Dehydration if fluid losses are more rapid than they are being replaced (e.g., emesis, diarrhea, high-output ostomies or fistulas).

Drug toxicities/adverse effects
- Toxicities and adverse effects are drug specific and should be monitored as such.
- Nephrotoxicity and ototoxicity associated with use of aminoglycosides.
- Neutropenia from using antifungals and antineoplastics.

Fatigue (patient and/or caregiver)
- While possibly secondary to the underlying disease process, medication schedules that require frequent dosing and/or sleep interruption may interfere with patients and their caregivers getting adequate rest.

Social isolation (patient and/or caregiver)
- Cumbersome equipment or frequent or continuous dosing schedules may unnecessarily confine the patient and caregiver to the home.

CLINICAL/DIAGNOSTIC FINDINGS

Serum chemistry
- Albumin levels monitored to evaluate overall nutritional status.
- Weekly renal function tests [i.e., blood urea nitrogen (BUN), creatinine] for patients receiving agents that can be nephrotoxic.
- Random, mid and postinfusion glucose levels to evaluate how the concentrated glucose loads in hyperalimentation formulas are being tolerated. Fingerstick glucoses may be utilized in place of venipuncture.

Heme status
- Complete blood count (CBC) with differential is assessed to identify neutropenia or evaluate the effectiveness of blood product infusions.

Drug levels
- Random levels and scheduled peaks and troughs are assessed to evaluate for therapeutic blood levels. Monitoring is usually done weekly on stable patients.

Coagulation studies
- Partial prothrombin time (PTT) assessment is done to evaluate for therapeutic dosing of anticoagulants. Frequency of assessments depends upon the individual patient's status. Venipuncture is still more commonly used; however, bedside coagulation monitors are currently available.

Microbiology
- Blood cultures and swabs of catheter exit sites are obtained when there is suspicion of an IV catheter related infection.

Radiographic studies
- Chest x-ray is necessary to confirm placement of centrally placed IV catheters. A portable chest x-ray can be performed in the home.

▶ NURSING DIAGNOSIS: *Altered Nutrition—Less Than Body Requirements*

Related To decreased ability to absorb nutrients in the gastrointestinal tract, obstruction, decreased intestinal surface area, or the presence of severe malnutrition

Defining Characteristics
- Hypoproteinemia
- Decreased oral intake
- Hyperemesis
- High-output ostomy
- Significant loss or absence of small intestines

Patient Outcomes
Nutrient intake is adequate to meet needs for restoration and maintenance of body's needs, as evidenced by:
- weight gain.
- return of serum albumin to normal.

Nursing Interventions	Rationales
Instruct patient to maintain daily record of body weight, oral intake (if appropriate), and output (e.g., urine; stool frequency, volume, and consistency; emesis).	For patients receiving hyperalimentation, nutrition content is adjusted to match needs. Weight gain or loss, changes in oral intake, and changes in output must be balanced by intravenous intake to assure the patient is not being over- or undernourished. For other patients, drugs such as antineoplastic agents may result in anorexia, altered taste, dysphagia secondary to stomatitis, nausea, or vomiting. Any of

Nursing Interventions	Rationales
	these symptoms can cause or worsen an alteration in nutrition.
Monitor laboratory parameters as ordered. Usually these include serum chemistry, magnesium, and CBC.	There is a potential for fluid and electrolyte imbalances when administering intravenous products. Monitoring these values will identify problems early.
Compare label on hyperalimentation with the physician's orders, checking formula, total volume, and expiration date. Expired formula should be discarded or returned to the pharmacy.	This is done to prevent administration errors. This is particularly important if the patient has had recent formula changes.
Assist the patient and caregiver to integrate nutrition therapy into their daily routine.	Patients and their caregivers are more likely to be compliant if treatment does not create unnecessary barriers to daily living. Parenteral nutrition can be administered continuously or in cycles. A common cycle is an 8–12-h infusion every 24 h. The length of the cycle depends on the total volume of the daily formula as well as the patient's ability to handle the more concentrated glucose load that will occur with cycling. Cycled formulas are often administered at night, while the patient is asleep, to minimize interference with daytime routines. Continuous infusions, if necessary, can be administered via an ambulatory pump that permits patients to move more freely inside and outside the house.

▶ NURSING DIAGNOSIS: *Fluid Volume Deficit*

Related To increased fluid loss and/or decreased oral intake

Defining Characteristics
- Emesis
- Diarrhea

- High-output ostomy
- Anorexia
- Decreased urine output/concentrated urine

Patient Outcomes

Patient will attain/maintain normal fluid volume, as evidenced by:
- urine output greater than 720 cc/24-h period.
- moist, pink mucous membranes.
- improved skin turgor.
- decreased fluid loss.

Nursing Interventions	Rationales
Administer maintenance IV fluids as ordered. Usually 5% dextrose in normal saline is given at a rate of 1 L over 8 h or less. Acute fluid loss may require more rapid administration.	Volume, rate, and frequency of IV fluids administration depends on the patient's hydration status and their ability to handle fluid volumes.
Instruct patient or caregiver in maintaining a daily record of weight, intake (oral and IV), and output.	This helps to evaluate the patient's response to treatment and need for further treatment.
Assess integument for signs of improved fluid balance (i.e., skin turgor, oral mucosa).	This assesses patient's response to treatment and ongoing need for IV fluids.

▶ NURSING DIAGNOSIS: *High Risk for Infection*

Risk Factors
- Immunosuppression
- Neutropenia
- Exposure to blood and body fluids
- Central venous catheter or other centrally placed venous access device
- Poor nutritional status

Patient Outcomes

Patient/caregiver will:
- correctly return-demonstrate sterile technique.
- verbalize rationale for handwashing.

Patient will maintain:
- a normal temperature.
- a normal white blood cell count.

Nursing Interventions	Rationales
Use sterile technique when accessing venous access devices for specimen withdrawal or medication/fluid administration.	Venous access devices provide a port for infectious agents that can result in a systemic infection. Also, patients receiving infusion therapy may be immunocompromised secondary to their underlying disease process or the adverse effects of the therapy itself, thus increasing their risk for infection.
Assess temperature and venous access site every visit.	Elevated temperature and redness and drainage at the catheter exit site are cause to suspect a line-related infection.
Instruct patient/caregiver in proper handwashing.	Handwashing is the first line of defense in preventing infections.
Instruct the patient or caregiver to report signs or symptoms of infection immediately, such as elevated temperature, redness, or drainage around the IV catheter exit site.	Signs or symptoms of infection may occur between the nurse's home visits. Delaying identification until the next home or clinic visit will also delay needed treatment.

▶ NURSING DIAGNOSIS: *High Risk for Injury*

Risk Factors
- Administration of cancer chemotherapeutic agents capable of causing or forming a blister or tissue destruction

Patient Outcomes
The patient will not experience local tissue damage as the result of extravasation of a vesicant agent.

Nursing Interventions	Rationales
Vesicant administration should be done ideally through a centrally placed IV catheter. If a peripheral IV catheter must be used, the infusion should be administered IV push through the side arm of a running	Vesicant agents are effectively diluted by infusing into either the larger volume of blood in the central circulation or a running IV. Directly infusing into the peripheral line is contraindicated because

Nursing Interventions	Rationales
IV. Do not administer vesicants by continuous infusion into a peripheral vein.	the agent would be too concentrated with too high a risk of tissue damage if extravasation occurred.

▶ **NURSING DIAGNOSIS:** *High Risk for Injury (Caregiver)*

Risk Factors
- Exposure to contaminated blood and body fluids, sharps, and toxic agents
- Use of needles and other sharps in the home setting
- Administration of antineoplastic agents

Patient Outcomes
Patient/caregivers and others in the home will:
- demonstrate correct use of all equipment for IV administration.
- demonstrate correct disposal of all sharps.
- verbalize actions to be taken in the event of a chemotherapy spill.
- demonstrate correct use of universal precautions.

Nursing Interventions	Rationales
Provide patient with a container for sharps disposal.	Sharps disposed directly into the general family trash create a risk of needle stick to the patient, caregivers, and trash collectors.
Use needleless systems for IV administration.	Needleless systems minimize caregiver and nurse risk of needle sticks.
Instruct home caregivers in using universal precautions when they administer IV therapy and/or care for venous access devices.	Family caregivers are placed at risk for exposure to blood-borne pathogens when they are providing this care.
Instruct patient/caregivers how to double bag soiled dressings and bed pads before placing in the general trash. Soiled linens should be washed in hot water with bleach.	This helps to protect caregivers and others from exposure to body fluids that may be infected.

Nursing Interventions	Rationales
Provide all patients receiving anti-neoplastic agents with a spill kit and a chemotherapy disposal bucket.	Spill kits provide materials for cleaning accidental spills with minimal exposure. Buckets are used to isolate any antineoplastic materials, including used IV bags and tubing. Full buckets should be disposed of by the home health agency or the home infusion pharmacy according to their agency's policies.
Instruct patients and caregivers to wash linens and clothing that are soiled with the patient's body fluids separately within 48 h postchemotherapy.	Body fluids carry traces of these agents for up to 48 h. Handling soiled materials separately minimizes caregiver exposure.

▶ NURSING DIAGNOSIS: *Knowledge Deficit*

Related To adapting infusion therapy to the home setting

Defining Characteristics
- Home infusion therapy is new for the patient.
- Patient/caregiver expresses lack of understanding of IV administration and in-home monitoring.
- Patient/caregiver expresses lack of understanding of venous access device care.
- Patient/caregiver expresses lack of understanding of problems to report to the home health nurse.

Patient Outcomes
Patient/caregiver will return-demonstrate:
- care of IV site.
- correct operation and troubleshooting of infusion pump or other infusion devices.
- correct technique for connecting and disconnecting an infusion.

Patient/caregiver will verbalize:
- monitoring to be done at home [e.g., temperature, intake and output (I&O)].
- problems to be immediately reported to the home health nurse.
- correct storage of IV medications and fluids.

Nursing Interventions	Rationales
Initiate teaching prior to hospital discharge.	Whenever time permits, initiating the teaching plan early helps to minimize patient and caregiver anxiety at home. Also, patients and caregivers who are independent in home care will require fewer home visits, making home care more cost effective.
Schedule the initial home visit to coincide with the first at-home administration.	Even if predischarge teaching occurred, the home care nurse will need to assess that the patient and/or caregiver are competent once in the home setting. Also, supplies delivered to the home may differ somewhat from those used in the hospital, possibly confusing the patient/caregiver.
Plan subsequent home visits based on the patient/caregiver need for additional instruction and supervision.	The frequency of home visits should be based on the patient and caregiver need for supervision from the nurse. Those that are more competent should require fewer home visits.
Review teaching objectives at least weekly and whenever there is a change in the home regimen.	The patient and caregiver must be able to demonstrate that they have assimilated any changes in the home care routine. Also, the nurse will want to assure that compliance is ongoing in order to prevent complications. Occasionally, patients and caregivers may become lax in their technique as they become more comfortable with the procedures.
Provide patient/family with access to staff after hours.	Problems, such as venous access site complications and equipment malfunctions, can occur at any time between home visits. The home care nurse and agency should be able to accommodate these needs at home as a part of the home care plan. Nurses who are familiar with the plan of care and equipment can

Nursing Interventions	Rationales
	manage problems, bring more satisfaction to the patient, and keep the overall costs of care down.

DISCHARGE PLANNING/CONTINUITY OF CARE
- The patient has completed the prescribed course of infusion therapy and is no longer in need of skilled home care services.
- If infusion therapy will be lifelong, ensure that the patient and/or caregiver can:
  - independently administer infusion therapy.
  - troubleshoot equipment.
  - care for the venous access device.
  - work with the home care pharmacy to assure regular delivery of supplies.
  - travel to the clinic for regular follow-up with the physician and other health providers
- Use case management principles to maintain regular contact with patients who are not in need of nurse home visits but may need access to the nurse in the event of a problem or change in their status.
- Refer patients to support groups to help in coping with their disease process (e.g., I Can Cope, Crohn's and Irritable Bowel Syndrome Foundation).

BIBLIOGRAPHY

Bernstein, L. H. (1992). Marketing home IV antibiotic therapy to physicians. *Caring, 11*(5), 50–56.

Hayes, N. N., & Lovetang R. (1991). Home infusion therapy options for patients with AIDS. *Caring, 10*(7), 20–26.

Hinkle, J. L. (1990). Home antibiotic therapy for brain abscesses. *JIN, 13*(3), 172–176.

Rosen, G. H. (1990). Home parenteral nutrition. *Caring, 9*(5), 34–36.

Strumpfes, A. L. (1991). Lower incidence of peripheral catheter complications by the use of elastomeric hydrogel catheters in home intravenous therapy patients. *JIN, 14*(4), 261–267.

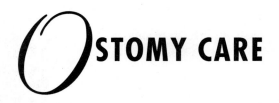

OSTOMY CARE

Jennifer A. Dore, RN, MSN, CETN

An ostomy is a surgically created opening into a hollow organ of the body. This opening may be temporary or permanent. The stoma refers to the portion of the bowel or urinary tract brought to the abdominal surface through which stool or urine drains. The terms *stoma* and *ostomy* are used interchangeably. There are three common types of ostomies: ileostomy, colostomy, and urinary diversion.

An ileostomy is an opening into the ileum, or final portion of the small intestine. A colostomy is an opening created anywhere along the length of the colon and is further identified by the specific site in the colon (i.e., ascending, transverse, descending, and sigmoid colostomies). Urinary diversion refers to any surgical procedure which diverts urine away from an obstructed area of the genitourinary system or a diseased bladder. The most common type is the ileal conduit.

Three main nursing interventions are teaching stoma management, identifying and treating complications, and providing emotional support for patient and family.

ETIOLOGIES

Ileostomy
- inflammatory bowel disease (ulcerative colitis and Crohn's disease)
- familial polyposis
- trauma
- necrotizing enterocolitis in the neonate

Colostomy
- colorectal cancer
- diverticular disease
- abdominal trauma
- congenital conditions (e.g., Hirschsprung's disease and imperforate anus)

Urinary diversion
• bladder cancer
• neurogenic bladder
• congenital anomalies (e.g., prune-belly syndrome, bladder exstrophy)

CLINICAL MANIFESTATIONS
Normal stomal signs and symptoms include:
• stoma pink to beefy red in color
• stoma round or oval in shape
• optimal protrusion 2 cm beyond abdominal surface
• peristomal skin intact and clear

Problems include:

Ileostomy
• thirst, dry skin, dry mucous membranes
• low urine output (<30 per hour), concentrated urine
• fatigue, weakness
• dizziness, orthostatic hypotension
• crampy abdominal pain
• change in character of output (e.g., more or less than usual amount, watery, foul odor)
• nausea/vomiting
• stomal swelling
• abdominal distention
• bloody output

Colostomy
• hard stool, less than normal amount
• abdominal pain
• prolapsed/herniated stoma

Urinary diversion
• cloudy, malodorous urine
• flank pain

CLINICAL/DIAGNOSTIC FINDINGS

Ileostomy
• blood electrolytes that show imbalances: sodium, potassium
• complete blood count (CBC) that shows dehydration or bleeding
• abdominal x-ray (KUB) that shows an obstruction
• guiac output for occult blood (positive for internal bleeding)

Colostomy
• digital examination that shows impaction
• guiac stool for occult blood that shows internal bleeding
• KUB that shows obstruction

- colonoscopy and barium enema that show obstruction, perforation, or recurrent tumor

Urinary diversion
- urine culture and sensitivity that shows infection

▶ **NURSING DIAGNOSIS:** *Knowledge Deficit*

Related To ostomy management

Defining Characteristics
- New ostomy patient
- New caregiver (i.e., patient can no longer accomplish care)
- Verbalizes uncertainty in managing ostomy, equipment, and lifestyle changes
- Recurrent appliance failure or frequent ostomy complications

Patient Outcomes
Patient verbalizes and demonstrates ability to manage ostomy, equipment, and lifestyle changes and experiences infrequent complications.

Nursing Interventions	Rationales
Assess current knowledge base about ostomy care and management.	This helps determine educational needs.
Teach patient/family proper removal of ostomy appliance. When removing old appliance, carefully support abdominal skin and gently loosen appliance seal.	This minimizes skin trauma.
Teach patient/family how to cleanse peristomal skin using mild soap and carefully dry with clean cloth or towel.	Cleaning skin removes ostomy effluent, skin barrier, and adhesive residue and prevents skin irritation/pain.
Teach patient/family how to properly measure stoma diameter and prepare skin barrier/pouch with each pouch change.	The skin barrier/pouch should match the stoma size, allowing no more than ⅛ in. clearance around stoma to prevent skin irritation and promote pouch seal. Stoma shrinks dramatically the first 6–8 weeks postoperatively and must be measured with each pouch change to ensure proper fit and skin protection.

Nursing Interventions	Rationales
Assist patient in visualizing and properly centering and applying pouch in both a sitting and standing position. Use mirrors if necessary. When patient finds comfortable position, encourage patient to use this position for future appliance changes.	This maximizes proper fit and seal.
Assess patient's visual acuity and manual dexterity when choosing a clamp. Make sure patient/family can properly secure the clamp.	This maximizes ease of use and proper application.
Teach patient to fold pouch tail up once around bar of clamp.	Folding the pouch tail more than once makes it difficult to close clamp and increases the probability of the clamp falling off.
Teach patient/family to empty pouch when no more than one-third full. Teach patient/family with urinary diversion to use a night drainage system to prevent pouch overfilling during sleep.	A heavy pouch can pull away from the skin, causing leakage and skin irritation.
Discuss lifestyle changes. Patient may bathe and shower with or without pouch. Reinforce that the pouch seal will remain intact. Patient can swim, but suggest using waterproof tape around edges of pouch in a "picture-frame" fashion. No change in clothing is necessary.	This promotes psychological health and decreases anxiety/fear.
Discuss types of foods that cause gas (bowel ostomy) and odor. Suggest optimal diet to minimize and treat constipation, diarrhea, and blockage for bowel ostomies. (See table 49-1).	This promotes psychological health and reduces risk of complications.
Encourage colostomy patient to drink at least 6–8 glasses of fluid a day; 10–12 glasses are recommended for the ileostomy and the ileal conduit patient unless medically contraindicated.	Fluid intake will decrease chance of constipation for colostomy patient and will ensure adequate fluid replacement for ileostomy patient. High fluid intake maintains an acidic urine, which decreases

Nursing Interventions	Rationales
	bacterial growth and prevents infection for ileal conduit patients.
Insure patient/family are able to maintain all necessary supplies. Discuss any financial issues related to securing supplies and equipment.	Patient and family awareness of convenient and economic supply sources can prevent complications related to inappropriate substitution or overusing supplies and equipment.

▶ NURSING DIAGNOSIS: *Impaired Skin Integrity*

Related To appliance leakage, improper pouch application, weight loss/gain, stomal retraction, peristomal hernia, overgrowth of yeast

Defining Characteristics
- Red, irritated, broken, weepy skin
- Complaints of pain, itching, burning

Patient Outcomes
- Patient's skin will be intact.

Nursing Interventions	Rationales
Assess any changes in self-ostomy care, equipment, weight, medication changes, chemotherapy, and radiation therapy.	These can change the integrity of the pouching system.
Remove appliance. In lying, sitting, and standing positions, assess stoma, peristomal area, and overall abdominal contours for irregularities (e.g., creases, folds, stomal retraction).	Determining the cause of the problem leads to correct treatment.
Modify equipment, add skin barrier wafer, use skin barrier paste, or change pouching system to maintain or create appliance integrity. For example, build up or fill in abdominal dips, folds, and crevices with	Skin will heal itself under a correctly fitted and applied pouch.

Nursing Interventions	Rationales
additional pieces of skin barrier wafer or skin barrier paste. Add an ostomy belt if needed. This may require a different pouching system and consultation with an enterostomal therapy (ET) nurse. Call the Wound Ostomy Continence Nurses Society (WOCN) for a list of local ET nurses.	
Assess for yeast (*Candida*) infection. Patient reports itching, and/or burning of peristomal area. Skin is erythematous with pustules. Assess if on antibiotic therapy, on chemotherapy, or in warm weather.	Yeast infections are treated differently and must be correctly identified. Yeast commonly grows in a dark, moist, warm environment or when normal flora is altered by medications.
If patient has a yeast infection (*Candida*), apply antifungal powder to peristomal skin. Brush off excess powder before applying pouch.	Too much powder remaining on skin will interfere with pouch seal.

▶ NURSING DIAGNOSIS: *Ineffective Individual Coping*

Related To body image changes, lifestyle changes, overall diagnosis (cancer, Crohn's disease, or other chronic illness), financial distress.

Defining Characteristics
- Verbalizes inability to cope
- Anger/denial/depression
- Social isolation
- Tearful

Patient Outcomes
- Patient will resume previous activities, integrating ostomy lifestyle changes.
- Patient/family will verbalize ability to cope.

Nursing Interventions	Rationales
Encourage patient/family to discuss feelings and ventilate anger.	This gives patient/family permission to identify and express feelings.

Nursing Interventions	Rationales
Contact United Ostomy Association (UOA) for local support groups and ostomy visitor information.	Support groups/ostomy visitors provide encouragement and role modeling to help successfully adapt following ostomy surgery.
Refer to social services for financial assistance.	Some health insurance plans may not cover the cost of ostomy supplies.
Contact physician for psychiatric referral, if needed.	An ostomy may overwhelm the patient's coping ability or exacerbate preexisting psychological problems.

DISCHARGE PLANNING/CONTINUITY OF CARE
- Reinforce need for follow-up physician appointment(s).
- Refer to local ET nurse.
- Provide a list of necessary equipment and source of suppliers.
- Provide name and number of local ostomy or other relevant support group(s).

Table 49-1 • Ostomy Dietary Considerations

Foods that may cause gas	Foods that may cause odor	Foods that thicken stool	Foods that loosen stool	Ileostomy blocking foods
• Beans	• Asparagus (urinary ostomy)	• Applesauce	• Alcohol	• Celery
• Beer	• Beans	• Bananas	• Beans	• Chinese vegetables
• Cabbage family vegetables (broccoli, brussel sprouts, cabbage, cauliflower)	• Cabbage family vegetables	• Bread	• Beer	• Coconut
• Carbonated beverages	• Cheese	• Cheese	• Chocolate	• Coleslaw
• Cucumbers	• Eggs	• Marshmallows	• Coffee	• Corn
• Dairy products	• Fish	• Pasta	• Fried foods	• Mushrooms
• Onions	• Garlic	• Peanut butter	• Prune or grape juice	• Nuts
• Radishes	• Onions	• Rice	• Raw fruits and vegetables	• Popcorn
		• Tapioca	• Spicy foods	• Raisins
			• Spinach	• Raw vegetables and fruits
				• Seeds

OTHER PLANS OF CARE TO REFERENCE
- Grief/Loss
- Human Sexuality
- Social Isolation
- Caregiver Burden/Support/Conflict Resolution
- Skin Care

BIBLIOGRAPHY

Black, P. K. (1994). Hidden problems of stoma care. *British Journal of Nursing, 3*(14), 707–711.

Burt-McAliley, D., Eberhardt, D., & van Rijswijk, L. (1994). Clinical study: Periostomal skin irritation in colostomy patients. *Ostomy Wound Management, 40*(6), 28–30.

Hampton, B. G., & Bryant, R. A. (1992). *Ostomies and continent diversions: Nursing management.* St. Louis: Mosby Year-Book.

Krol, M. A. (1994). Commentary on ostomy patient managment: Care that engenders adaptation. *ONS Nursing Scan in Oncology, 3*(2), 9.

National Resources

Adult Children of Alcoholics
(ACOA)
PO Box 3216
Torrance, CA 90510
(310)534-1815

Alanon/Alateen
Midtown Station
PO Box 862
New York, NY 10018
(800)344-2666

Alcoholics Anonymous
475 Riverside Drive
New York, NY 10115
(212)870-3400

Alexander Grahm Bell Association
for the Deaf
3417 Volta Place NW
Washington, DC 20007
(202)337-5220

American Cancer Society and
Reach to Recovery
1599 Clifton Rd. NE
Atlanta, GA 30329
(800)ACS-2345

American Diabetes Association
1660 Duke St.
Alexandria, VA 22314
(800)232-3472

American Foundation for the Blind
15 W 16th St.
New York, NY 10011
(800)232-5463

American Heart Association
7272 Greenville Ave.
Dallas, TX 75231
(214)373-6300

American Lung Association
1740 Broadway
New York, NY 10019
(212)315-8700

American Parkinson's Disease
Association
60 Bay St.
Staten Island, NY 10301
(800)223-2372

Arthritis Foundation
1314 Spring St. NW
Atlanta, GA 30309

Asthma and Allergy Foundation of
America
1125 15th St. NW #502
Washington, DC 20005
(202)466-7643

Centers for Disease Control
1600 Clifton Rd NE
Atlanta, GA 30333
(404)639-3311

Health for Incontinent People
PO Box 544
Union, SC 29379
(803)579-7900

Juvenile Diabetes Association
432 Park Avenue South
16th Floor
New York, NY 10016
(800)223-1138

La Leche League International
(800)LaLeche

Mended Hearts Club
7320 Greenville Ave.
Dallas, TX 75231
(214)706-7442

Narcotics Anonymous
PO Box 9999
Van Nuys, CA 91409
(818)780-3951

National Association of Area
Agencies on Aging
1112 16th St. NW, Suite 100
Washington, DC 20036
(202)296-8130

National Cancer Institute
Bldg. 31
9000 Rockville Pike
Bethesda, MD 20892
(800)4-cancer

National Parkinson's Disease
Association
1501 NW 9th Ave.
Bob Hope Rd.
Miami, FL 33136
(800)327-4545

Overeaters Anonymous
PO Box 92870
Los Angeles, CA 90009
(310)657-6252

Simon Foundation
PO Box 815
Wilmette, IL 60091
(800)237-4666

United Parkinson Foundation
220 S State St.
Chicago, IL 60604
(312)922-9734

United Ostomy Association
36 Executive Park #120
Irvine, CA 92714
(800)826-0826

INDEX

clinical/diagnostic findings in, 312
clinical manifestations of, 312
discharge planning/continuity of
care in, 318
etiologies of, 311–312
food guide pyramid and, 318
infusion therapy and, 352–353
nursing diagnoses
knowledge deficit, 316–318
weight gain, 314–316
weight loss, 313–314

O

Occupational Safety and Health
Administration (OSHA), 9, 300
Occupational therapy (OT)
arthritis/osteoporosis and, 201, 204
cerebral insult and, 167
exercise programs and, 328, 329
grief and loss and, 59
inadequate personal hygiene
and, 332
joint replacement/fractures and,
209, 213
medication compliance/
noncompliance and, 348
referral to, 29, 30
spinal cord injury and, 173
visual deficit and, 115
Older people. *See* Elder abuse/neglect
Oral hygiene
inadequate personal hygiene and,
331, 333
taste and smell deficits and, 117
tuberculosis and, 297
Osteoarthritis, 198
clinical/diagnostic findings in, 199
clinical manifestations of, 199
incidence of, 204
See also Arthritis/osteoporosis
Osteoporosis, 198
clinical/diagnostic findings in, 200
clinical manifestations of, 199
etiologies of, 198
incidence of, 204
See also Arthritis/osteoporosis
Ostomy care, 360–367
clinical/diagnostic findings in,
361–362
clinical manifestations of, 361
dietary considerations in, 366
discharge planning/continuity of
care in, 366

etiologies of, 360–361
nursing diagnoses
impaired skin integrity, 364–365
ineffective individual coping,
365–366
knowledge deficit, 362–364
sexuality pattern changes and, 75
Overeaters Anonymous, 314, 371
Overflow incontinence, 241, 242
See also Urinary incontinence
Overweight, 311
clinical/diagnostic findings in, 312
clinical manifestations of, 312
etiologies of, 311–312
See also Nutrition problems

P

Pain, 267–271
arthritis/osteoporosis and, 201–202,
204
breast cancer/treatment and, 190
cardiovascular disease and, 143–145
clinical/diagnostic findings in, 268
clinical manifestations of, 267–268
death and dying and, 54
discharge planning/continuity of
care in, 270–271
etiologies of, 267
nursing diagnoses
anxiety, 269–270
pain, 268–269
postpartum home care and, 222–223
primary cause of, 267
rating scales for, 268
Pain clinic, 204
Paraplegia. *See* Spinal cord injury (SCI)
Parenteral nutrition therapy, 349–350
See also Infusion therapy
Parenting. *See* Child abuse/neglect; Elder
abuse/neglect; Failure to thrive;
Ineffective parenting
Parents Anonymous, 88, 89
Parkinson's disease, 180–187
age of onset of, 180
clinical/diagnostic findings in, 181
clinical manifestations of, 181
discharge planning/continuity of
care in, 186
etiologies of, 180–181
nursing diagnoses
altered gastrointestinal function,
181–183
injury, 184–185

Vascular disease. *See* Peripheral vascular
  disease
Venous disease, 154, 155, 156
  See also Peripheral vascular disease
  (PVD)
Ventilation systems, home, 4, 12
Vermin infestation, 4, 11
Violence
  self-directed, 34–35
  substance abuse and, 337–338
Violence against women, 94–100
  clinical/diagnostic findings in, 95
  clinical manifestations of, 95
  discharge planning/continuity of
    care in, 100
  etiologies of, 94–95
  nursing diagnoses
    knowledge deficit, 97–98
    physical injury, 95–97
    self-esteem disturbance, 98–100
Visual deficit
  clinical/diagnostic findings in, 113
  clinical manifestations of, 112
  discharge planning/continuity of
    care in, 118
  etiologies of, 111
  nursing diagnosis of, 113–115
  See also Sensory deficit

W

Weakness, and death and dying, 50–51
Weight control, and sexuality pattern
  changes, 75
Weight gain, by baby in breastfeeding,
  230, 237–238
Weight loss, HIV/AIDS and, 286,
  288–289
  See also Underweight
Weight Watchers, 314
Women
  breast cancer/treatment and,
    188–197
  violence against. *See* Violence
    against women
Women's shelters, 96
Wood stoves, emissions standards
  for, 11
Wound Ostomy Continence Society
  (WOCN), 365
Wounds, healing phases, 255
  See also Skin care

Y

Yeast infections, and ostomy care, 365